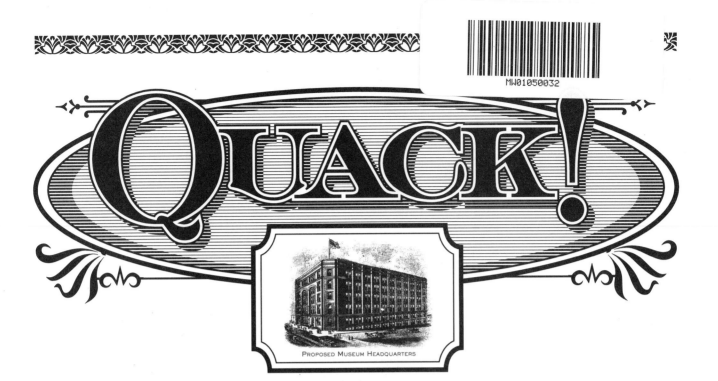

PROPOSED MUSEUM HEADQUARTERS

TALES OF MEDICAL FRAUD
FROM THE MUSEUM OF QUESTIONABLE MEDICAL DEVICES.

BOB MCCOY
CURATOR OF THE MUSEUM OF QUESTIONABLE MEDICAL DEVICES

SANTA
MONICA
PRESS

Published by:
Santa Monica Press LLC
P.O. Box 1076
Santa Monica, CA 90406-1076
1-800-784-9553
www.santamonicapress.com

SANTA
MONICA
·PRESS

Printed in the United States

Santa Monica Press books are available at special quantity discounts when
purchased in bulk by corporations, organizations, or groups. Please call our
special sales department at 1-800-784-9553.

*This book is intended to provide general information. The publisher, author, distributor,
and copyright owner are not engaged in rendering health, medical, legal, financial, or
other professional advice or services, and are not liable or responsible to any person or
group with respect to any loss, illness, or injury caused or alleged to be caused by the
information found in this book.*

ISBN 1-891661-10-8

Library of Congress Cataloging-in-Publication Data
McCoy, Bob, 1927-
        Quack! : tales of medical fraud from the Museum of Questionable
Medical Devices / by Bob McCoy
        p. cm.
        Includes bibliographical references.
        ISBN 1-891661-10-8 (pbk.)
        1. Quacks and quackery–United States. 2. Consumer protection–
United states. I. Museum of questionable Medical Devices. II. Title.

        R730 .M44 2000
        610–dc21

99-059928

The author would like to thank the following people for their outstanding
contributions to this book:

Shawne FitzGerald, Associate Curator
James Satter, Assistant Curator
Margaret McCoy, Medical Consultant

Museum web page: www.mtn.org/quack. Includes ordering information
about museum video tape, posters, and other publications.
Office Phone: 763-545-1113
Fax: 763-540-9999
Museum address: 201 Main St., Minneapolis, MN 55414
Museum phone: 612-379-4046

Book and cover design and production by Ken Niles
Additional interior production by Lynda Jakovich, Cooldog Design

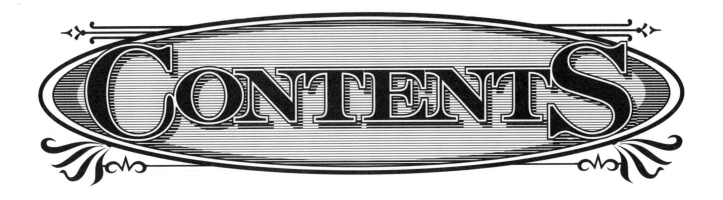

CONTENTS

PREFACE IV

INTRODUCTION *Here a Quack, There a Quack* 7

1. QUACKERY
—— *Common Questions and Their Answers* 17

2. MECHANICAL
—— *Simple Machines to Set You Straight* 25

3. MAGNETISM
—— *The Curative Magic of Magnets* 33

4. ELECTRICITY
—— *Flipping the Switch to Good Health* 49

5. RADIONICS
—— *Albert Abrams, Ruth Drown, and the Miracle of Vibrations* 71

6. RADIUM
—— *Good for What Ails You* 95

7. RAYS
—— *Let the Sun Shine In* 115

8. PSYCHOLOGY
—— *Use Your Head—The Bumpy History of Phrenology* 135

9. SENSORY
—— *Devices to Clear Your Head* 157

10. BEAUTY
—— *From Quack Straps to Nip & Tuck* 175

11. SEX
—— *Sex ex Machina* 207

CONCLUSION 237

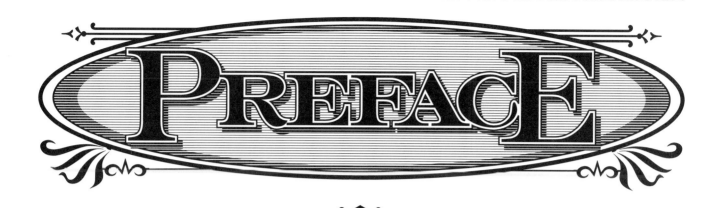

PREFACE

The Museum of Questionable Medical Devices can trace its origins to an accidental encounter in the mid-1960s with John White at a fundraiser for the Minneapolis Institute of Art. He was trying to operate a phrenology machine known as the Psycograph which supposedly would read the bumps on a person's head and print out a personality reading on a paper tape by rating the client's personality on a one-to-five scale. John was having trouble getting the machine to print out the tapes, and being mechanically inclined I offered to help him to get it running again, which we did. After this, we would occasionally operate the machines for fun at parties or other fundraisers.

Some time later John offered me the remaining machines from a warehouse where his father, Frank White, the financial backer of the "Psycograph" business in the 1920s, had stored them since the 1930s when the Psycograph went into eclipse. I spent a summer in the early '70s fixing the machines and got several into good working order.

In September 1984, Riverplace, a shopping and entertainment complex, opened on the east bank of the Mississippi River in Minneapolis and it seemed an ideal place to set up the Psycographs and charge for readings.

The Phrenology Company was born and provided after-school employment for my children. My wife, a bit skeptical, thought we would only be open a few weeks, for by then everybody who wanted their head examined would have done so.

A chance encounter with some television producers led to a live appearance on a national television morning show which led to other appearances and a request to demonstrate more goofy devices. The American Medical Association in Chicago, the Food & Drug Administration in Minneapolis, and the St. Louis Science Center had quack items in storage which they were willing to lend, so I transported these items back and forth for television appearances.

Ultimately, a permanent display location opened up and the Museum of Questionable Medical Devices was established in the late 1980s. New finds, many from the attics of the inventors' relatives, are constantly being acquired and the museum has grown steadily, now containing more than three hundred items of medical quackery. The first national article about the museum was written

by Ryan Ver Berkmoes and appeared in the *American Medical News* in September 1990.

Donald Aird, Director of Consumer Affairs in the Minneapolis FDA office, has been one of our champions both in supplying items and making contacts around the country. Dr. Suzanne Junod, Dr. John Swan, and Dr. Wallace Janssen, FDA historians in Washington D.C., have been enormously helpful. Victoria Davis, the AMA's former director of the Department of Archives, History, and Policy Information, arranged the loan of several large devices from the AMA and gave me duplicates from their substantial archives. Materials from this collection substantiate much of the information in this book.

Other staff who were working for the AMA at this time and were quite helpful were Marguette Fallucco, Dr. John Zwicky, Dr. Jim Carson, and Dr. Arthur Haffner. This division of the AMA is presently operated by Allen Podraza and Robert K. Willamson III who continue to assist us. The AMA Archives Department continues to operate as a resource about the history of the AMA and American medicine in general at (312) 464-4083.

Ron Beer of the St. Louis Science Center, Dr. Ellen Kuhfeld, Dr. David Rhees of the Bakken

Library and Museum in Minneapolis, and Dr. William Jarvis of the National Council for Reliable Health Information Inc. in Loma Linda, California have all been invaluable sources and have loaned the museum several items from their collections. Ms. Martha Dillegas of the California Department of Health Services Food & Drug branch cleaned out an old closet before the department moved and gave us several devices.

Graham Ford, a private collector, has loaned and supplied us with several extraordinary devices and is a knowledgeable and willing volunteer. His brief history of phlebotomy is included in Chapter Two. Kevin Horan took all of the draped background photogaphs included in the book. Dr. Olgierd Lindan of Cleveland, the most outstanding private collector, has been most generous in his advice and encouragement and I appreciate his friendship. I thank Ken Raines, publisher of the *JW Research Journal,* for allowing me to use his materials on Dr. Albert Abrams, as well as Jack Coulehan for allowing me to reprint his poem on Abrams, "The Dynamizer and the Oscilloclast."

I also thank Jeff Behary, curator of the virtual Turn of the Century Electrotherapy Museum who knows more about violet ray generators than one could imagine, for the information in that section.

Most of the ephemera and quoted articles in this book originated with the American Medical Association. An index of the Association's holdings, the *Guide to the American Medical Association's Historical Health Fraud and Alternative Medicine Collection,* was published in 1992. Duplicates from this collection were provided to the Museum of Questionable Medical Devices in 1994.

Historically, the AMA's documentation of fraudulent medical practices began in earnest in 1906 when Arthur J. Cramp, M.D. joined the editorial staff of the *Journal of the American Medical Assocition* and began publishing regular items concerning health fraud and quackery. In 1913 the Association formally established a separate "Propaganda Department" with Dr. Cramp as the first Director, to gather and disseminate information concerning health fraud and quackery. The Department's name was changed in 1925

to "Bureau of Investigation," and again in 1958 to "Department of Investigation." Oliver Field held the title of Director of Research from 1948 to 1965.

The only document approaching a bibliography on the AMA's collection is *Nostrums and Quackery,* a four volume, out-of-print American Medical Association Press publication. The volumes appeared in 1911, 1912, 1921, and 1936. *Nostrums and Quackery* is available at many public and academic institutions and also from some rare book dealers.

This book would not have been possible without the incredible energy and enthusiasm of my long time associate Shawne FitzGerald. She, together with James Satter, graduate student in the History of Science and phrenologist extraordinaire, have put much of this book together. I thank them from the bottom of my heart. And finally, thanks to my wife Margaret, who retired as a physician last year and thought she had finished reading pseudo-medical texts.

–Bob McCoy

INTRODUCTION

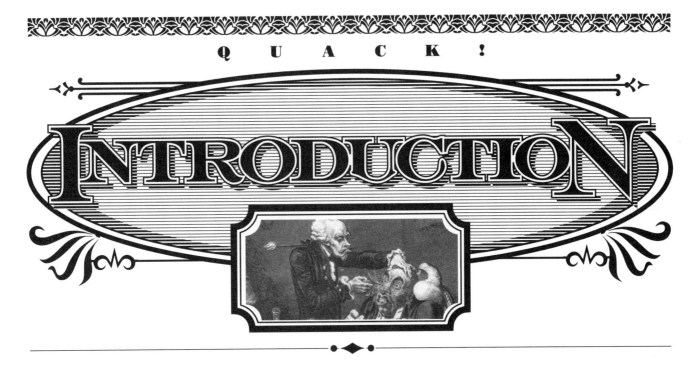

HERE A QUACK, THERE A QUACK . . .

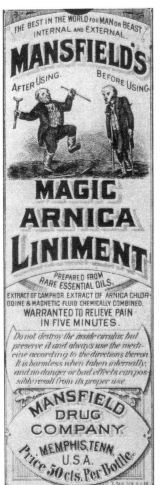

You don't have to go far these days to find ads for medical devices that look . . . questionable. Many of these so-called cures claim to have special metals or energies. Others, supposedly, will shock, rattle, or shake you to better health. These devices are often sold by the mail, via the Internet, or at special outlets by people who may or may not be able to explain how in the world these contraptions actually work.

Quackery, however, is nothing new. Over the years people have spent countless amounts of money on questionable medical devices to treat everything from arthritis to baldness to cancer. Many of these gadgets use special lights, heat, vibrations, metals, shockers, rollers, shakers, radio waves, or chemicals to cure illnesses. Some machines look technologically sophisticated on the outside, while some look amazingly simple. A few treat only one or two symptoms, but others supposedly cure just about everything. It's little surprise that many so-called devices that sound too good to be true actually are too good to be true.

People have been concerned about fraudulent or unethical physicians since ancient times. After

Perhaps the "magnetic fluid" in this product gave the user his lively step.

Touted as a women's tonic, Cardui had twice the alcoholic content of champagne.

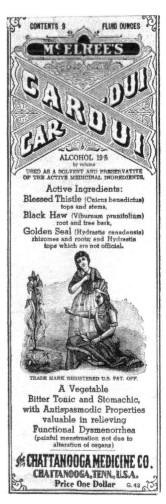

all, the Hippocratic oath, which discusses the importance of honesty in medicine, dates back to the fifth century B.C. In the famous oath, Hippocrates wrote, "The regimen I adopt shall be for the benefit of my patients according to my ability and judgment. . . . Whatsoever house I enter, there will I go for the benefit of the sick." But, not everyone heeds those words.

Professional medical associations and universities were in place during the Middle Ages when concern over medical standards continued. The term "quack"– meaning someone who pretends to be a physician or who claims to have medical knowledge that they don't really possess–dates as far back as the 1600s. A wide assortment of misguided or misleading medical practitioners have helped to keep the term in use ever since. The term "quackery," meanwhile, includes any objects or practices used by a quack. Because medical information has increased substantially over the centuries, medical assumptions and practices considered valid in the past are now considered "quackery."

Quackery Comes to America

In the eighteenth century, quack medical treatments traveled from Europe to North America, as many colonists ordered bottled elixirs, oils, tonics, or special pills intended to cure anything from arthritis to rheumatism. By today's standards, many of these treatments were scientifically contestable. Soon after the American Revolution, inventors in the United States could patent their devices– including inventions that turned out to be quack medical devices. One of the best remembered

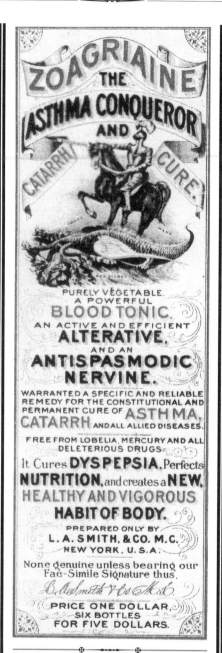

A typical patent medicine label, with grandiose claims to cure widely disparate disorders, without disclosing the contents.

examples of this concerned Connecticut physician Elisha Perkins, who received a U.S. patent in 1796 for his "Metallic Tractors." The Perkins tractors were two rods made of different metals to treat patients through the dubious effects of "animal

magnetism." The Tractors were popular at first, and Perkins seems to have been sincere in his belief that his device really worked.

Physicians continued to grow concerned about the reputation of the medical profession and questioned the benefits of generations-old treatments, such as bloodletting, in which diseases were "cured" by removing significant amounts of the patient's blood. Meanwhile, people continued to develop new ideas about how people might be treated. For example, in 1810 Samuel Friedrich Hahnemann introduced homeopathy, which suggested that patients could be treated using highly diluted quantities of a substance. Other popular treatments involved a combination of mesmerism and magnets. Over the years, a parade of magnetic devices came onto the market claiming to improve physical strength, stamina, and resistance to disease. Many magnetic devices were designed as apparel, including magnetic belts and magnetic shoe insoles.

In the nineteenth century, many physicians in the United States were trained through apprenticeships instead of at medical schools. Because of this,

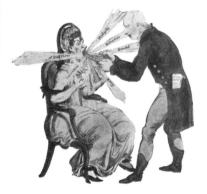

CARTOON SHOWING NOXIOUS ENERGY BEING RELEASED BY THE USE OF PERKINS TRACTORS.

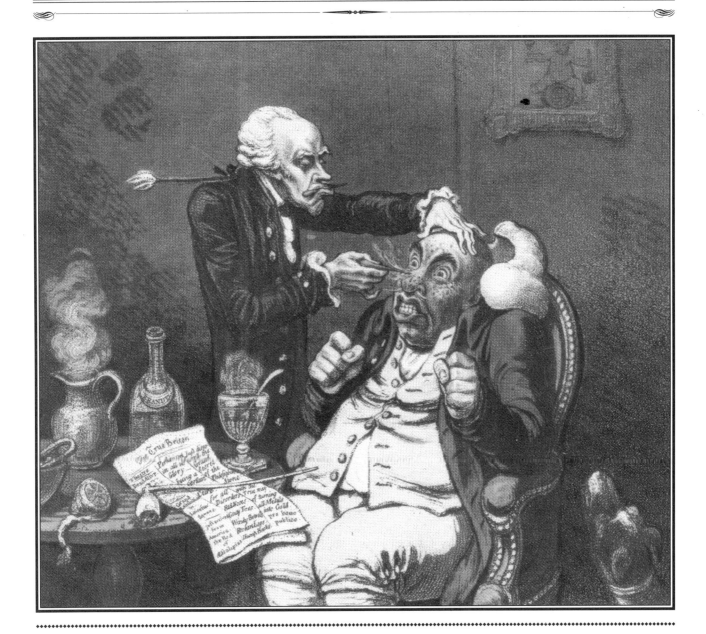

patients did not necessarily expect their doctors to have formal credentials. Instead they relied on a sense of trust—of which numerous quacks and nostrums took advantage. Many charlatans advertised their products readily and sold them through the mail. Others traveled from town to town selling so-called medicines with exotic cures. Tricks of the trade became well known. They included bold advertisements making false statements about the effectiveness of a treatment, claims that cures included a secret ingredient (perhaps

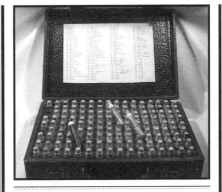

164 vials of common substances (peanut butter, Lea & Perrins sauce, etc.) that were placed in the Pathoclast to effect cures.

known only to Native Americans), or the practice of hiring an assistant who pretended to have been cured by the treatment.

    Other quacks, meanwhile, sold counterfeit versions of legitimate medicines. An often overlooked consequence of quackery is that charlatans who make false claims about their remedies scare legitimate scientists from looking seriously into any treatment that reminds them of the work of a well-known quack. In addition to harming patients, quackery can hinder

"A MINE OF HEALTH"

By Using the KICKAPOO REMEDIES.

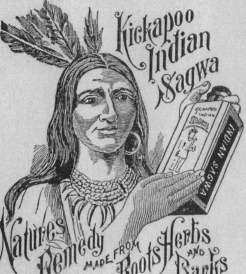 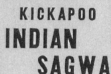 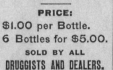 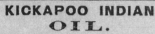

LONG LIFE AND GOOD HEALTH.

FOR THE KIDNEYS, LIVER and STOMACH.

A COMPOUND of the virtues of Roots, Herbs, Barks, Gums and Leaves. Its elements are Blood-Making; Blood Cleansing and Life Sustaining. It is the Purest, Safest, and Most Effectual Medicine known to the world. By its Searching and Cleansing Qualities it Drives Out the Foul Corruption which contaminates the blood and causes Derangement and Decay. Stimulates and Enlivens the Vital Functions, Promotes Energy and Strength, Restores and Preserves Health, and Infuses New Life and Vigor throughout the Whole System. There is probably no class of Complaints which Occasion so much misery as those connected with the Kidneys, including Backache, Lumbago, Sciatica, Diabetes, Bright's

Disease, Inflammation of the Bladder, Gravel, Womb Complaints and Uterine Affections, which are the Outgrowth of a Disordered Stomach and Liver, and cannot be cured without first regulating these organs For all these troubles

KICKAPOO INDIAN SAGWA

is a Sovereign Remedy, and *Never* Fails to restore the Kidneys to Health.

PRICE:
$1.00 per Bottle.
6 Bottles for $5.00.

SOLD BY ALL DRUGGISTS AND DEALERS.

KICKAPOO INDIAN MEDICINE CO., NEW HAVEN, CONN.

Kickapoo Indian Sagwa — Nature's Remedy MADE FROM Roots Herbs AND Barks

---

KICKAPOO INDIAN OIL.

An Absolutely Certain Remedy for all Pains whether External or Internal; Stomach Disorders, Bruises, Sprains, Toothache, Rheumatism, and the countless thousand pains of daily suffering promptly yield to its application. It is known everywhere as a

QUICK CURE FOR ALL PAINS.

Remember that it is equally good for Man or Beast, and no Household should be without it.

PRICE, 25 CENTS PER BOTTLE.

KICKAPOO INDIAN SALVE.

The most Soothing, Cleansing and Healing preparation known. Made of the Choicest Roots and Herbs, combined with the Purest of Tallow. It Quickly Cleanses and Heals all Sores, Cuts, Wounds and Bruises. This preparation should be in every household, as it is daily needed for common accidents like Burns, Scalds, Etc.

PRICE, 25 CENTS PER BOX.

KICKAPOO INDIAN WORM KILLER.

The Safest and Most Effective Remedy of the kind in the world. It is made from Roots and Herbs, and furnishes a Pleasant, Reliable and Prompt Remedy for the Removal of Stomach Coat or Pin Worms from Children or Adults. It has been truly called

The Adult's Friend.
The Children's Savior.

PRICE, 25 CENTS PER PACKAGE.

KICKAPOO INDIAN COUGH CURE.

A Famous Indian Vegetable Remedy for the Cure of All Diseases of the Throat and Lungs. Coughs, Colds, Sore Throat, Influenza, and all similar troubles yield like magic to Kickapoo Indian Cough Cure. A single trial is sufficient to convince, and once used you will never be without it in the house.

PRICE, 50 CENTS PER BOTTLE.

KICKAPOO INDIAN PILLS.

For SICK HEADACHE, CONSTIPATION, NERVOUSNESS and COMPLEXION.

PURELY VEGETABLE.
PRICE, 25 CENTS.

ALL THESE REMEDIES SOLD BY DRUGGISTS EVERYWHERE.

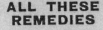

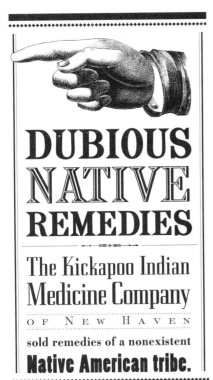

DUBIOUS NATIVE REMEDIES

The Kickapoo Indian Medicine Company

OF NEW HAVEN

sold remedies of a nonexistent **Native American tribe.**

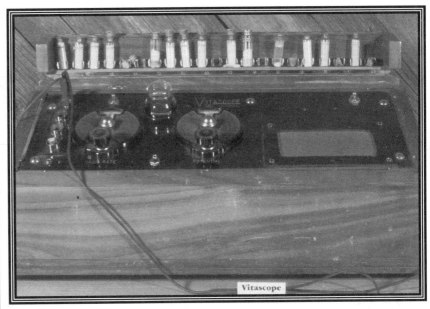

VITASCOPE.

The Vitascope of California, used for absent treatment, contained a built-in rack for storing homeopathic remedies.

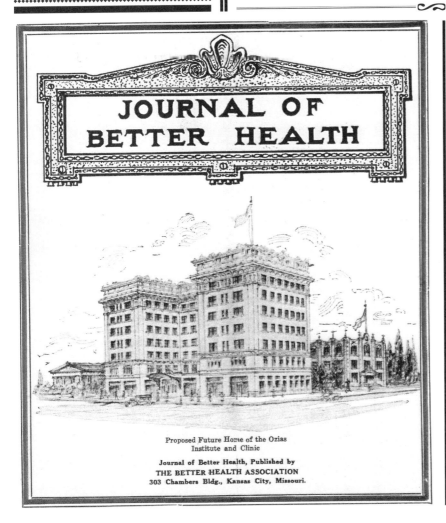

Proposed Future Home of the Ozias Institute and Clinic

Journal of Better Health, Published by
THE BETTER HEALTH ASSOCIATION
303 Chambers Bldg., Kansas City, Missouri.

beneficial advancements in medicine.

Early Attempts to Stop Quackery

In the United States, the movement against quacks was aided by the formation of the American Medical Association in 1847. (Today the AMA is the largest and most active medical organization in the world.) By the 1880s, large numbers of charlatans and other wanna-be doctors could purchase fraudulent medical degrees from one of several "diploma mills" without ever attending a day of medical school. Putting an end to diploma mills was one of the AMA's objectives during the early twentieth century.

ELABORATE proposed building by "Dr." Charles Ozios, a quack whose activities included alleged cures for cancer and paralysis.

CALIFORNIA UNIVERSITY
OF LIBERAL PHYSICIANS
CHARTERED·MAY·18th·1914·BY·THE·STATE·OF·CALIFORNIA

TO·ALL·TO·WHOM·THESE·LETTERS·SHALL·COME·GREETING
THE·DIRECTORS·OF·THE·COLLEGE·ON·THE·RECOMMENDATION·OF·THE·FACULTY
AND·BY·VIRTUE·OF·THE·AUTHORITY·IN·THEM·VESTED
HAVE·CONFERRED·ON

ERYN SKYE DEWEY

WHO·HAS·SATISFACTORILY·PURSUED·THE·STUDIES·AND·PASSED
THE·EXAMINATIONS·REQUIRED·THEREFOR
THE·DEGREE·OF

MASTER IN DENTAL SURGERY, ANESTHETICS & EXTRACTION

WITH·ALL·THE·RIGHTS·PRIVILEGES·AND·HONORS
THEREUNTO·APPERTAINING
GIVEN·AT·LOS·ANGELES·IN·THE·STATE·OF·CALIFORNIA
ON·THE·_____·19___

Carl Schultz, M.D. D.C. D.O.
PRESIDENT

Karl M. Pretz, N.D.
SECRETARY

During the late nineteenth century, numerous people visited health spas or "sanitariums." John Harvey Kellogg, the inventor of granola, established one of the most famous sanitariums of this period. Patients who visited his Michigan-based Battle Creek Sanitarium would exercise, get fresh air, eat special diets, and use "mechanotherapy" devices to improve their health. A special vibratory chair, for example, was designed to prevent constipation—by rapidly shaking the patient up and down! With "mechanotherapy,"

This degree was conferred upon students and apprentices in dentistry who paid a small fee for a pamphlet on dentistry. Most had no training in the art.

patients were supposed to use devices to maintain their health even if they weren't sick.

In addition to trying to improve their physical health, many early Americans consulted phrenologists who would assess their "mental constitution" by measuring the size and shape of a person's head. Although phrenologists initially did not use devices, that changed in 1905 when Henry C. Lavery invented the Psycograph, which gives personality printouts based on the size and shape of a person's head.

Beginning in the 1870s, a number of states began to pass general food safety laws, but most of these laws did not effectively

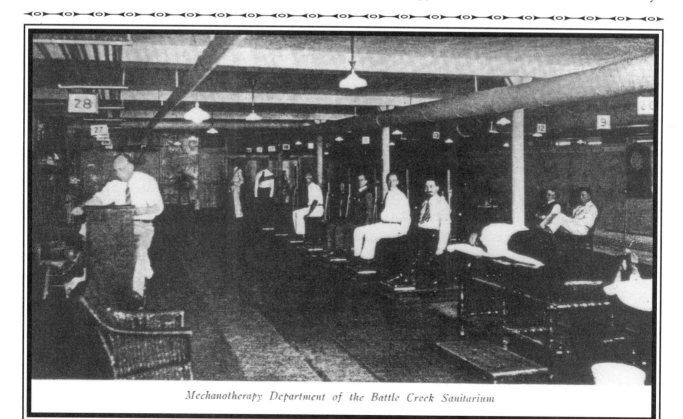
Mechanotherapy Department of the Battle Creek Sanitarium

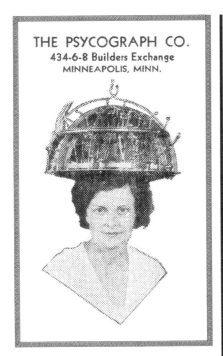

THE PSYCOGRAPH CO.
434-6-8 Builders Exchange
MINNEAPOLIS, MINN.

prevent the sale of harmful or worthless "medicines," including Hunt's Remedy for liver and kidney troubles, and Lydia Pinkham's syrup for women. By 1906, more than one hundred food and drug bills had been introduced in the U.S. Congress. Dr. Harvey Wiley, chief chemist of the U.S. Department of Agriculture from 1883

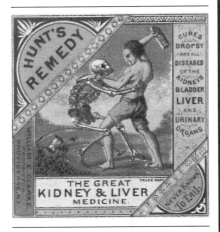

to 1912, was one of the most active proponents for federal laws governing food and drug safety. Wiley's efforts helped lead to the 1906 Pure Food and Drug Act, which prohibited the movement of adulterated foods and drugs in

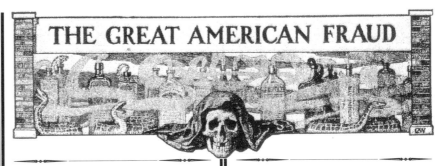

THE GREAT AMERICAN FRAUD

interstate commerce and required honest food labeling. This was a major strike against the patent remedy industry.

Public concern over these issues was evident in an influential series of articles that Samuel Hopkins Adams wrote for *Collier's* magazine from 1905 to 1907. "The Great American Fraud" was a multi-part exposé that documented the careers of numerous medical fakes who lied about their credentials, made false advertising claims,

took advantage of the gullible and the desperate, and often prescribed dangerous medicines containing opium, cocaine, and radium. In the January 13, 1906 installment in the series, Hopkins opened with the following remarks about the desperation of people:

"Incurable disease is one of the strongholds of the patent medicine business. The ideal patron, viewed in the light of profitable business, is the victim of some slow and wasting ailment in which

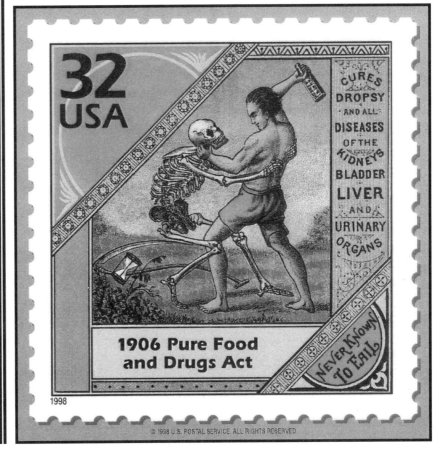

32 USA

1906 Pure Food and Drugs Act

1998

recurrent hope inspires to repeated experiments with any 'cure' that offers."

And in the September 1, 1906, article, Hopkins wrote these poignant words:

"Specializing is the modern tendency in medical practice. Hence the quack, who is but an exaggerated and grotesque imitation of the regular practitioner, smells money in devoting himself to specific fields of endeavor. Sedulously he perfects himself in his own department; not by acquiring knowledge of the nature and treatment of diseases, indeed, but by studying how most effectively to enmesh the sufferer from a certain class of ailments in the net of his specious promises."

The FDA and the Rise of Questionable Medical Devices

The early twentieth century saw the rapid rise of questionable medical practitioners who used devices instead of consumable medicines. This was a time when the United States experienced the success of automobiles, radios, and electric lights. Many writers dreamed of utopian futures, in which technology made the world spotless, healthy, and problem-free. The discoveries of X-rays and radium during the 1890s added to this excitement about the promise of new devices that used radiation to treat diseases— although a number of these new treatments turned out to be life-threatening.

As Americans' faith in new technology and new forms of energy grew, self-styled medical

inventors capitalized on the public's optimism. Many families purchased vibratory belts intended to shake off extra pounds, or hand-held electric or ultraviolet ray devices to boost fitness levels or cure just about everything. One of the most successful charlatans of this period was Albert Abrams, who was undoubtedly the "King of Quackery." Covered with knobs, switches, and dials, Abrams's furniture-sized

ALBERT ABRAMS

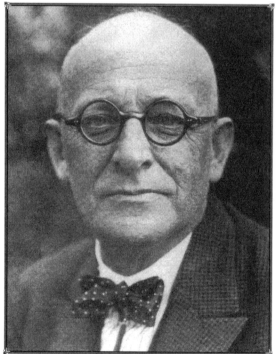

KING OF QUACKERY

machines apparently could diagnose and cure just about anything. Though impressive looking from the outside, these devices were essentially hollow on the inside— and utterly worthless.

The federal government's authority to regulate medical devices grew in 1928 when Congress authorized the Food, Drug and Insecticide Administration to work with the Pure Food and Drug

Act. In 1931 the unit's name changed to the Food and Drug Administration. The FDA had the power to inspect factories, scientifically test foods and drugs, and disseminate legal advice to prevent violations. The FDA's ability to police medical devices was granted in 1938 with the Federal Food, Drug and Cosmetic Act, which defined a medical device as "an instrument, apparatus, implement, machine, contrivance, implant, in vitro reagent, or other similar article that is intended for use in the diagnosis of disease or other conditions, or in the cure, mitigation, treatment or prevention of disease." This covered a lot of territory.

The Federal Food, Drug and Cosmetic Act had the following lasting effects:

- Cosmetic and therapeutic devices are regulated by the FDA.

- Drug manufacturers must provide scientific proof that new products are safe to use before putting them on the market.

- Companies cannot "misbrand" products with false or inaccurate labels.

- The FDA has the authority to inspect factories that produce medical products.

- Most drugs and certain medical devices must be approved by the FDA.

- The FDA has the authority to seize illegal medical devices and bring charges against those involved.

One of the first devices the FDA investigated was the

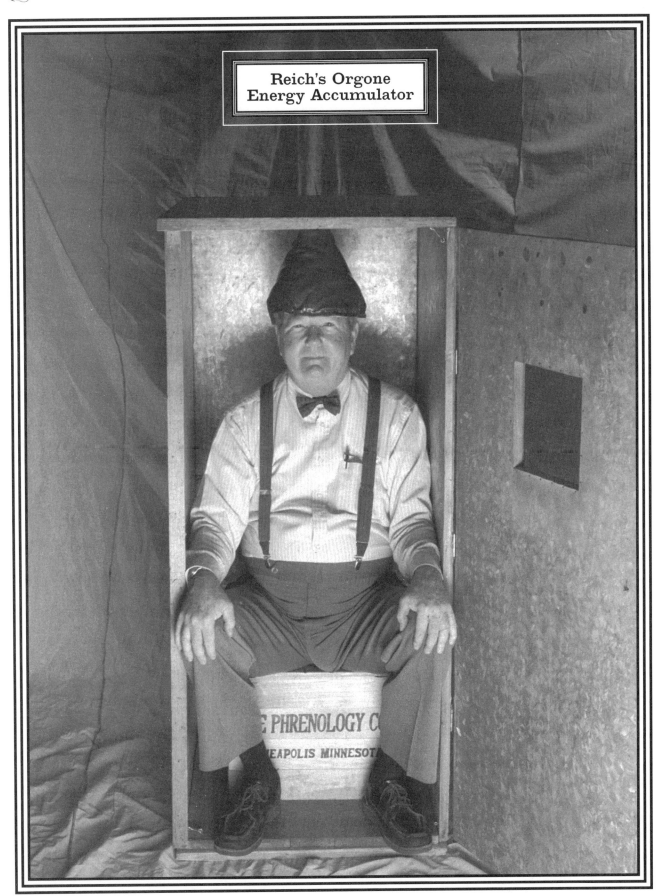

Reich's Orgone
Energy Accumulator

PROOF PRESS

Miles Medical Co.

· 1900 ·

Dr. Miles' Nervine was originally bottled in 1884 in the home of Elkhart, Indiana physician Dr. Franklin Miles. By 1890 the company formed by Dr. Miles was advertising in eight hundred

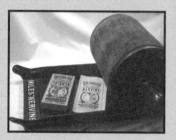

small town newspapers. The company promoted advertising in ingenious ways. In exchange for advertising space, they sent small newspapers such useful items as the proof press, electrotype ad, and ink brayer exhibited in this photo. His company later developed Alka-Seltzer and is now a part of Bayer AG of West Germany, the world's third largest pharmaceutical manufacturer.

It pays to advertise!

Dr. Miles' Restorative Nervine — Shipped by Charles Franklin Miles, Andrew H. Beardsley, and Albert R. Beardsley, traded as the Dr. Miles Medical Co. of Elkhart, Ind. Analysis showed the product to consist essentially of a watery solution of sugar, benzoic acid, arsenic, and bromide and chlorides of ammonium, calcium, potassium, and sodium, colored and flavored. Falsely and fraudulently advertised, C.F. Miles was fined $300 and costs, and A.R. and A.H. Beardsley were each fined $200 and costs.— (notice of Judgment No. 5892).

Spectrochrome. Invented in 1938 by "Doctor" Dinshah Ghadiali, the Spectrochrome projected different colored lights, each intended to treat a particular ailment or

—— DINSHAH GHADIALI ——

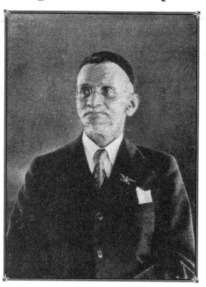

HUMBLE SERVANT OF SUFFERING MANKIND

strengthen the body in a particular way. But all of the colors of the Spectrochrome were equally ineffective, and Ghadiali was found guilty of fraud when he went on trial.

One of the most famous devices outlawed by the FDA was the Orgone Energy Accumulator. Invented in 1940 by noted psychoanalyst Wilhelm Reich, this uncomplicated-looking device supposedly used an undetectable form of energy to improve health. But the power of Orgone couldn't prevent Reich from going to prison for contempt in 1956–or from dying there a year later.

Over the years, the Federal Food, Drug and Cosmetics Act has been amended to further regulate medical devices. For example, in 1976 Congress amended

the act to require that new medical devices be proven safe and effective before going on the market. Previously, the law had been limited to action against hazardous or falsely represented devices after they went on sale. In 1990, the law was again amended with the Safe Medical Device Act, requiring medical facilities and product distributors to report to the FDA the number of deaths, serious illnesses, and serious injuries related to medical devices. Over the years, other nations have adopted similar laws to stop dangerous medicines and medical devices from reaching the public.

The maximum fine for individuals who violate the Federal Food, Drug and Cosmetic Act is now $100,000 per offense for conviction of a felony or of a misdemeanor resulting in death. For corporations, the maximum fine is twice that amount. In some instances, fines have been as high as $10 million for multiple offenders. In spite of these efforts, experts estimate that each year Americans spend $100 million on untested or quack medical cures that will not help them at all, and in some cases might worsen their condition.

Even though most quack devices eventually go off the market, many of these gadgets seem to reappear in one form or another a generation later, as there always seems to be plenty of new questionable medical devices to take the place of those that have been discredited.

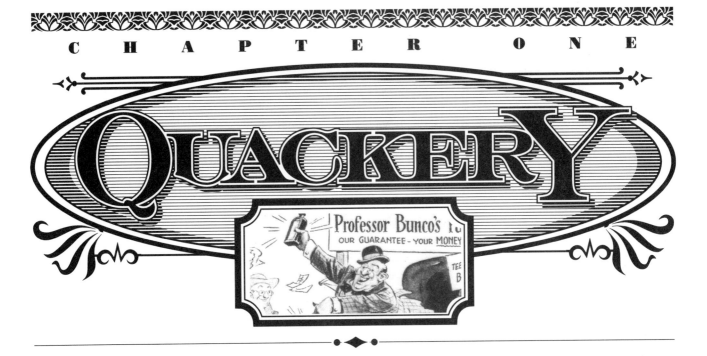

QUACKERY

Professor Bunco's
OUR GUARANTEE - YOUR MONEY

COMMON QUESTIONS AND THEIR ANSWERS.

What is a quack?

A quack is someone who offers medical treatments and medical advice that are not based on established medical knowledge or scientific principles. Quacks may provide questionable psychological advice as well. And quacks often have charismatic and reassuring personalities, heartwarming testimonials, or complicated charts and graphs. But not all quacks are alike. Here are three general types of quacks:

1. CHARLATANS. These con artists know that their cures don't work. Crooks at heart, they don't mind lying about their credentials or fabricating success stories to persuade people to pay for their fake cures. They are likely to have polished, well-scrubbed appearances, which hide their selfish motives.

2. WISHFUL THINKERS. These quacks often have a poor understanding of scientific principles and may sincerely believe that their remedies work. They can also seem like the most honest souls you've ever met. If you catch them exaggerating or misleading their patients, they'll say that it's only because modern science hasn't yet been able to prove that their remedies work.

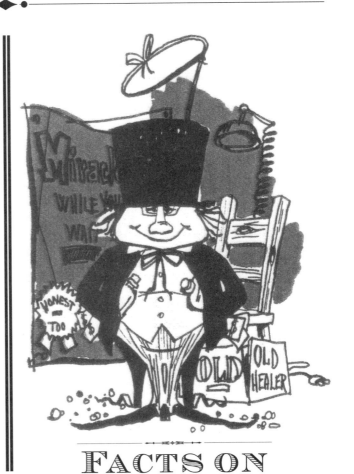

FACTS ON QUACKS

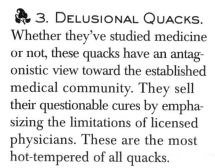

3. DELUSIONAL QUACKS. Whether they've studied medicine or not, these quacks have an antagonistic view toward the established medical community. They sell their questionable cures by emphasizing the limitations of licensed physicians. These are the most hot-tempered of all quacks.

What types of problems do people see quacks for?

People consult quacks for the same reasons they see licensed physicians or psychologists—to look and feel better. Here are some common reasons:

❦ To lose weight, cure baldness, or improve appearance.

❦ To relieve recurring headaches or back pain.

❦ To cure life-threatening illnesses.

❦ To relieve anxiety or depression.

❦ To increase overall strength and vitality.

❦ To enhance sexual pleasure and passion.

Why do people see quacks instead of certified physicians?

Quacks often have a knack for seeming sympathetic, dedicated, and optimistic. This helps them to convince patients that their cures may work, in spite of plenty of evidence to the contrary.

How do quacks try to look legitimate?

1. Many quacks use technological devices that look impressive—at least from the outside. This has been particularly true in

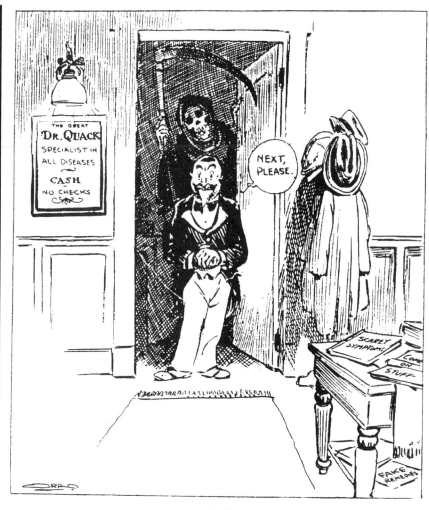

HIS SILENT PARTNER.

the twentieth century. These questionable medical devices may use colored lights, make mechanical noises, produce electric shocks, shake a patient's body, or contain numerous dials, switches, and knobs (which, in reality, may or may not do anything at all!).

2. Other quacks claim to use mysterious ingredients from far away lands, from under the ocean, or even from outer space. Exotic cures were a selling point in many of the traveling medicine shows that were popular in the nineteenth century. Some people today are still attracted to cures that sound like magic.

3. Quacks of all kinds try to manipulate language to increase sales. Some rely on "common sense" explanations and avoid jargon that could intimidate customers. Other quacks use complicated terms that might sound scientific to the general public. Different approaches work best for different types of quackery.

4. To appear trustworthy, quacks often rely on testimonials and personal stories from people who claim to have been cured. "If this worked for me," they say, "it can work for you." The authenticity of these testimonials, however, may be in question.

How can you tell if a new treatment is quackery?

Whether simple sounding or complex, quack explanations are based on principles that don't hold up under scientific scrutiny. Here are some examples:

1. The remedies rely on a substance or scientific process that doesn't exist or can't be proven in well-controlled laboratory studies done by impartial researchers.

2. The remedies ignore well-established laws of physics, chemistry, or biology.

3. The cures have explanations that contain fancy buzz words yet lack any scientific basis of their own.

4. The remedies utilize equipment that doesn't work mechanically, much less medically.

5. The treatment is based on the idea that if some type of treatment can help people under some circumstances than it can cure almost any physical or psychological problem.

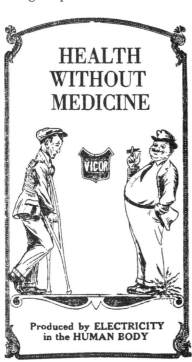

HEALTH WITHOUT MEDICINE

VIGOR

Produced by ELECTRICITY
in the HUMAN BODY

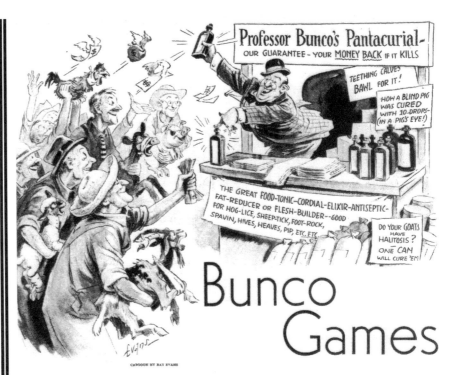

Bunco Games

Before there were infomercials and tabloids, hucksters sold their bogus cures through medicine shows. This 1920s-era cartoon parodies the one-bottle-cure-all claims touted by charlatans of the day.

Why do some forms of quack medicine seem to work?

1. Many physical symptoms are inherently temporary or cyclical; they naturally come and go. Because of this, patients may inaccurately conclude that a remedy was responsible for alleviating pain when it goes away for a brief period of time.

2. Using any type of cure may lessen a patient's fear and make them feel better emotionally—even while their physical symptoms persist.

3. Because patients believe they will get better, quack cures may alleviate psychosomatic symptoms, if only temporarily.

4. Due to optimism or stubbornness, patients may convince themselves that they feel better even if their symptoms persist or get worse.

5. Quacks often rely on real or fake testimonials from patients who say they have been cured. (But they won't tell you about the people who didn't get better!) This can give the impression that the quack treatment has a better track record than it really does.

Are quack medicines harmful?

Yes, some quack treatments are dangerous. But even those questionable remedies that don't cause direct physical harm can have negative consequences. Here are a few more things to keep in mind:

1. Quackery does cost money. Paying for a questionable medical treatment can inflict aches and pains to the checkbook.

2. Quack remedies often take a large amount of time. Who wants to spend 30 minutes a day

trying out a remedy that doesn't really work?

3. In addition to promoting their own pet cures or devices, many quacks give out misinformation about general health issues. They may pretend or presume they are knowledgeable about medical topics they really know nothing about–to the detriment of their patients.

4. Using unconventional remedies may prevent patients from seeking out established cures with a better chance of working. And some quack treatments may even interfere with existing medical treatments.

Mind over Matter?
—The Placebo Effect

People familiar with quackery are well aware of the term "placebo," as it helps to explain the persistence of many questionable remedies that provide no reliable medical benefits–even if true believers claim that they do.

Medical researchers use the term "placebo" to refer to harmless substances (such as sugar tablets) given to research subjects to test the results of new drugs or medical remedies given to other research subjects. In short, if enough people trying out the new drug get better than those who unknowingly take the placebo, the drug might work.

The "placebo effect," however, takes place when a patient appears to get better by using an unconventional remedy that actually has no scientific basis for working. In many cases, the "placebo effect" appears to alleviate psychological problems or psychosomatic ailments, if only temporarily. Through the placebo effect, patients might get better (or

You Might Be a Quack if...

☞ **You call yourself "Doctor" even though you don't have a medical degree.**

☞ **Your medical degree (and perhaps your high school diploma) comes from a mail-order diploma mill.**

☞ **You compare yourself to renowned scientists of the past.**

☞ **You promise quick results and easy answers.**

☞ **You ignore scientific evidence that contradicts your claims.**

☞ **You lack any concrete evidence to support your claims.**

☞ **You hire people to pretend that they've benefited from your cures.**

☞ **You offer your medical services door-to-door or through the mail.**

☞ **You offer information about medical topics you know nothing about.**

☞ **You complain that other physicians and scientists aren't taking your work as seriously as they should.**

☞ **You've been arrested several times.**

☞ **You advise your patients to use new machines, secret formulas, or undetectable chemicals "more advanced" than modern medicine.**

☞ **Large numbers of patients have died under your care.**

☞ **You claim that most conventional medical procedures actually cause people harm.**

☞ **You tell your patients to trust no one but you.**

☞ **Countless other doctors call you a "quack."**

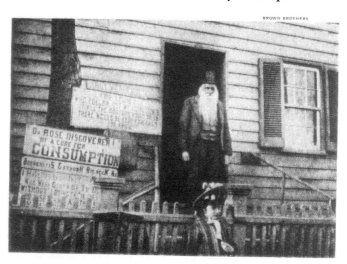

DR. ROSE, TIME AND PLACE UNKNOWN, SAID, "NOT MY PATIENT," AS FUNERALS PASSED BY.

It Might Be a Quack Device if . . .

☛ The machine apparently uses little-known energies that are undetectable by ordinary scientists.

☛ The device can diagnose or cure people living miles away.

☛ The machine has a convoluted yet "scientific-sounding" name.

☛ The device was invented by a "world famous" doctor that no one has ever really heard of.

☛ The manufacturer isn't exactly sure how or why the apparatus works.

☛ The machine has bright lights that serve no practical purpose.

☛ The device has knobs and dials that don't work.

☛ The gadget shakes, rattles, rolls, sucks, shocks, or warms your body.

☛ To get results, patients must face a certain direction or use the machine only at unusual times.

☛ The device can cure just about anything.

☛ You're supposed to use the machine even if nothing's wrong with you.

☛ The Food and Drug Administration has outlawed the device.

☛ The machine is available only through the mail or at special outlets.

☛ You can never find the contraption in a regular doctor's office.

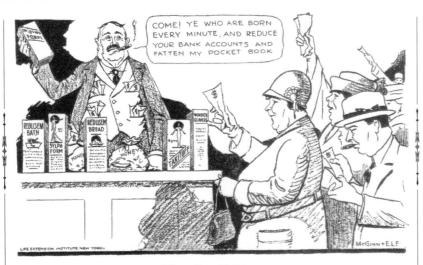

The Fat Fakirs

rather, think they are getting better) simply because they believe they will be cured—not because the treatment actually works. This can become very dangerous when patients talk themselves into thinking they are getting better—when in fact they are getting worse—and thus forgo proper medical treatment.

"Prof." Bragg—Food Faddist and Sexual Rejuvenator

Another hallmark of quacks is their use of common, everyday items as both the source of health problems as well as their cures. Nothing in this category is more prevalent than food quackery, a current trend spurred by deregulation of nutritional supplements. The Depression-era tale of Paul C. Bragg bears an eerie resemblance to some in the nutritional supplement business today.

The AMA on several occasions pointed out that the activities of "Prof." Bragg flouted many existing laws, and while he was sometimes fined and even declared a fraud by the post office, local authorities were often reluctant to do anything about his activities. These reports appeared in the "Bureau of Investigation" column of the *AMA Journal* on January 24, 1931 and April 18, 1936:

For years it has been known that those sections of the country in which elderly people and invalids congregate have more than their share of quacks and faddists. For this reason southern Florida is beginning to challenge the eminence of other resorts for this doubtful honor. This winter Miami has been visited by the quack who calls himself "Professor Paul C. Bragg." Readers of *The Journal*

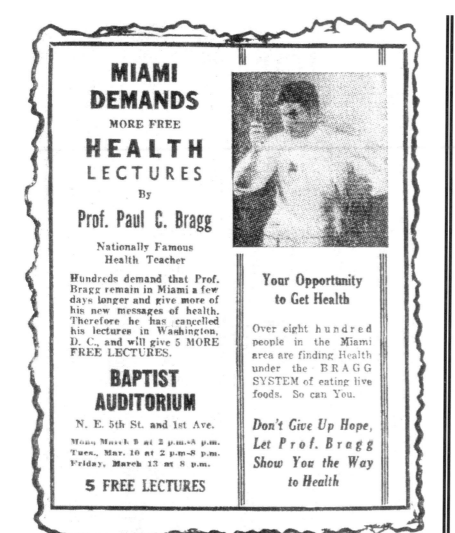

may remember what has been published regarding Bragg, who was described as a "food faddist and sexual rejuvenator." Bragg is one of those ignoramuses with a flair for public speaking who confer on themselves ornate titles and give "free lectures," which are really come-on advertisements for the books, the nostrums and the so-called private courses that they have for sale.

Bragg has worked particularly along two lines: food fads and sex, two subjects that are perennially popular with the type of intelligence that is impressed by charlatans of the Bragg type. Following the "free lectures," it has been Bragg's habit to take up collections, offer his books and "patent medicine" for sale, as well as suggest that the audience subscribe for his special classes.

Bragg seems to have found Miami

a lush field this winter, but toward the end of the season he began to talk of going back north. A Miami paper, however, in a March 8 advertisement stated that because of hundreds of demands, Bragg would remain in Miami a few days longer, and that he had "canceled his lectures in Washington, D.C.," and would give five more "free lectures."

Bragg's cancellation of his lectures in Washington, D.C. may have been due to the fact that suckers were still biting in Miami: but is quite as probable that his action was at least partly predicated on the fact that when he conducted his lecture in Washington a year ago he was charged with practicing the healing art without a license, found guilty and fined a hundred dollars. He violated the law of the District of Columbia by attempting to diagnose diseases, by prescribing a "patent medicine" of his own devising and by attempting to relieve certain diseases.

He is estimated to have taken about $7,000 out of Washington, for he charged $20 a person for a series of so-called classes which some 350 persons attended. Observers from the office of the Commission on Licenses and from the District medical Society attended Bragg's "classes" and obtained enough evidence to bring action against him in the police courts.

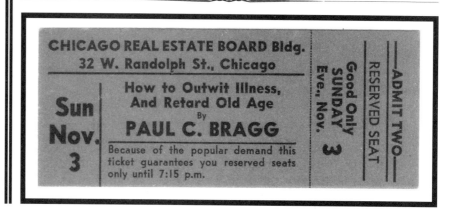

A report made by a physician regarding a talk Bragg gave on May 20, 1930 at the Trinity Church, Denver makes an interesting study. According to this report Bragg declared that the tonsils are spongy organs located in the throat, that tonsillitis is due to eating "mucus-forming foods," and the mucus so produced is caught by the spongy tonsils, causing them to swell up. He also claimed that cancer is caused by eating "gooey, slimy foods," that tuberculosis is due to the fact that young girls smoke cigarettes, that colds are caused by the eating of white bread or ice cream, and that asthma, "gas on the stomach," "pink tooth brush," etc., are caused by formations of mucus due to eating white bread! Of course, "Bragg Laboratories" had a white bread substitute for sale along with something called "Live Sprinkle"—a substitute for salt that contained sodium chloride!

As another of his activities, Bragg went into the mail-order business, selling a "patent medicine" called "Glantex." Some of the claims made for Glantex were:

"No matter how old you are or how weak and run down you are from abuses or other causes, Glantex never fails. It is used by men and women the world over. Glantex works wonders!"

One month's supply of Glantex sold for five dollars though the United States mails. In November, 1930, the postal authorities called on Mr. Bragg. They pointed out in their memorandum that Bragg, who was not a physician, was promising that his various preparations would produce cures. It was brought out in the investigation that those who purchased Glantex, both men and women, received a circular-letter advising them to take cold sitz baths daily—whether the patient suffered from inflammation of the prostate or from painful menstruation. The Postmaster issued a fraud order and notified local postmasters that they were forbidden to pay any postal money orders drawn to the order of Bragg's outfits and were to return all letters and other mail matter addressed to Bragg and his concerns to the senders, with the word "Fraudulent" stamped on it.

This of course did not prevent Bragg from continuing his much more profitable schemes of "courses and lectures" in person. He just changed his name!

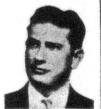

PROF. BRAGG

Will Bring You Back to

Health Nature's Way

PROF. PAUL C. BRAGG
America's Foremost Lecturer Teacher and Writer on Scientific Living Principles

NOT with medicines, not with surgery, not with vaccines and drugs; but he will teach you how to banish all disease and build abundant, glorious health through following the unfailing principles of Nature. In past years you have disregarded Nature and her rules by wrong habits of living, by inactivity and the over-rich, devitalized foods of civilization. In consequence you have become sick. Prof. Bragg will instruct you how to overcome this mistake and be completely rid of all your ailments by living in accordance with Nature's great inviolable laws. He will teach you how to revitalize and rejuvenate your body, step by step, internally and externally. He has done this for hundreds of others, and he can do it for you, through his scientific and never-failing application of the natural laws governing the physical body.

Free Lectures Now Going On
TEMPLE THEATRE
January 15-22—8:15 P. M.

REMEMBER THAT—
SICKNESS is *ignorance!*
OLD AGE is *unnecessary!*

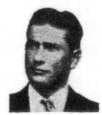

Great New Message of

HEALTH

"How to Banish Disease and be Strong and Healthy at Any Age"

By PAUL CHAPPIUS

Internationally Known Health Writer, Lecturer and Research Worker

Hear the man who has rebuilt thousands by his System of Scientific Blood Cleansing and Tissue Purification.
Learn how you can banish disease and outwit old age by following his simple new drugless, natural-living methods.

7 FREE LECTURES
PALACE THEATRE
March 22nd to 28th Inclusive, 8:30 P. M.

Paul C. Bragg was declared a fraud, December 30, 1930. On March 23, 1931, one "Paul Chappius," describing himself as an "Internationally Known Health Writer, Lecturer and Research Worker," appeared in Houston, Texas. Above right is reproduced the first page of a Chappius leaflet; on the left, the first page of a Paul C. Bragg leaflet.

MECHANICAL

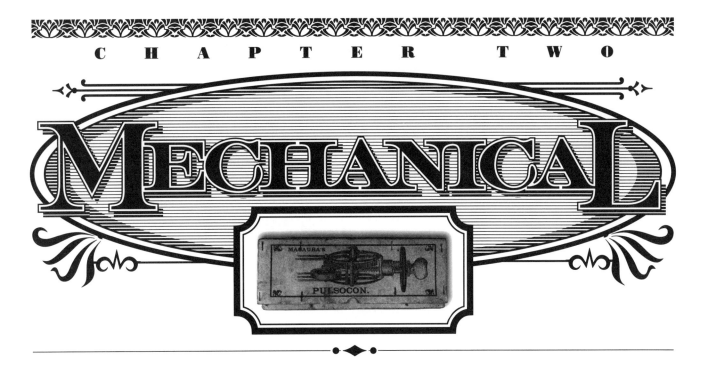

PULSOCON.

SIMPLE MACHINES TO SET YOU STRAIGHT.

While quacks often claim their devices are a part of a new and emerging technology, some classic quack devices are actually very simple machines. Bloodletting devices were wedges designed to cut into veins; of these, the spring operated 12 blade scarificator was the most complex. Of course, bloodletting devices are not truly quackery, for in their time they were considered to be on the "cutting edge" of modern medical practice. Perkins Tractors, the first quack medical device in the U.S., were levers with a point. By the twentieth century, hand-cranked gears operated a vibrator, a clamp with nasty wedges controlled nocturnal emissions, and a hand-operated rescue pump was powerful enough to collapse the lungs of a child. With the arrival of electricity, a small electric motor and a belt could transform everyday objects into vibratory cures.

Phlebotomy: The Ancient Art of Bloodletting

The practice of bloodletting seemed logical when the foundation of all medical treatment was based on the four body humors: blood, phlegm, yellow bile, and black bile. Health was thought to be restored by purging, starving, vomiting, or bloodletting.

The art of bloodletting was flourishing well before Hippocrates in the fifth century B.C. By the

Middle Ages, both surgeons and barbers were specializing in this bloody practice. Barbers advertised with a red (for blood) and white (for a tourniquet) striped pole. The pole itself represented the stick squeezed by the patient to dilate the veins.

Bloodletting came to America on the Mayflower. The practice reached unbelievable heights in the eighteenth and early nineteenth centuries. The first U.S. president, George Washington, died of a throat infection in 1799 after being drained of 9 pints of

The Spring Loaded Lancet

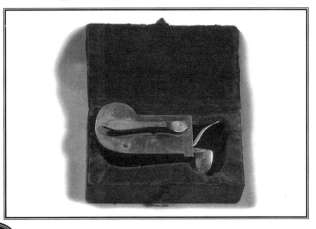

Spring loaded lancets appeared in the eighteenth century.

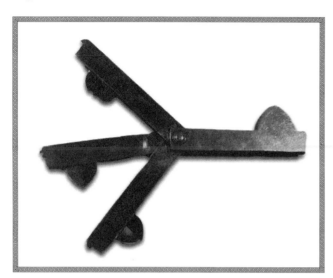

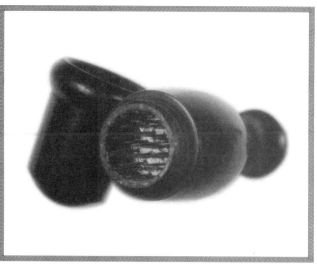

BLOODLETTING. An all-steel fleam with three different size blades that fold up into the handle. The fleam was extremly popular in the eighteenth and nineteenth centuries. A wooden "fleam stick" was often used to hit the back of the blade to drive it further into the vein.

BAUNCHEIDT'S LEBENSWECKER (1851-1915). Lebenswacker is German for "Life Awakener." The hollow ebony tube contained a handle with coiled springs attached. When pushed, the 30 sharp needles punctured the skin. This would "awaken" anyone.

blood within 24 hours. The draining of 16 to 30 ounces (1 to 4 pints) of blood was typical. Blood was often caught in a shallow bowl, and when the patient became faint the "treatment" was stopped. Bleeding was often encouraged over large areas of the body by multiple incisions. By the end of the nineteenth century, phlebotomy was declared quackery.

A variety of devices were used to draw blood:

• The lancet was first used before fifth century B.C. The vein was manually perforated by the practitioner. Many shallow cuts were sometimes made.

• Spring loaded lancets came into use during the early eighteenth century. The device was cocked and a "trigger" fired the spring-driven blade into the vein.

• The fleam was heavily used during the eighteenth and nineteenth centuries, and many varieties existed. Sometimes a wooden "fleam stick" was used to hit the back of the blade and drive it into the vein. The fleam was also often used by veterinarians.

• The scarificator, a series of twelve blades, was also in vogue during the eighteenth century. This device was cocked and the trigger released spring-driven rotary blades which caused many shallow cuts. The scarificator seems more merciful than the other bloodletting instruments.

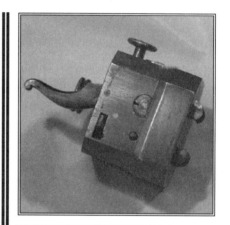

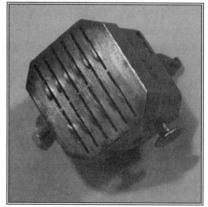

The Scarificator (CA. 1790) USED FOR TOPICAL BLEEDING, ALLOWED THE PHLEBOTOMIST TO REGULATE THE DEPTHS OF THE CUTS.

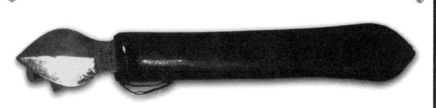

Fleams CAME IN TWO SIZES: LARGE FOR ANIMALS AND SMALL FOR PEOPLE.

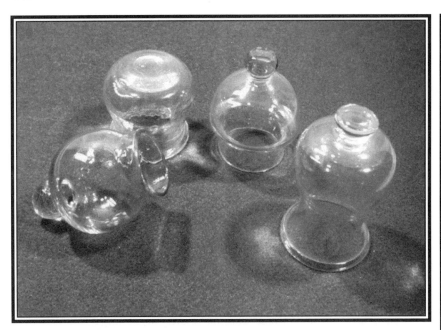

Alcohol was burned in glass cupping cups to create a vacuum. As soon as the flame burned out, the cup was applied to the wound to accelerate bleeding.

• Blood was caught in shallow bowls. During the seventeenth to nineteenth centuries, blood was also captured in small flint glass cups. Heated air inside the cups created a vacuum causing blood to flow into the cup—a handy technique for drawing blood from a localized area. This practice was called cupping.

Perkins Tractors

Ironically, the first medical device patented in the United States in 1796 was Perkins Metallic Tractors, a quack device. The metallic tractors were used for the relief of pain and disease by Dr. Elisha Perkins (1745–1799), an American physician and, for a long time, president of the Connecticut Medical Society. The tractors, pairs of rods about three inches long and pointed at one end, were hammered out of iron and brass ("the white" and "the yellow") though their "formula" claimed that one rod

contained copper, zinc, and gold, while the other contained iron, silver, and platinum.

The rods were used as levers pressed against the skin to draw

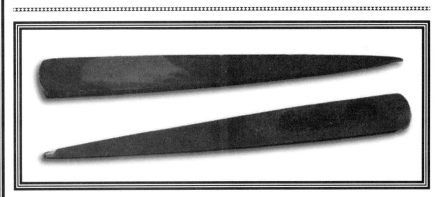

☞ These reproductions of Perkins Tractors are on permanent loan from the U.S. Food and Drug Administration.

harmful "electricity" out through the extremities, for Dr. Perkins believed that toxic electricity caused disease. His belief was rooted in the concept of "animal magnetism," or organically generated electricity. This concept was the result of scientist Luigi Galvani's

1791 discovery that a frog muscle would twitch when touched with an electrically charged scalpel. Galvani believed the electricity was in the muscle, but Italian physicist Alessandro Volta repeated the Galvani experiment and discovered the source of the current was dissimilar metals. Count Volta went on to build his "voltaic pile" of dissimilar metals which generated an electric current, an accomplishment today recognized as the first chemical battery.

Dr. Perkins may have noticed that a muscle touched with a metal pointer would twitch. He claimed that the Tractors could draw out the pains of headache, rheumatism, and other ills. Later, he added paralysis, lameness, and deformities to the list. Application of the Tractors varied with the condition.

The Metallic Tractors was the fad device of their day–high government officials, including the family of President George

Washington (who signed the Tractors patent) were said to use the device. Benjamin Douglas Perkins, Elisha's son, brought the tractors to London where a pair sold for five pounds to doctors and for ten pounds to the general public. A physician in Chester,

Dr. John Haygarth, became interested in the device and, enlisting the aid of his friend, William Falconer, conducted tests on the effectiveness of Tractors. Dr. Haygarth made a pair of "Wooden Tractors of nearly the same shape as the metallic, painted to resemble them in color" and applied them alternately with Perkin's Metallic Tractors to five patients with "Chronik Rheumatism." The "ligneous Tractors" were found to have the same effect as the "metallick" and Haygarth concluded that both acted by "the impression . . . made upon the patient's imagination." Dr. Haygarth published his findings in the tract, "Of the Imagination as

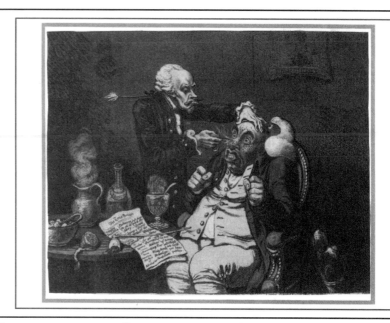

AN ENGRAVING BY GILRAY SHOWING PERKINS "TERRIBLE TRACTORS" IN USE.

OF THE

IMAGINATION,

AS A CAUSE AND AS A CURE OF DISORDERS OF THE BODY;

EXEMPLIFIED BY

FICTITIOUS TRACTORS,

AND

EPIDEMICAL CONVULSIONS.

" DECIPIMUR SPECIE." HOR.

Read to the Literary and Philosophical Society of Bath.

BY

JOHN HAYGARTH, M.D.

F. R. S. LOND. AND EDINB.
OF THE ROYAL MEDICAL SOCIETY AT EDINBURGH, AND OF THE AMERICAN
ACADEMY OF ARTS AND SCIENCES.

BATH, PRINTED BY R. CRUTTWELL;
AND SOLD BY
CADELL AND DAVIES, STRAND, LONDON.

1800.

Price One Shilling.

FRONT COVER OF DR. HAYGARTHS' PAMPHLET DECRYING THE EFFECTIVENESS OF THE PERKINS TRACTORS.

a Cause and as a Cure of Disorders of the Body" in 1800.

Back in the United States, the Connecticut Medical Society, of which Elisha Perkins was a founder, became suspicious of the sensational Tractors cure. Members built wooden tractors of their own and duplicated the Haygarth experiments. The tractors were considered "faith medicine" and Dr. Perkins was expelled from the society as "a patentee and user of nostrums."

The Macaura Pulsocon

While Gerald Macaura called himself a "vibrotherapist," his true gift was a genius for advertising. In 1908, he founded an "institute" in Manchester, England, that featured many drugless cures. It was here that he devised the Pulsocon (originally called the Pulsator). The Pulsocon was a simple machine that worked like an egg beater, with a hand-turned crank that operated gears which in turn caused a vibratode to vibrate. The alleged benefits of

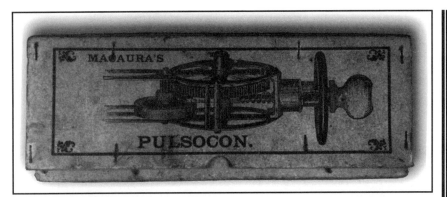

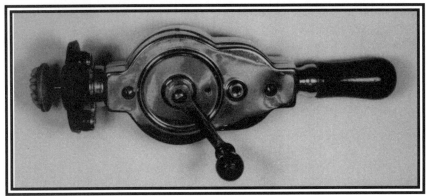

Macaura Pulsocon.

the Pulsocon were increased circulation, loosened joints, and elimination of chronic pain.

Mr. Macaura rented theaters and put on popularly attended lectures to advertise his device. His greatest marketing achievement was persuading the influential and prestigious social reformer, journalist, and reviewer, W. T. Snead, to "test" and endorse the Pulsocon during a lecture. The event received excellent free coverage in British newspapers. Mr. Snead later reversed his position and disavowed the efficacy of the Pulsocon, an announcement barely mentioned in the press. Mr. Macaura also had a hefty print advertising budget.

Mr. Macaura's success in England was short-lived; by 1911, he was working in continental Europe. In 1912, he was expelled from Prussia on the charge of

"attempt to cheat." In Paris, he was charged with practicing medicine illegally and swindling; a Paris

court sentenced him to three years and a $600 fine. Meanwhile, the Cirkulon Institute of Kansas City, Missouri distributed the device in the U.S. under the brand name of "Cirkulon." The 1914 U.S. price was $15, a cost $5.50 higher than Pulsocons sold for in Great Britain.

The Timely Warning

In his 1888 book, *Plain Home Talk*, Dr. Edward B. Foote expressed his concerns about amorous dreams, today called nocturnal emissions:

"An amourous dream is indeed practically an involuntary act of masturbation. It has often been remarked that no exercise is so tiresome to the muscular system as to kick or strike at nothing. All know, too, how it wrenches one to step down a foot or two while walking. What this wrench is to the muscular system, an amative dream is to the nervous system. A volley of

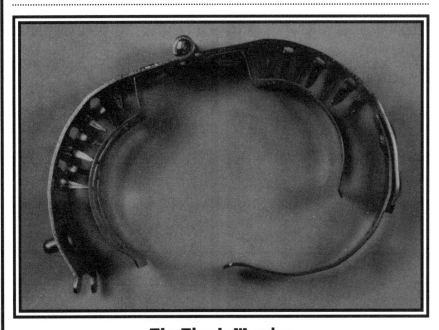

The Timely Warning.

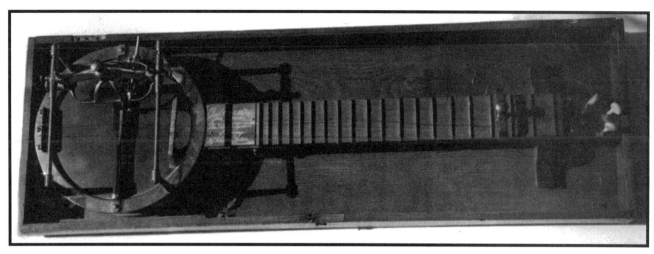

THE VIBROMETER.

nervous force is gathered up from all parts of the body, and directed with the greatest impetuosity toward a supposed companion in the sexual embrace, and it passes off with violence and is lost, while the compensative nervous or electrical volley from the supposed companion is not received. In men this nervous loss is accompanied with an expenditure of some of the most vital fluids of the system—those secreted by the testicular glands, and which are composed of the most vital elements of the blood. This nervous waste—the nervous shock—the wrench of the magnetic system, as such as will, if frequently repeated, prostate the nervous energies, destroy the memory, and weaken all the faculties of the mind."

Dr. Foote seems to have pondered this problem for well over a decade, for in 1905 he patented the Timely Warning, his solution to the problem of amorous dreams. The device is basically a two-inch hose clamp, albeit very unusual with the addition of triangular teeth with the points facing inward. And yes, the two dollar contraption—"made of aluminum weighs but two drams and saves pounds of drugs and worry"—was designed to be worn around the penis. As stated in the promotional material, upon erection the Timely Warning "prevents night emissions by arousing the wearer."

The Vibrometer

The Vibrometer was used for applying "Dr. Garey's System of Massage by Vibratory Motion" according to a silver plate attached to the device. A motor powered a small wheel containing tacks which "plucked" the strings of the banjo-like instrument. The wheel was mounted within the chrome casing. The instrument sounds like a sitar and appears to have "cured" ailments using the vibrations of musical notes.

The Battle Creek Combination Vibratory Chair

The Battle Creek Vibratory Chair was extolled as four machines in one: a vibrating chair, a vibrating footstool, a vibrating bar, and a foot vibratory. The wood in the chair is sturdy mahogany, and slats in the back of the chair are curved to promote optimal posture. Vibration is caused by an electrical motor attached to the seat of the chair with belts. The chair is elevated from the floor and cushioned on vibrating coil springs—this prevents transmission of vibration to the floor so that the patient receives the full effect! The chair does vibrate rather violently.

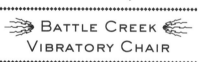

BATTLE CREEK VIBRATORY CHAIR

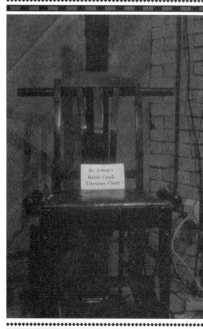

The Vibratory Chair was marketed to hospitals, institutions, clubs, gymnasiums, private homes, and steamship companies. Physicians, it was suggested, might install a Vibratory Chair in their waiting rooms to entertain patients "weary of waiting."

Standing on the rubber-coated mahogany platform at the front of the chair was recommended for increasing circulation to the feet and the legs. Localized treatment for the lower limbs was achieved by placing the patient in a stationary chair situated behind the Vibratory Chair with her feet resting in two metal foot plates attached to the rear of the apparatus. In addition to increased circulation, this position was claimed to draw the blood to the lower extremities thereby relieving congestion (such as congestion of the lungs) in all parts of the upper body.

The greatest impact of the vibration was experienced while sitting directly on the chair seat. The headrest was designed to vibrate the head and neck and on either side of the seat were handles to increase vibration to the hands and arms. Claims for the chair included increasing volume of blood supply and lymph flow, enhancing cell nutrition, improving respiratory function, stimulating body secretion, curing constipation, toning muscles, improving metabolism, aiding in production of animal heat, improving excretion and elimination, and relieving muscle contraction, engorgement, congestion, varicosity, eruption, and pain. A treatment of three to four minutes was said to renew vigor while a slightly longer treatment of four to five minutes would stimulate peristalsis. Prolonged treatments were required to increase body temperature.

The chair was manufactured by the Sanitarium and Hospital Equipment Company ("The Home of Physiotherapy") in Battle Creek, Michigan, a sideline of the Battle Creek Sanitarium and its chief of staff, Dr. John Harvey Kellogg. For the curious, the Vibratory Chair can be seen in action in the 1993 film, *The Road to Wellville.*

Res-Q-Aire
Emergency Respirator

Individuals aren't the only purchasers of quack medical devices. Organizations have supported quacks after listening to a high-powered sales pitch. During the 1960s, Crown Products of Cleveland made such pitches to service clubs and organizations urging them to purchase emergency equipment for groups and institutions in their communities. They were selling the Res-Q-Aire Emergency Respirator, a resuscitation device. According to Crown Air, the device was effective for "every breathing difficulty."

The Battle Creek Vibratory Chair in action.

The easy-to-read instructions failed to warn that the device was inappropriate for emergencies involving obstructions, aspirated objects, and dentures. No warning explained that the pump generated an air volume which might damage the lungs of a small child or infant. The labeling was charged as false and misleading and the FDA argued that the directions were inadequate, as adequate instructions could not be written. A default decree ordered that the devices be destroyed.

THE RES-Q-AIRE.

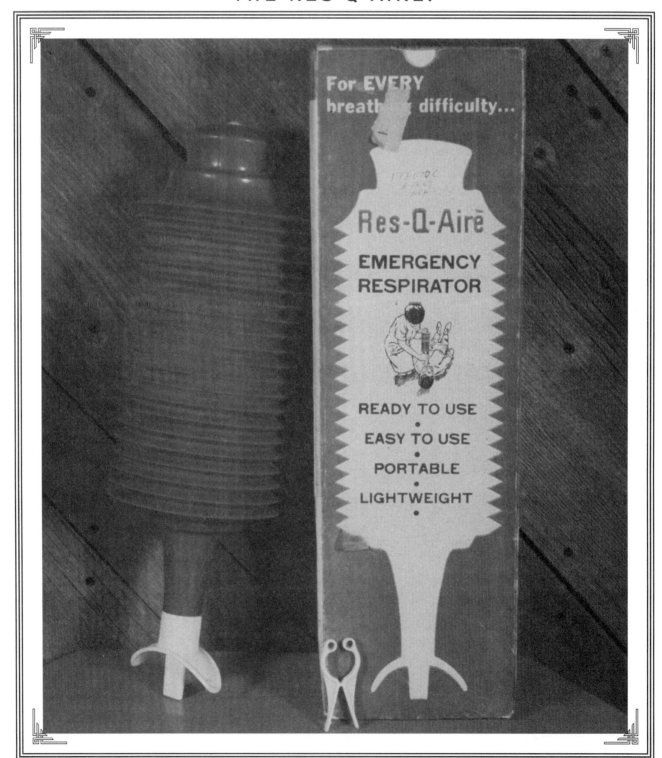

For EVERY breathing difficulty...

Res-Q-Aire

EMERGENCY RESPIRATOR

READY TO USE
•
EASY TO USE
•
PORTABLE
•
LIGHTWEIGHT
•

MAGNETISM

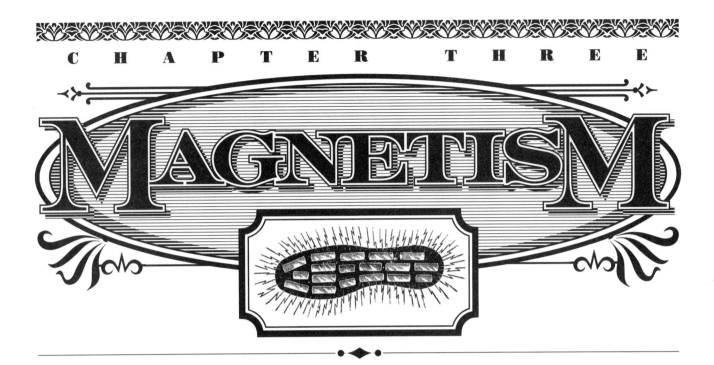

THE CURATIVE MAGIC OF MAGNETS.

Magnetism has fascinated people for hundreds of years, ever since the discovery of lodestones–rocks containing magnetite. Because lodestones had the unusual ability to attract iron, philosophers speculated that these materials might have other wonderful properties as well. Interest in the healing properties of magnets became widespread during the Middle Ages, when many European physicians thought that lodestones might work as an aphrodisiac or serve to cure such ailments as gout, arthritis, poisoning, and baldness.

In the sixteenth century, Swiss alchemist and physician Paracelsus became one of the most famous scientists to test the healing potential of lodestones, investigating if they could treat epilepsy, diarrhea, hemorrhages, and other problems. Early surgeons sometimes used magnets to help remove shattered blades or other weapons from victims, and during the nineteenth century, some physicians and more than a few charlatans combined the notions of magnetic healing with forms of hypnotism when treating patients, although this idea fell out of favor over time.

Rising Popularity in the Twentieth Century

Despite the fact that the AMA's first alert to its members about what they called "mechanical fakes" occurred in *The Journal* in 1910, a long list

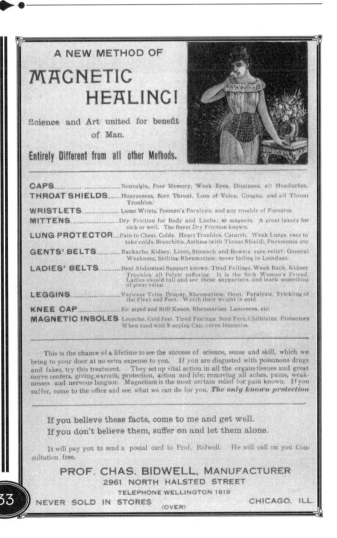

of magnetic products, making a wide variety of claims, have been available on the market over the past one hundred years. A 1922 ad for several magnetic devices made this ambitious announcement:

"This is the chance of a lifetime to see the success of science, sense and skill, which we bring to your door at no extra expense to you. If you are disgusted with poisonous drugs and fakes, try this treatment. They set up vital action in all the organs, tissues and great nerve centers, giving warmth, protection, action and life; removing all aches, pains, weakness and nervous languor. Magnetism is the most certain relief for pain known. If you suffer, come to the office and see what we can do for you. The only known protection."

In spite of such bold claims, there was plenty of reason to believe that magnets were not as effective as the advertisements claimed. For example, the February 17, 1929, edition of *The Detroit Free Press* carried an advertisement for the Theronoid, a magnetic belt that purportedly removed harmful waste from the body and treated chronic ailments. According to the ad, the Theronoid had cured Peter J. Clemens of a life-threatening gall-bladder infection. But the following day, *The Detroit Free Press* carried an obituary for Mr. Clemens, reporting that he had died of pneumonia! (See right.) Clearly the Theronoid's powers were limited.

Although interest in magnetic devices faded in the decades that followed, the 1990s saw a new surge of interest in the healing powers of magnets, motivated in part by Major League baseball players who told reporters that

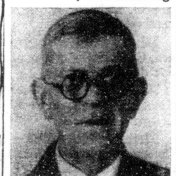

WHAT ARE TESTIMONIALS WORTH?

The Detroit Free Press

SUNDAY, FEBRUARY 17, 1929.

Gall Bladder and Stomach Trouble

Detroit man finds relief after two years suffering

PETER J CLEMENS, 325 Drexel Ave, Detroit, Mich

Mr. Clemens suffered a severe attack of stomach pains two years ago, belched large quantities of

gas. The diagnosis by his own physician was infection of the gall bladder, but treatment for that condition did not give satisfactory results. Could scarcely eat anything whatever. Lost 34 pounds weight and suffered a continuation of his symptoms until November 27th, 1928, when he purchased a Theronoid. Improvement was noted during first month's use and in January, 1929, he reports normal appetite and digestion, 10 pounds increase in weight, health and strength restored so that he can walk 10 miles with ease

Try Theronoid Free

A safe, easy, pleasant method of applying magnetic energy to the body in a form which has proven effective in most chronic ailments. Call at our nearest office or phone for free home demonstration.

Theronoid of Detroit

MONDAY, FEBRUARY 18, 1929.

PETER J. CLEMENS DIES AFTER WEEK'S ILLNESS

Peter J. Clemens, 64, 325 Drexel avenue, died yesterday at his home following a week's illness of pneumonia.

Clemens was born at Eagle River, Mich. He came to Detroit when five years old. For many years he was head brewmaster at the East Side brewery in Detroit and later was brewmaster at the Pontiac brewery. About 13 years ago he opened a billiard hall at 12856 East Jefferson avenue. He was a member of the Elks lodge of Pontiac.

Surviving are his widow, Elizabeth; two sons, Raymond and Gilbert; a daughter, Mrs. Fred Rachwitz, and a brother, Raymond.

wearing magnets improved their strength, speed, and overall performance. Others have said that magnets can help treat a wide variety of physical ailments, including arthritis, rheumatism, asthma, headaches, writer's cramp, gout, varicose veins, insomnia, stress, general aches and pains, skin legions, sore muscles, cancer, warts, or problems in the kidneys, liver, lungs, stomach, and bowels.

Today, numerous magnetic devices are on the market, often selling for anywhere from $25 to $100 (and sometimes a lot more). Many of these devices fit like

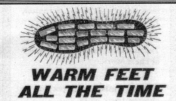

clothing, jewelry or apparel, such as magnetic belts, bracelets, and shoe insoles. There are also magnetic seat cushions, magnetic coils, and adhesive magnetic patches. And then there are magnetic body pads, knee braces, mattresses, mittens, back braces, eye masks, thigh supporters, elbow tubes, wrist bands, ankle wraps, and back supporters. The list goes on and on.

Many of these products are washable or stretchable, or include copper plating, building on folk medical beliefs that copper bracelets can reduce the effects

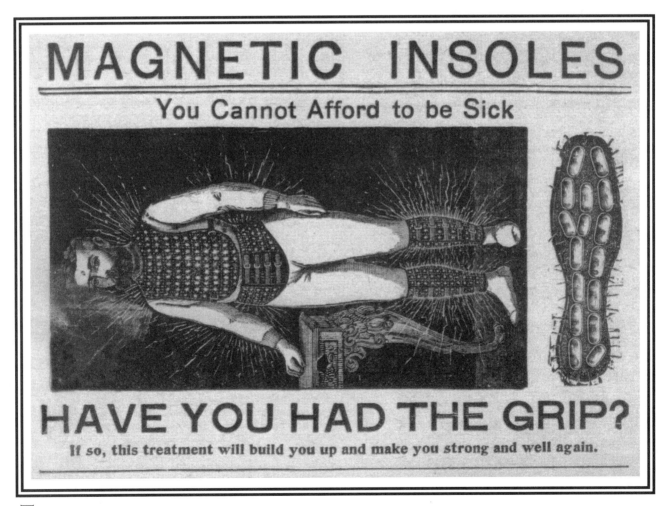

Typical of the grandiose ads touting magnets that continue to this day. Most of these products claim to heal illness with magnetic force. Modern proponents claim that magnets can be used for diagnosis of "magnetic deficiency states."

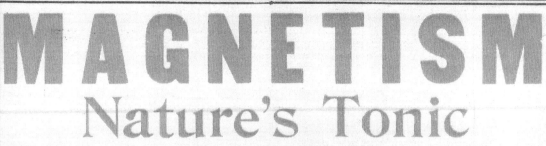
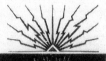
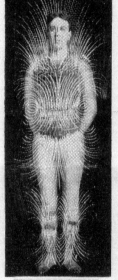
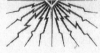
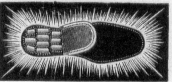

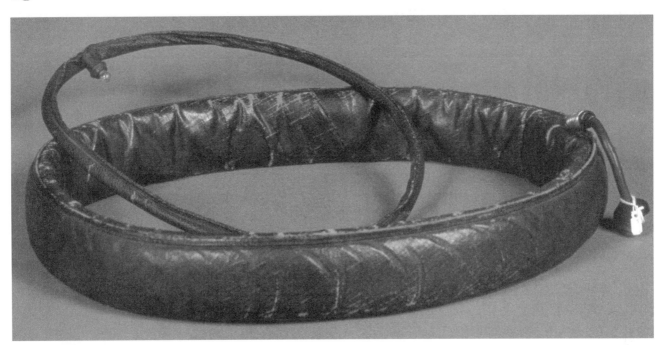

The Wilshire I-ON-A-CO was dubbed the "Magic Horse Collar," and was the first magnetic belt on the market. The I-ON-A-CO—for I Own A Company—was made by Gaylord Wilshire. It was simply a coil of insulated wire about 18 inches in diameter, with an electric plug. It was placed over the neck of the patient, and would supposedly magnetize the iron in the patient's blood. There was a smaller coil that played no part in the alleged curative use the belt, but did play an all-important part in the magical features of the scheme. The smaller coil was also of insulated wire, having its two free ends attached to a miniature light socket containing a flashlight bulb. When the larger coil was plugged into the light socket, the small coil lit up when it was brought in close proximity to the large coil, supposedly demonstrating the power of the larger coil.

of arthritis and alleviate other aches and pains. Some magnetic devices allegedly use some of the principles of acupuncture as well.

Here is a list of some common magnetic devices that have been on the market over the years, plus the types of problems they allegedly cure:

Copper Bracelet: alleviates arthritis, neuritis, and general soreness.

Magnetic Bandages: for arthritis and general aches and pains.

Magnetic Belt: treats back aches, removes fat from around the middle, gets rid of constipation, and treats kidney, liver, stomach, or bowel problems.

Magnetic Bracelet: prevents carpal tunnel syndrome.

Magnetic Cap: improves memory and eyesight, and prevents headaches and dizziness.

Magnetic Leggings: for varicose veins and gout.

Magnetic Lung Protector: prevents colds, asthma, and heart trouble.

Magnetic Mattress: relieves

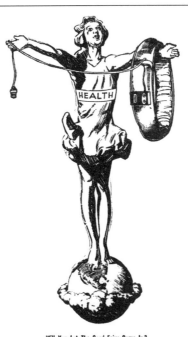

Will You Let The Good Fairy Come In?
THERONOID
Brings Health to Your Home   Keeps Health in Your Home

stress, improves blood circulation, and gives you a good night's sleep.

Magnetic Patches: alleviate pain, reduce stiffness and swelling, and improve blood circulation.

Magnetic Shoe Insoles: treat hot, sweaty, cold, and sore feet—and in some cases cure colds, rheumatism, neuralgia, and the swelling of the limbs.

Magnetic Throat Shield: prevents sore throats.

Science Speaks Out

Scientific researchers have debated whether magnets ever have any permanent effect on patients, or if the benefits are nothing more than the "placebo effect" (in other words, "the power of suggestion"). Laboratory researchers have found that magnetic fields do have a minor biological effect, but increasing the dosage beyond a certain point

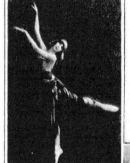
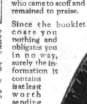
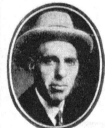
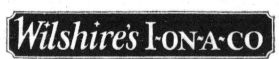

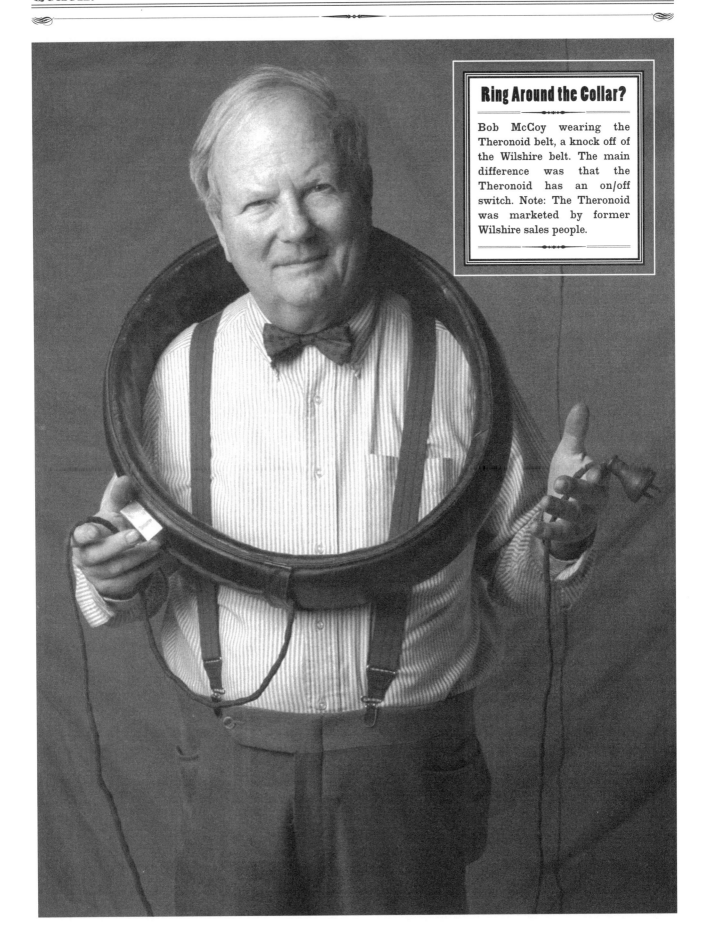

Ring Around the Collar?

Bob McCoy wearing the Theronoid belt, a knock off of the Wilshire belt. The main difference was that the Theronoid has an on/off switch. Note: The Theronoid was marketed by former Wilshire sales people.

does not appear to increase benefits. According to some research, magnets are not effective unless they have a gauss measurement of magnetic strength of at least 500–much stronger than a regular refrigerator magnet, which has a gauss measurement of only 10. But many magnetic devices on the market aren't much stronger than refrigerator magnets.

Concluding that there is no scientific evidence that magnets have a permanent, beneficial effect in the treatment of cancer, or that they will relieve pain beyond a placebo effect, the Food and Drug Administration has made efforts to stop the sale of several magnetic devices promoted for

pain relief, including Acu-Dots and the Magnetic Ray Belt.

In 1991, the International Medical Research Center of Murrieta, California, paid $40,000

in fines and court costs and agreed to stop selling magnet devices as medical aids designed to permanently cure patients. The company had placed a billboard at the

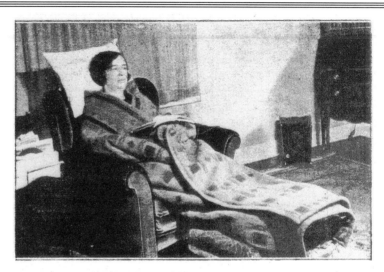

The Magnecoil Tonic Treatment.

Tonic treatments may be taken as here shown or by spreading the MAGNECOIL on bed or couch and lying on it. These treatments are taken while fully dressed and as often as possible. Backaches, fatigue, "that tired feeling" are thus treated.

Acu-Dot Magnetic analgesic patches falsely claimed to provide temporary relief from occasional minor aches and pains of muscles and joints. Multiple FDA Seizures. (1980)

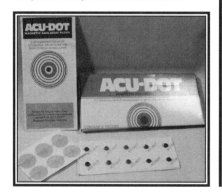

the MAGNECOIL

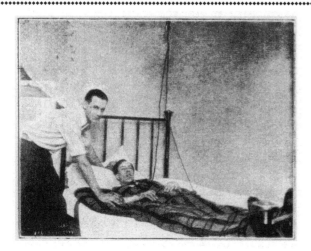

Magnecoil in Severe Illness.

In using MAGNECOIL in cases of desperate illness spread it over one half of the bed, cover with rubber sheet, place patient on it, fold over—and it is ready at once with no fatigue to the patient. During the treatment the U-COIL is used to thoroughly warm the other side of the bed—the treatment finished, the patient is rubbed—rough towel or alcohol—placed on the warmed side of the bed and the U-COIL applied to the extremities or to any desired portion of the body. If emergency arises—chill, high fever, shock, "sinking spell," or sleeplessness—MAGNECOIL and U-COIL are right there—always ready—any member of the family may apply it and meet the emergency instantly.

intersection of two Interstate highways declaring "Curing Cancer with Super Magnets." Promotional materials pictured the company's owner with a cancer patient who claimed she had "experienced recovery and remission from her cancer with the supermagnet." But that was not the case. Tragically, the woman died of cancer, and the company's owner was prosecuted under California's law that forbids the marketing and use of unapproved devices for cancer treatment.

Even if they are used only for temporary relief, how exactly are magnets supposed to work? Here are some of the ideas that theorists have proposed:

Magnets make people healthier by improving their connection to the earth's magnetic field.

Magnets "align" the elements in the human body.

Magnets increase blood flow by dilating blood vessels and attracting oxygen.

Magnets block pain signals sent by nerves to the brain.

Magnets alter the pH balance (acid/alkaline) of bodily fluids.

Magnets attract the iron in the blood, which stimulates blood circulation.

Magnets change the migration of calcium ions in the body to heal broken bones faster or move calcium away from arthritic joints.

Some manufacturers of magnetic products argue that people are weaker than they were in the past because our contact with the earth's magnetic field has grown weaker since we moved into cities (animals in the wild, supposedly, don't get sick). And, they claim, magnets can improve fitness and strength in seconds!

Franz Anton Mesmer —A Masterful Magnetizer

Franz Anton Mesmer attracted a lot of attention during the late eighteenth century. First positive attention . . . then negative attention. Born in 1734 in Swabia (Germany), Mesmer received his medical degree from the University of Vienna in 1766. But Mesmer wasn't like most physicians of his day. When patients arrived at his clinic, Mesmer attempted to treat them through the unconventional process of "animal magnetism," an idea that Mesmer adapted from Maximillian Hell, an astronomer working in Vienna at the time.

A firm believer in astrology, Mesmer thought that planets affected human health through a universal force that influenced an invisible fluid in living bodies. Mesmer also believed that, like magnets, the human body has two poles. By waving magnets

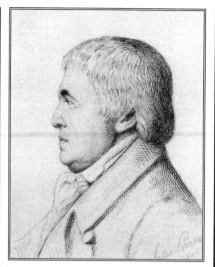

FRANZ MESMER

over a patient's body–from head to toe–Mesmer thought that he or another trained practitioner could improve the circulation of this invisible fluid and make patients feel better. Later, Mesmer tried using magnetized water to help his patients and then went on to claim that he could influence this invisible fluid by moving his hands over patients without the direct assistance of magnets. Patients' symptoms included vomiting, toothaches, blindness, paralysis, urinary retention, and melancholy (depression).

During treatments, Mesmer tried to create a rapport with his patients by placing them in a state of waking sleep (through the process now called "hypnotism"). Some patients reported that Mesmer cured them of various illnesses, and in retrospect many of them may have suffered from psychosomatic illnesses instead of physical diseases. Mesmer, after all, had plenty of unsatisfied customers who did not get better through the process of "animal magnetism." In 1778, as reports that Mesmer was a fraud increased, the master magnetizer fled Austria for France.

In Paris, Mesmer continued practicing his unique form of medicine, which brought him financial success. He earned a reputation for having an intelligent mind, sharp appearance, and striking gaze. But the new location did not solve all of his problems. As Mesmer's popularity in France increased, so did the complaints of Parisian physicians who were skeptical of Mesmer's techniques.

In 1784, King Louis XVI appointed a commission of scientists to investigate Mesmer's claims. The commission, which included French chemist Antoine-Laurent Lavoisier and Benjamin

These shoe insoles had tiny magnets imbedded into the surface and were supposed to ground you to the earth's magnetic field to prevent disease. They sold for $60 in 1994. The two combs are claimed to be magnetic, but since they are aluminum this would be a difficult task!

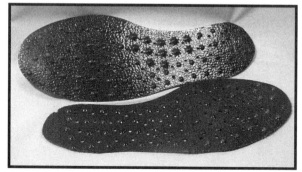

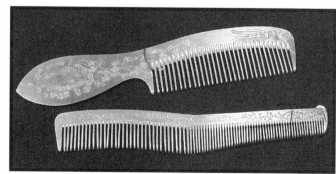

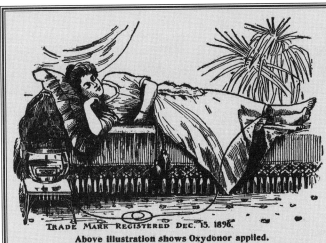
Franklin (who was representing the United States in France at the time), discredited the magnetizer by concluding that there was no such thing as invisible "Mesmeric fluid." Mesmer's popularity declined from that point on, and he spent his final days living in Germany.

During the late nineteenth century, when trained psychologists began using hypnotism as a therapeutic technique, some worried that they would be negatively associated with Mesmer. Since then, as public curiosity about the healing powers of magnets has gone up and down, few people remember the shaky career of the foremost magnetic healer, Franz Anton Mesmer.

The Electropoise, Oxydonor and Similar Fakes

The AMA strongly criticized these devices. This section consists of excerpts from reports of the time.

It is sometimes hard to decide which is the greater—the impudence of the quack or the credibility of his victims. The comparative ease with which the medical faker is able, by the most preposterous of

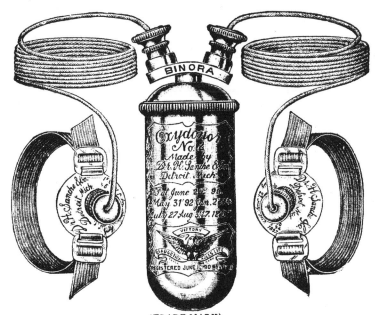
The Binora attachment is designed for two people. The Post Office condemned these devices on the basis that they claimed to cure all diseases—many of which, if allowed to continue without immediate medical or surgical treatment, could prove fatal to the patient.

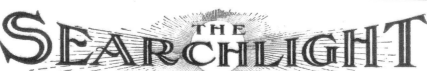

THE SEARCHLIGHT
— JOURNAL OF OXYPATHY.

Published by The Oxygenator Co.

Buffalo, N.Y. U.S.A.

Vol. 1   BUFFALO, N. Y., U. S. A., December, 1909.   No. 2

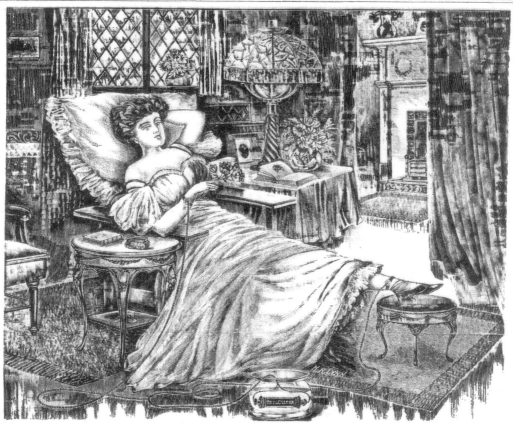

Simply Two Small Clasps To Adjust — Nature Does The Rest.

Sold on its record of results.

Drugs are never used in Oxypathy.
A sick person cannot be made well by giving him something that would make a well person sick.

THE OXYGENATOR

Restores to Health Regardless of the Kind of Disease— Its Severity—Duration—or Failure of Previous Systems of Treatment.

SIMPLY—SAFELY—SURELY—SPEEDILY

Without Further Cost than Its Purchase Price.

Sold most where best known.

"OXYPATHY," our beautiful 72-page book, in colors, is yours for the asking. It costs nothing to cultivate a receptive mind with our literature.
If appearances were the only judge diamonds would never have been found.

THE ALTERNATIVE.

Of late years the utter fraud and worthlessness of drug medication has become more and more known, owing to the praiseworthy pioneer work done by certain magazines and other independent interests.

When people are sick, however, they demand that SOMETHING be done.

Until recently no general alternative was known.

With the OXYGENATOR a new day dawns for the sick and afflicted.

Under the searchlight of public enlightment, the drug-sham is rapidly withering.

THE VICTORY.

For many years science has searched in vain for a perfect disease oxidizer.

Peroxides and similar preparations have accomplished much good, but their use is confined almost entirely to the surface of the body.

OXYGEN from tanks is extremely costly, in many instances cannot be obtained at all, and at best reaches but few diseases.

The trouble with these methods is principally that they do not convey OXYGEN and in quantities to the seat of the trouble.

By means of the OXYGENATOR

the problem is solved—great quantities of OXYGEN are induced into the human system where needed and when needed, and without cost.

CUTTING THE CHAINS.

Every one of OXYPATHY'S representatives is a volunteer in this great international fight to free the world from the delusion of drug-medication and the slavery it entails.

All of OXYPATHY'S brave fighters are contending for the common good and are pledged to carry on its great work to the glorious finish.

Until drug-medication has been

relegated to the unfortunate past, will this fight go on.

Not until then will OXYPATHY'S deserving crusaders cease the struggle and the world's people indeed be free.

HANDS ACROSS THE SEA

Mr. Harold S. James, manager of The Warwick Oxygenator Co., Stratford-on-Avon, England, tells us about a case of severe bilious attack which the Oxygenator cured in just 25 minutes by the watch.

THE PHILADELPHIA OXYGENATOR CO., WM. NELSON, Mgr.,   1007 Spruce St., Philadelphia, Pa.

claims, to separate the fool from his money indicates the enormous potentialities in advertising. It might be supposed that an individual who set out to sell, as a panacea for most fleshly ills, a piece of brass pipe with one or two wires attached to it and falsely labeled it a magnetic cure, would have a hard and rocky road before him. But such a supposition would be incorrect. Not only would the enterprising faker find customers for his pseudo-magnetic gas pipe, but there would be such a demand for this most insane of "therapeutic" devices, that two or three imitators would immediately enter the market.

The original exploiter of what may be called "magnetic gas-pipe therapy," was one Hercules Sanche, who modestly described himself as the "Discoverer of the Laws of Spontaneous Cure of Disease." Of course, Sanche did not "discover" this long-known truth at all, but he did appropriate its commercial value. Starting with the premise that a certain proportion of sick people—and of

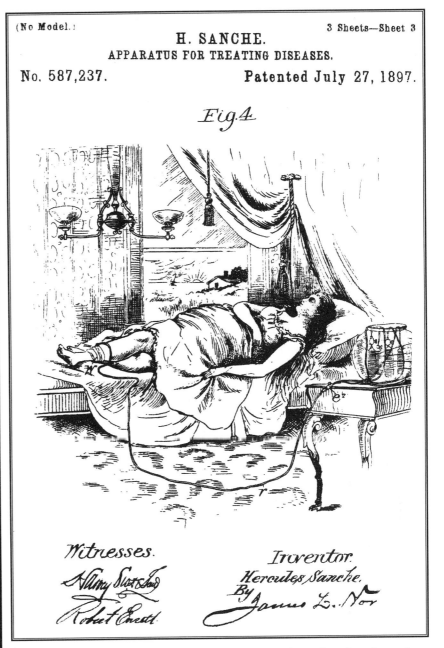

(No Model.)　　　　　　　　　　　　　3 Sheets—Sheet 3

H. SANCHE.
APPARATUS FOR TREATING DISEASES.

No. 587,237.　　　　　　　　　Patented July 27, 1897.

Fig. 4

Witnesses.　　　　　　　　　Inventor.
Hercules Sanche.
By James L. Nor

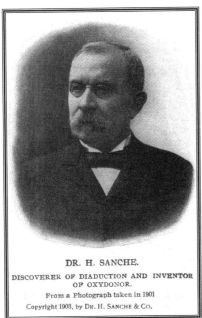

DR. H. SANCHE.
DISCOVERER OF DIADUCTION AND INVENTOR OF OXYDONOR.
From a Photograph taken in 1901
Copyright 1903, by DR. H. SANCHE & CO.

HERCULES SANCHE

those who think they are sick—will get well without treatment, or in spite of it, he cast about to devise a means of reaping a pecuniary reward from the operation of this natural law.

Sanche might, of course, have used some harmless or medicated tablets and, after describing at great length the marvelous properties inherent in them, sold them at a substantial profit. This method of fleecing the public, however, besides being old and threadbare,

was not altogether free from the probability of legal complications. He might have also offered to sell "absent treatments" and have discoursed learnedly on the benefits and virtues of this wonderful therapeutic force. But "absent treatment" does not appeal to the average man who wants something tangible in exchange for his dollars.

Sanche finally hit on a device that was perfectly harmless—and worthless—and yet theoretical enough to make the purchaser feel that he was getting something for his money. He called it the "Electropoise," and it consisted of a piece of metal pipe, closed at each end, with a flexible wire attached. It sold for ten dollars.

So popular did this humbug become that Mr. Sanche extended his operations by introducing the "Oxydonor"—a modification of the Electropoise that was shorter, contained a stick of carbon (instead of being empty), and sold for $35 instead of $10.

Coincident with his invention of the Oxydonor, Sanche also invented a "force" or "power" which he christened "Diaduction." The Oxydonor was the instrument by which the "force" was supposed to be created. To operate the Oxydonor, the distal end of the wire attached to it was applied to the wrist or ankle of the fool who used it. The Oxydonor itself was placed in cold water and the "diaduction force" would thus be generated.

The commercial success

attending the proliferation of this fake was such that many imitations appeared under various names, such as the "Oxygenor" or the "Oxygenor King."

These devices differed little from the Oxydonor—so little, in fact, that Sanche brought suit against the Oxygenor concern for infringement of patent. The court held, however, that such a palpable humbug as the Oxydonor was not entitled to legal protection.

Possibly the worst fake, called the "Oxygenator," was sold through booths at fairs. In many ways this type of charlatanry is the worst, inasmuch as claims are made for it that are not only absurd, but dangerous. For instance, the following statements occur in literature accompanying the Oxygenator:

"DIPHTHERIA. This overwhelming child's disease finds its supreme master in the Oxygenator. No earthly power except the Oxygenator can take the slowly choking child, and with speed,

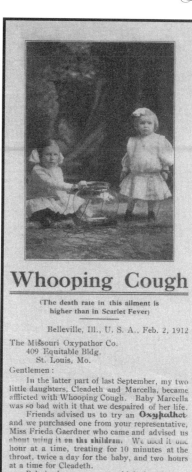

Whooping Cough

(The death rate in this ailment is higher than in Scarlet Fever)

Belleville, Ill., U. S. A., Feb. 2, 1912

The Missouri Oxypathor Co.
409 Equitable Bldg.
St. Louis, Mo.

Gentlemen :

In the latter part of last September, my two little daughters, Cleadeth and Marcella, became afflicted with Whooping Cough. Baby Marcella was so bad with it that we despaired of her life.

Friends advised us to try an Oxypathor and we purchased one from your representative, Miss Frieda Gaerdner who came and advised us about using it on the children. We used it one hour at a time, treating for 10 minutes at the throat, twice a day for the baby, and two hours at a time for Cleadeth.

Baby's fever was very high but in two treatments it was broken and in one week's time every vestige of cough had disappeared.

Both children are now rosy and healthy as their pictures will show.

I can surely give your machine a hearty recommendation and hoping for your continued success, I beg to remain,

Yours most sincerely,
MRS. PETER M. ABEGG.
435 West Ninth St.

AN EXAMPLE OF THE Oxypathor's WORK
When baby is sick accept no one's opinion.
Decide on the Oxypathor and be safe.

→ The Oxydonor →

OXYDONOR
No. 2   No. 2

simplicity and safety, bring it back to health. Don't jeopardize the health and life of your children by allowing to be injected into their veins and blood the often fearfully contaminated and death-dealing serum of an animal, otherwise known as antitoxin."

It is difficult to restrain one's indignation at the thought that such viciously cruel lies as these are permitted to be broadcast. Let the neurotic and neurasthenic adult, if he can convince himself that a nickel-plated piece of gas-pipe possesses curative properties, experiment with it on his own person if he wishes. But that a helpless child in the throes of a fearfully dangerous—and yet, rightly treated, curable—disease, should be allowed to suffer and die because ignorant parents have been persuaded to rely on these mechanical frauds, is no less than criminal. As for the miserable harpies who for a few filthy dollars will write such cold-blooded untruths as those quoted above, the safety of society demands that they be put with the thieves and murderers, where they can do no further harm.

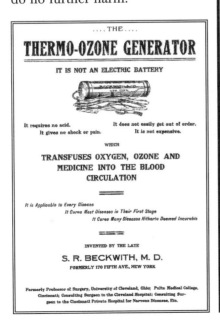

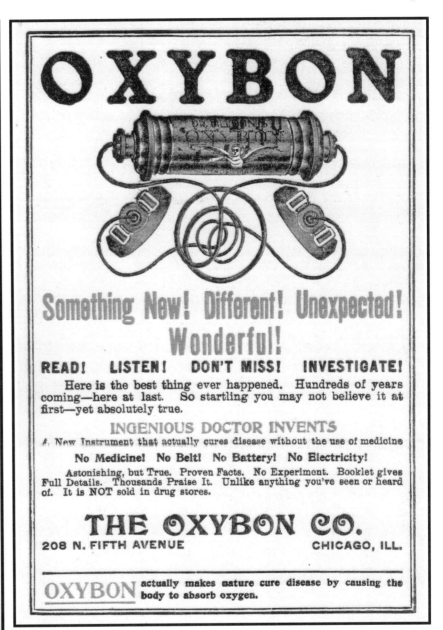

The Electropoise, the Oxydonor, the Oxygenor, the Oxygenator, and all of the other imitations are utterly worthless except as a means of enriching their exploiters. Their therapeutic value, aside from the element of suggestion that may be induced in those simpletons who are willing to pay from $10 to $35 for a piece of nickel-plated tubing, is absolutely nil.

If adults wish to squander their money on such foolishness and are content to confine the "treat-ment" to their own persons, well and good. If they have nothing much the matter with them they may believe they have received benefit; if they are dangerously ill, nature will probably exterminate them as unfit. But let no person try to "cure" the helpless child with such frauds; as soon as that is attempted, such an individual ceases to be a harmless idiot and becomes a dangerous one

The AMA pulled no punches in the 1920s.

ELECTRICITY

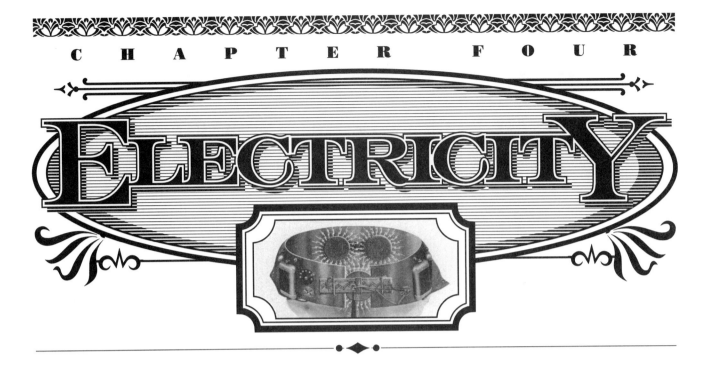

FLIPPING THE SWITCH TO GOOD HEALTH.

66 It is related of Ben Johnson, a revolutionary soldier, of Milford, Massachusetts, that he was struck with lightning several years ago" wrote Dr. Edward B. Foote, "and remained insensible for two days, when two doctors were called, who said he would die; but just at that moment his speech returned, and he ejaculated: 'I have stood cannon, musket-balls, and bayonets, and I can stand thunder and lightning if only the doctors will let me alone.' The old man recovered. Now no one supposes that such an overwhelming dose of mercury would have ever let the veteran soldier speak again." Dr. Foote, sharing this anecdote in his *Plain Home Talk* (1888) seems to have captured the mood of the nation, for after decades of "heroic medicine," of bleeding and leeches and massive doses of the purgatives like calomel or mercury salts, the American public was ready for electrical cures.

Electricity was more than the new technology, electricity was magic! The power of lightning was captured in a small box or small jar. Unlike other "magic" cures, electricity could be felt. Something was happening! Beginning in the middle of the nineteenth century, a medical battery was considered essential equipment by many physicians. It took about 50 years, until 1916, for a committee of the AMA to disparage the quackery in electro-therapeutics. It would be another 24 years

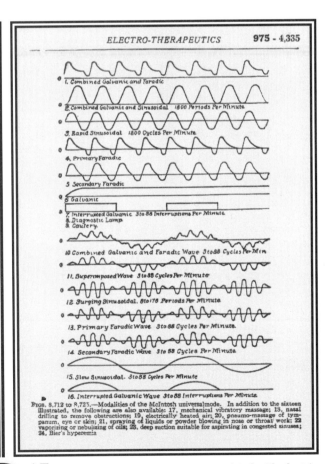

49

THE **ABOVE WAVE FORMS** associated with electric currents bamboozled many into thinking that the treatments promoted were scientifically based.

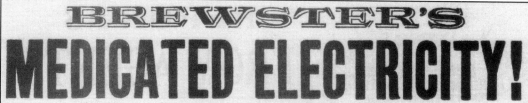

"The Electreat Mechanical Heart" consisted of flashlight batteries, a small electrical coil equipped with a door bell buzzer, and attachments for applying electricity to various parts of the body. It was one of the first devices seized by the FDA.

before the government was granted the power to review and regulate medical devices under the 1938 Food, Drug and Cosmetic Act.

The new technology of electricity in medicine was not confined to physicians. First, the public was in a mood to reject the heroic medicine which had been in vogue since the U.S. Colonial period. Secondly, the combination of the egalitarian legacy of the Jacksonian era plus the social reform movements of the middle and late nineteenth century opened the door for lay healers to enter the field of electro-therapeutics.

For decades, the field of electro-therapeutics was experimental.

How much current? From what source–galvanic or faradic? In what combination? At what interval and frequency? How often should treatments be given? In 1912, the National College of Electro-therapeutics in its manual, *The Electro-Therapeutic Guide*, included these "Condensed Facts for the General Practitioner Who Uses Electrification":

- *P.P.P.–Positive pole for pain.*
- *Electrolysis is chemical, galvanic only.*
- *Phoresis is mechanical, galvanic and static.*
- *Catalysis is physiological, galvanic,*

faradic, static.

- *Never use a bare electrode on dry skin.*
- *The faradic has a mechanical and catalytic action.*
- *The galvanic is the only mode having a chemical action.*
- *Mild doses only should be applied to the sensitive parts.*
- *The best method of irritation is by rapid change of polarity.*
- *Use iodine preparations under negative pole in cataphoresis.*
- *Use cocaine and alkaloids under positive pole in anaphoresis.*

☞ *All modes and either pole have a great influence upon nutrition.*

☞ *Do not make long exposures to the X-ray, with the tube close to the patient.*

☞ *Never leave a galvanic or faradic battery turned on, or short-circuited.*

☞ *The electrodes should always be in position before the mode is turned on.*

☞ *Don't try experiments on patients. Try them on yourself first and see how it goes.*

What was known was that electricity was efficient for cauterization. Physicians discovered that electrical treatments were sometimes effective when treating pain and paralysis. Some experimented with using electricity for resuscitation. Soon, electricity was being used as a cure-all. It was even thought by some to cure mental illness. Most of the earliest devices were batteries producing galvanic electricity, and so "galvanic treatments" came to be synonymous with medical electricity.

One of the earliest U.S. electrotherapeutic devices was the 1854 Davis Kidder Magneto, which generated electricity using a magnet. A hand-turned crank operated gears connected by a thin leather belt which spun a velvet-covered armature. This generated an electric flow conducted over cloth-insulated lead wires to the electrodes—using the machine briefly was not unpleasant. Use caused involuntary muscle contractions. The device came with two hand electrodes, about two and one-half inches long, and a rectangular metal plate electrode. The doctor could attach the plate to one part of the body, have the patient hold a hand electrode, and send current between the two locations.

The D'Argence and Other Chemical Batteries

Chemical batteries were also for sale in the mid-1800s. The Nonpareil Co., founded in 1855, recommended a formula of eight ounces sulfuric acid mixed in five

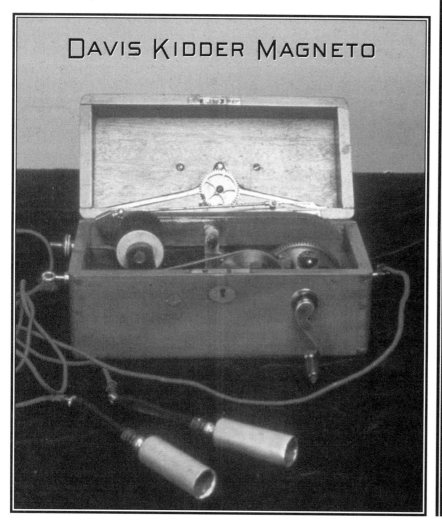

DAVIS KIDDER MAGNETO

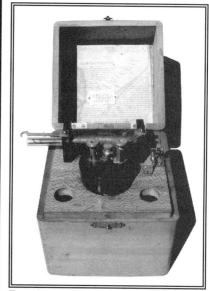

THE NONPAREIL CHEMICAL BATTERY.

pints water. Into this was dissolved seven and one-half ounces of pulverized bichromite potassa. The mixture was placed in the glass container inside the battery box. The D'Argence Electric Brush was actually an elegant and compact chemical battery. The oval wood case was six and one-half inches long and three and one-half

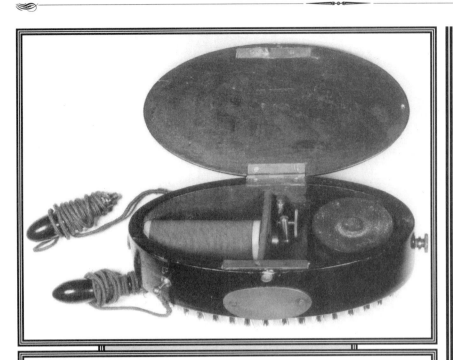

THE D'ARGENCE ELECTRIC BRUSH

inches at the widest section. A hinged cover opened to reveal a container and two small wooden electrode handles wrapped in their cords. Most of the brush bristles were wire. The set included a small circular sponge electrode handsewn to a thin metal plate. The D'Argence was sold as a baldness remedy and a body battery.

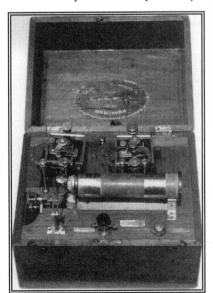

THIS FARADIC BATTERY, PATENTED IN 1870, ENABLED PATIENTS WITHOUT ELECTRICITY TO STILL RECEIVE TREATMENT.

By the 1880s, dry cell batteries were available and "battery boxes" became common. While these devices had legitimate medical applications, battery boxes soon were a cure-all recommended for, but not limited to, weak or lame back, cramps, writers' cramp, cold feet, contracted muscles, nervous cough, circulation, general debility, headache, hysteria, neuralgia, palsy, paralysis, rheumatism, sciatica, chilblains, and hair loss. The boxes, often made of oak, came with a variety of electrodes: a hair brush with wire bristles, cylindrical metal hand electrodes about three inches long, rectangular "foot plates," and sponge electrodes which were inserted into wooden handles. These boxes are common in antique stores today.

The Roche Electric Hygienic Machine, patented in 1915, is a late example of a battery box. Its inventor, Professor J. B. Roche, declared that electricity is the spark of life and that many diseases "originate in the waste of

that wonderful vital force upon which every nerve and organ of the body exists." His Hygienic Machine was one such device. Ingeniously designed, the varnished wood case opened to reveal an assortment of batteries and attachments: a ten inch long wood and aluminum comb, a nine inch brush with metal bristles, and a bath appliance—a fifteen inch dowel of oak permanently wired to the box with the final four inches covered in natural sponge.

The consumer stood barefoot on a pair of eleven inch metal conductor foot plates built into the fold-out top of the box. The machine was turned on and the moistened sponge was then rubbed over those parts of the

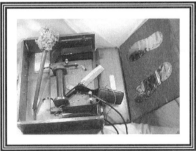

THE ROCHE ELECTRIC HYGENIC MACHINE.

body needing treatment. Glowing testimonials attest to the wonderful results achievable. What were Professor Roche's credentials? Advertisements called him "a well known Hygienic Instructor in Physical Science." Close examination of the 1915 patent reveals that it is for the design of the box only!

Electric Belts Become All-the-Rage

Electric belts were so popular at the turn of the twentieth century that the Sears catalogue featured

continued on page 56

Sears, Roebuck and Co., Chicago, ILL.

Directions for Operating the Three-Cell Medical Battery

from Medical Electricity at Home by Sears, Roebuck and Company

The Three-Cell Medical Battery when received will be connected up ready to generate a current as soon as the switches (t-1) and (t-2) are turned on. This medical battery is supplied with

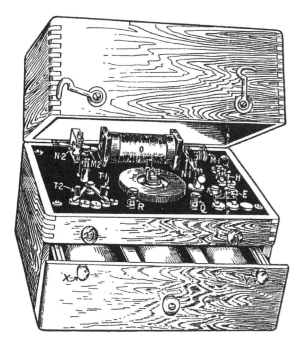

three cells of dry batteries, so that a very strong current can be produced. To start the battery working, move the switch (T-1) to point 1, and switch (T-2) to point 0. The medical battery will then be working on one cell. Move switch (T-1) to point 2, and it will then work on two cells, giving a stronger current. When switch (T-1) is moved on point 3, then it is working on three cells, giving the full capacity. Never cover two points

at once with switch, as this will short circuit the battery and wear out the dry cells in a very short time. When through using, turn the battery off by putting switch (T-2) on the point marked (off), and the switch (T-1) on point marked (0).

FAST INTERRUPTIONS. When the switches are turned on ready to use the battery see that the switch (H) is on the point (S). The rheotome (N-1) should begin to vibrate. Sometimes the rheotome does not start at once. It is then necessary to start it vibrating with the finger. If then it does not work it is because the tension screw (M-1) is not properly adjusted. Adjust this screw by turning it slowly in and out, continuing to vibrate the rheotome with the finger. When the tension is just right the rheotome should begin to vibrate and the position of the tension screw can be set with the auxiliary screw attached thereto.

SLOW INTERRUPTIONS. Put the switch (H) on point (W), which should cause the wheel rheotome (N-2) to revolve. If it does not start at once, start it with the finger. The speed of these interruptions can be regulated by raising or lowering the adjusting screw (M-2). By lowering this adjusting screw the spring is forced down until it will hit all of the pegs on the wheels. As the adjusting screw is raised the spring will only hit the longer pegs and finally the longest peg, thus making the interruptions slower.

STRENGTH OF CURRENTS. The strength of the current can be greatly increased by turning the rheostat switch (P) in the same direction as the hands on a clock move, that is, when the spring

Sears, Roebuck and Co., Chicago, ILL.

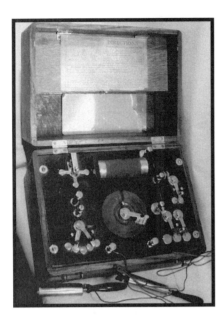

rests on the right hand side of the peg, the current is the weakest, and when it is swung around and the switch is on the left hand side of the peg, then the current is the strongest. The strength of the current is also regulated by running the battery on one, two or three cells as directed in the first paragraph.

THE POLARITY of the current can be changed by means of the switch (E). When the switch is turned to the extreme right, then the left hand bing post is positive and the right hand binding post is negative. Reverse the switch (E) by throwing it to the extreme left and this makes the left hand binding post negative and the right hand binding post positive.

IN FASTENING THE BATTERY CORDS to the binding posts, put one end of each cord in each of the binding posts and then tighten by turning down the screw. The other end of each cord is fastened to the various electrodes as used.

HOW TO PUT IN NEW DRY CELLS. Take out the two screws (X) and (Y) and then pull out the sliding drawer by means of the knob. This will expose the three dry cells and the connecting wires. These connecting wires, you will see, are marked at the connecting points by small tags. These tabs tell you where to fasten these points to the dry cells. The dry cells can be removed by simply unfastening the screws at the connecting points and then replace with fresh cells. Refasten the wires just as directed by the little tags. Replace the drawer to its original position and the battery is then ready for use again. With ordinary usage dry cells should last from eight to twelve months.

NEGATIVE AND POSITIVE POLES. When in doubt as to which binding post or contact hold is positive and which is negative proceed as follows: Connect the medical batter with the battery cords, the two metal sockets or hand electrodes. Let these two electrodes hang in a jar of water about 1/2 inch apart and then turn on the circuit. Air bubbles will collect on one of these electrodes, and the binding post or contact hole to which this electrode is connected is always negative.

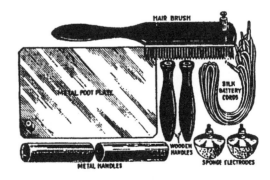

Electrodes.

them in five sizes, ranging from $4 to $18! Sears favored the Heidelberg Alternating Current Medical Electric Belts which, of course, contained no alternating current. Sears founder, Richard Warren Sears, and his second partner, Julius Rosenberg, vehemently disagreed over the appropriateness of including the Heidelberg belt in the Sears catalog. The dispute grew to embrace a full range of financial management issues and, in 1908, R.W. Sears quit his namesake company.

The belts had a copper disc in front and two to four chrome plated nickel discs towards the back. The alleged interaction between the copper and nickel was the source of the alleged electricity. In *The Story of Cures That Fail,* medical historian Dr. James J. Walsh (1865-1942) recalled the early days of his career when electric belts were customary:

"Once electricity became looked upon as possessing a potent force for good on the human system, the number of electrical appliances supposed to have medicinal value multiplied. Electric belts were advertised extensively and were evidently used far more extensively because the advertisements continued for years. They were made of chamois or other leather and contained a series of discs of metal supposed to be in contact and considered to be activated by the bodily electricity or by the warmth of the body—or by something. Men were represented wearing them with streams of electricity flowing up and down their backs and into all their members and presumably, of course, doing wonderful work in their abdominal region.

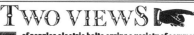

Two Views of popular electric belts curing a variety of common maladies, including gout, paralysis, epilepsy, asthma, constipation, kidney disorders and bronchitis.

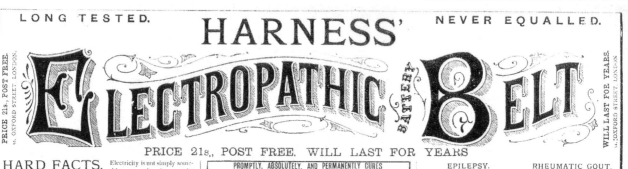

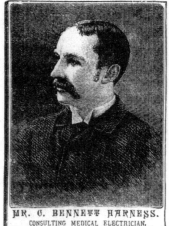

Heidelberg Alternating Current Electric Belts

At $4.00, $6.00, $8.00, $12.00 and $18.00

we sell the new improved and ONLY JUSTLY CELEBRATED HEIDELBERG ELECTRIC BELTS, guaranteeing them superior to belts that others sell at $10.00 to $40.00 . . . .

...SUPERIOR TO ANY OTHER ELECTRIC BELT MADE...

OUR FREE TRIAL OFFER. Select any belt wanted (state number inches around body at waist), we will send the belt to you by express C.O.D., subject to examination, we will send it in a plain sealed box so the express agent, or no one can see, tell the contents; we will instruct the express agent to collect from you our special price and express charges and **HOLD THE MONEY 10 DAYS**; you can give the belt 10 days trial, and if at the end of 10 days, you are not perfectly satisfied, if you have reason to believe the belt will not effect a speedy and permanent cure, pack the belt back in the same plain unmarked box it came in and take it back to the express agent and he **WILL RETURN YOUR MONEY** and will return the belt to us at our expense; otherwise, after 10 days if you do not bring the belt back, he will send the money to us.

10 DAYS' FREE TRIAL gives you every chance to see, examine and buy the belt and satisfy yourself that the HEIDELBERG ELECTRIC BELT will do more for you than any belt made; will cure you if a cure by electricity is possible.

OUR NO MONEY C.O.D. TERMS. To show that our Heidelberg Electric Belt has no equal at any price, that our Heavy Battery $18.00 Belt is superior to belts that sell at $40.00 to $100.00. We offer to send any belt in plain unmarked box to any address (no money in advance) by express C.O.D., subject to examination, and with our 10 days' free trial privilege if desired.

THE ONLY CURE BELT MADE giving a self automatic, regulating, alternating, electric current reaching every nerve tissue of the body, giving life and strength instantly in every part of the body.

THE ONLY ELECTRIC BELT that will effectually take the place at once of every other kind of electric appliance and electric treatments for the cure of all the many diseases and weaknesses for which electricity is the only agent.

ARE YOU TIRED OF DRUGS? ARE YOU DISCOURAGED WITH DOCTORS? Have you tried other belts been looking for?

ARE YOU SICK, WEAK AND DISCOURAGED? THEN TRY OUR GIANT $18.00 BELT on our FREE 10 DAYS' TRIAL offer. You will ge more comfort in the 10 days than all else has given you.

THE ONLY ELECTRIC BELT in which the lightest or heaviest current of electricity is at all times under the instantaneous control of the patient and in which the current is alternating, ever building up those nerve tissues, never reached by the many other belts and appliances.

THE HEIDELBERG ELECTRIC BELTS combine every good, every new and improved feature of any other belt made, and in addition, you have a current of electricity alternating and farther reaching than in any other belt made.

HAVE YOU TRIED OTHER BELTS? If you have tried any other make of belt and you have not received the desired benefit let us send you our Giant Heidelberg $18.00 Belt on 10 Days Free Trial, and if you do not say it is such a belt as is furnished by no other house, if you do not find the alternating current instantaneous in its effect, giving you the sought for relief that no other belt will give you, do not pay one cent but return it at our expense.

HOW THE HEIDELBERG ELECTRIC BELT EXCELS ALL OTHERS.

FIRST—They are made of the best material that can be procured, regardless of expense.

SECOND—More evenly regulated current of electricity is furnished than in any other electric belt made.

THIRD—Our alternating electric current reaches nerve centers and restores weak parts than can be reached by no other electric appliance.

FOURTH—More distribution, with more and larger electrodes, than on other belts. We give a more evenly distributed current of electricity than can be had from any other belt.

FIFTH—Power Regulator. With the Heidelberg battery you can get from three to five times the power that can be had from any other belt made, and the power regulator attached to the belt is so arranged that by simply moving a lever, without removing the belt, you can instantly change it to six different degrees of power.

SIXTH—Finish. The Heidelberg Electric Belt is the handsomest belt made; easiest adjusted and most convenient electric belt made.

OUR GUARANTEE. Every Heidelberg Electric Belt is covered by a binding one year guarantee, during which time if any piece or part gives out, by reason of defect in material or workmanship, it will be replaced or repaired free of charge. With care it will last a lifetime.

ABOUT OUR PRICES. Our inside prices of $4.00, $6.00, $8.00, $12.00 and $18.00 are less than one-half the price charged by others for inferior belts; in fact, our $4.00 belt will give better satisfaction than any other belt made, regardless of price, while our giant $18.00 belt is much better than other belts you can buy at $40.00 to $50.00, as the difference is the electric current we give. Our special prices are made only to cover our cost from the manufacture who gives us the exclusive sale of the Heidelberg Belt in America, with but one small profit added.

WE TOO COULD GET $20.00 TO $50.00 for our belts if we would ask it, for we have the only 20 to 80 gauge electric current electric belt made the only belt to reach the nerve centers.

FOR NERVOUS DISEASES of all kinds in men and women, to reach the nerve centers for the cure of all nervous disorders the Heidelberg Electric Belt stands alone. For weakness in men and women, nervous exhaustion, bringing back lost strength and power, over brain work, vital weakness, impotency, rheumatism, sciatica, lame back, railroad back, insomnia, melancholia, kidney disorder, Bright's disease, dyspepsia, diseases of the liver, female weakness, poor circulation, weak heart action and almost every known disease and weakness. The constant soothing, alternating, electric current is ever at work touching the weak spots, building up the system, stimulating the circulation. ALL THAT ELECTRICITY WILL DO FOR YOU will be received through the use of our electric belt.

OUR $4.00 HEIDELBERG ELECTRIC BELT.

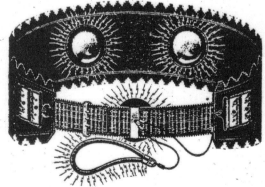

A HUNDRED LITTLE ACHES AND PAINS,
HEADACHES, BACKACHES and WEAK NERVE PAINS,
can be saved you by the use of one of these belts.
To Prevent Sickness, Save Doctor's Bills, and Preserve Health
DO NOT BE WITHOUT AN ELECTRIC BELT.

THIS Belt produces a 20-gauge current of electricity, and comes complete with stomach attachment and spiral suspensory.

This 20-gauge current belt is recommended for mild cases, and yet at 20-gauge, we believe it is superior to any other belt on the market, regardless of price.

Our $4.00 belt will be found in every way superior to that others sell at $15.00 to $40.00. It is the genuine Heidelberg 20-gauge belt full plated electrodes, best insulation, perfect alternating current.

No. 6482. 20-Gauge Current Belt. Our Price............$4.00

OUR $6.00 HEIDELBERG ELECTRIC BELT.

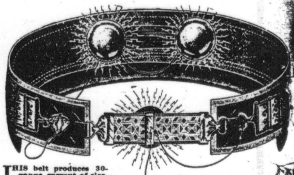

THIS belt produces 30-gauge current of electricity, and comes complete with stomach attachments and spiral electric suspensory.

This 30-gauge current belt is strong enough for all ordinary forms of disease and weakness, and is especially recommended for STOMACH, LIVER AND BLOOD DISORDERS, also for SICK HEADACHE AND DYSPEPSIA; the steady, soothing alternating current of electricity relieves you at once, and a cure in almost every case is soon effected.

IF YOU HAVE TRIED

OTHER BELTS

let us send you this 30-gauge belt on

TEN DAYS' FREE TRIAL,

and if you don't find it perfectly satisfactory, such a belt as you could not get elsewhere at any price, return it at our expense.

No. 6484. 30-gauge current belt. Our Price............$6.00

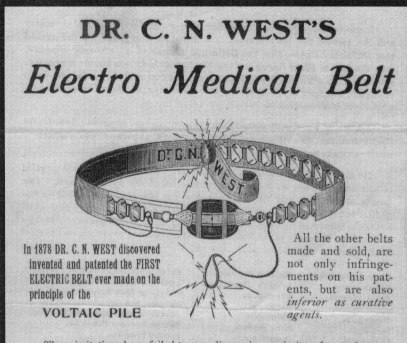

DR. C. N. WEST'S
Electro Medical Belt

In 1878 DR. C. N. WEST discovered invented and patented the FIRST ELECTRIC BELT ever made on the principle of the

VOLTAIC PILE

All the other belts made and sold, are not only infringements on his patents, but are also *inferior as curative agents.*

These imitations have failed to cure disease in a majority of cases, because they do not produce the kind of **current of Electricity** required.

This belt, being made to be charged by **water alone**, produces a *peculiar* current such as no other battery in the world can produce, and which perfectly adapts it to the human body, producing in it the same activity in all its various organs that the *vital* or *nerve* force usually performs in health. This belt is so made that every part of its battery can be opened, by swinging back two bands, and its decayed parts, within, removed and new metals put in by any child, thus making it last many years.

Its construction is so simple and perfect and its electricity is *so mild* that a *babe* can wear it, yet *so strong* that it will pass through a *No. 17* Copper wire, 10,000 miles in length, and *cauterize the skin*. But to prevent the possibility of burning, *wet sponge* or *chamois* electrodes are used. Besides the current producing battery, the belt has *10 stationary* batteries increasing the quantity of electricity ten-fold, by absorption, thus, passing into the human body a greater *quantity* of electricity than was ever done in any other manner. Thus making the belt the most curative appliance ever known.

Dr. West's Electro Medical Belt.

"Occasionally the belts were made to be worn as shoulder straps or in some other curious fashion and many, many people were cured by means of them. Electric belts and chest protectors [something like a muscle shirt sewn of red flannel worn next to the skin] were two forms of appliance cures that we young physicians in dispensary work a generation or so ago used to expect confidently to see at least one of whenever we asked a patient to strip. . . .

"It was simply surprising to see the faith they had in them and how confidently they would tell of the relief that had been afforded them, though they had to confess that there was still some trouble left for which they were applying to us for treatment. Wearers of the electric belts for which they had sometimes paid as high as $25 were quite sure in nearly every case that it was only a question of time until the electric belt would surely cure them,

only unfortunately they did not have the time to allow it to get in all its work, as yet, and therefore they had applied for the help that would be afforded by the doctors at the dispensary. After a while we came to be quite sure ourselves that if we did succeed in benefiting them in any way it would not be attributed to us but to the electric belt."

The Heidelberg belts pledged to "effectively take the place at once of every other kind of electric appliance and electric treatments for the cure of all the many diseases and weaknesses for which electricity is the only agent." Suggestive as the design was, the belts were cure-alls. The Heidelbergs promised to be effective "for Nervous Diseases of all kinds in men and women, to reach the nerve centers for the cure of all nervous disorders. . . . For weakness in men and women, nervous exhaustion, [to] bring back lost strength and power, over brain work, vital weakness, impotency, rheumatism, sciatica, lame back, railroad back, insomnia, melancholia, kidney disorder, Bright's disease, dyspepsia, diseases of the liver, female weakness, poor circulation, weak heart, and almost every known disease and weakness."

As technology changed, so did the electric belt. In 1915, the Lorenz Truss and Electric Works in Chicago advertised an electric belt which used dry cell batteries: "The Dr. Lorenz Electro Body Batteries are the only ones in the market which have the special feature of working without being constantly charged with vinegar or acids and have the patented anti-short rheostat; they are guaranteed to give 300% greater service, and that they are 400% easier

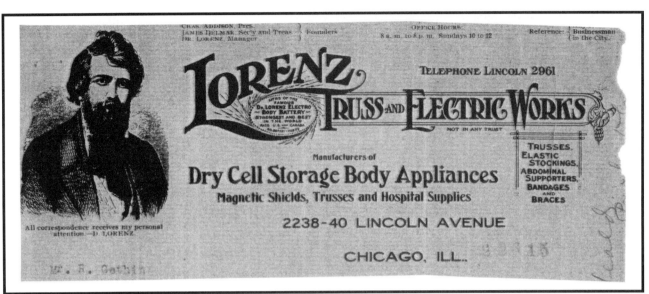

THE LORENZ TRUSS.

applied than the old style vinegar, so-called health belts, which are, if you wish to make a fair comparison, in no way nearer to our batteries, than the petroleum or coal lamp is to the electric light." The Dr. Bell Electro Appliance attached dry cell batteries to a girdle and allowed the user to adjust the amount of current. Despite their use of the dry cell batteries, the later electric belts were as ineffective as cure-alls as those of the 1880s.

Body Batteries: Wear Them Close to the Vest

Dr. Walsh asserted that electric metal batteries, extremely popular in the 1880s and 1890s, were almost as common as electric belts. He recalled, "The circular advertisements which described them always gave picture of a man with one of these on his chest and currents of electricity radiating in all directions from it. These were to be seen also in the newspaper advertisements of this wonderful electrical renewer of health and strength. Of course the only place

MIOXRLS Electric Body Battery

DIRECTIONS AND GENERAL REMARKS FOR THE MIOXRLS ELECTRIC BODY BATTERY

We naturally suppose that every purchaser of our Body Batteries desires to receive the greatest possible benefit therefrom:

Hence, we must in the strongest terms, request that these remarks and directions be **CAREFULLY READ AND FOLLOWED** *(New Label Adopted Jan 1, 1907):*

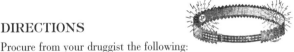

DIRECTIONS

Procure from your druggist the following:

BATTERY ACID—Chemically pure sulphuric acid, one fluid ounce; pure glycerin, two fluid ounces. Mix, and when cooled add one quart of water (good cider vinegar diluted with water is just as good a solution) to saturate the batteries when rolled up. The acid can be left standing in the cup (covered with a plate) for daily use, adding from the bottle as required. Observe how the belt is put together when received, so that you may be able to replace it properly.

Take the battery out of the pocket and saturate it in the above Battery Acid 10 minutes for the first time, and after that 5 minutes morning and night. To make sure that it has been Thoroughly Charged, touch the positive pole (one nearest the buckle) to the tongue, and place the negative pole (one on strap) between the eyes, when the electric current will be felt. Wear the belt around the hips. See that belt is properly connected as when received. In all ordinary cases the belt should be worn about two hours daily, or more. To prevent the plates from burning the skin, place a wet cloth between the plates and the skin. This cloth must be wet, otherwise it is a non-conductor. It is better to use several thicknesses of cloth, and they will retain more moisture.

The better care you take of the belt the longer it will last. If you will you can keep it clean; and with an occasional new set of batteries, it will last you for years. Wipe the batteries as dry as possible before placing in the belt. The acid will blacken the copper. Occasionally take a bit of rag, and, when you remove from the acid, while still wet with it, you can clean the batteries and keep them bright. When the belt is removed from the body, take the batteries out and leave the case of the belt open; thus keeping the whole dry, the belt will be preserved in better order. Once in three or four weeks soak the batteries in boiling water 15 or 20 minutes. If belt has been laid aside for a time, soak batteries as above before using again.

that the electricity flowed out of either the belt or the medal was in the newspapers and other advertising material." The major manufacturer of body batteries in the U.S. was J. C. Boyd of New York, whose pamphlet is reproduced below.

BOYD'S MINIATURE GALVANIC BATTERY

Professor Boyd is now offering to the public Batteries which are made on his newly discovered principle, and of metals, amalgamated in accordance with well-known principles and proportions which, by their *galvanic action* upon each other, produce results not less *startling* than *salutary*. A galvanic action (*i.e., electricity produced without friction*) *can* be obtained by the union of two or more metals, as was proved more than a century ago, by Galvani, the discoverer of Galvanism. This union of metals is characterized by a *soft and gentle action,* which, when applied to the body, is *perceptible only in its ultimate* RESULTS. For telegraphic purposes, it is necessary to intensify the galvanic action, and accordingly one of the metals is plunged into sulphuric acid, which, by corrosion, decomposes the parts exposed to it, thus facilitating their union with the other metal destined to form the amalgam. When, however, it is desired to apply the beneficial results of a *current of electricity to the human body,* no such intensity is required, as the simple action of the *natural humidity of the skin* is sufficient to set the chemical operations of nature in motion, and cause a constant but gentle flow of electricity to pass, from what we may term the BATTERY into the system.

There has been for many years back various apparatus manufactured, which produce a galvanic action, the inventors thereof applied for patents, and in many cases secured them, and a number of the leading physicians of this country and Europe endorsed what they then supposed to be meritorious inventions, and it has been only within the past year, that Professor Boyd convinced them without a shadow of doubt, that there could be no electricity whatever passed into the system by the use of what is called Electric Belts, Bands, Chains, Plasters, etc., etc.

Professor Boyd called a meeting of the leading physicians in order to demonstrate what he claimed which was done to the satisfaction of every one present. The Professor covered his entire body with Electric Bands, Pads, Chains, Plasters, Garters, and Belts, then stood in an upright position with his feet on a peculiarly constructed copper and zinc plate, then the Galvanometer test was applied, which showed that all of the electricity contained in those appliances had passed off over the surface at the Professor's feet. This demonstrated the fallacy of such contrivances.

Many of the physicians present had endorsed some of the Chains, Bands, and Belts used for this wonderful experiment, *supposing that the current did enter the system,* but now they are willing to acknowledge that they were mistaken in their views.

Then Professor Boyd produced his now famous Battery for the purpose of demonstrating to the profession his important discovery and his wonderful Miniature Battery invention. The Professor taking one of his small Batteries between his fingers, said: "Gentlemen, I will now convince you that I can pass more electricity into the system with this little

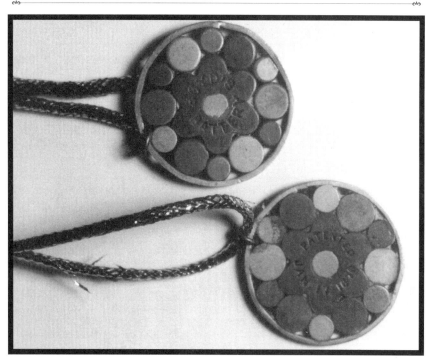

⇥ Boyd's Miniature Galvanic Battery ⇤

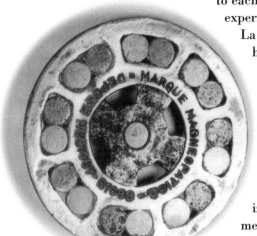

FRENCH BATTERY. This and the Boyd's battery on the previous page were given to the museum by Dr. Olgierd Lindan, a noted collector, who also observed the similarity between these two batteries.

invention than can be done with all this costly rubbish," pointing at the bands, belts, and chains, etc, that he had just taken off. The Professor stated that his Battery was now explained, which was to this effect: That the various blocks of metal were so placed that when the electricity was formed it would be formed in the gimlet shape, and he said it would enter the system in that form and pass on twisting until it spent its force. It is claimed that electricity formed by a Battery constructed in any other way, would pass off on the surface the same as a lightning rod. The Professor now took eight Batteries, held them on his chest, and within five minutes it was noticed, by the beating of the heart and pulse and the expression of the eyes, that the entire system was electrified to such an extent, that it was with difficulty that the Professor could keep from dancing. This concluded the experiment, which was satisfactory to all present. A Battery was then presented by the Professor

to each person who witnessed the experiments. When the great Dr. La Favels, of Paris, received his and examined its construction, he remarked that he was satisfied, after seeing what he had and from the wonderful ingenuity in constructing the Battery, that by putting it into general use, it would revolutionize the entire medical treatment, and added, that he had long been aware that nearly all diseases could be cured by electricity, if it could be passed through the blood. He also said that a large majority of ailments were brought on by an impoverished, poisonous and vitiated state of the blood, and those diseases could only be cured by the purification of that fluid; and it seems to me,

he said, that by the use of this little Battery, it will be decidedly the quickest, cheapest and most desirable way to accomplish that result. Professor Boyd, in answer, stated that it was his intention to give the public the benefit of his discovery and invention, and that he had put the price of his Battery so low that it would bring it within the reach of all suffering humanity, and that it was his desire to save neither labor nor expense in placing it properly before the American people in all parts of the United States.

The Professor said that he was glad to see, of late years, that there had been a radical change in the method adopted by the medical profession for the treatment and cure of nearly all diseases. He said it has been ascertained, beyond a doubt, that nine-tenths of all

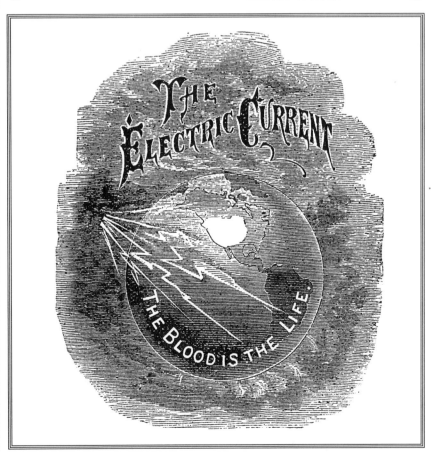

THE DR. BELL ELECTRO APPLIANCE
An Electro-Medical Dry Cell Body Battery
READY TO WEAR AS ARRANGED FOR MEN

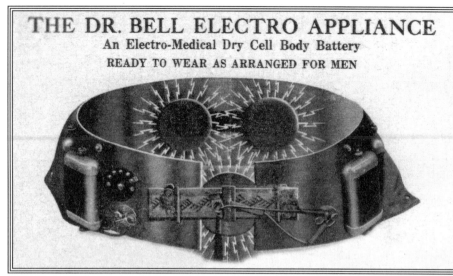

THE LATEST IMPROVEMENTS

Found only on the Dr. Bell Electro Appliance. Notice each improvement on the cut above. Read the reason why.

These improved Electro Medical Batteries last longer, give a stronger current, which is guaranteed 4 months, and can be recharged time and again at small expense.

There is no daily recharging with vinegar or acid; no smell or corrosion; no burning, blistering, irritating or shocking sensation. You feel a soothing glow.

All attachment wires, whether for head, neck, arms, legs or sexual organs, are reinforced with rubber insulation, as seen on the Stomach or Liver Disc and Loop Suspensory in the illustration.

the distressing maladies originate in a vitiated state of the blood, caused by the absence of a *proper proportion of electricity* in that fluid, and the remedies now used are generally applied with a view of supplying the blood with its *requisite quantity of electricity*, and thus restoring it to its normal condition.

The celebrated HARVEY, who discovered the circulation of the blood, stated that this fluid was expelled from the heart, completed its circuit of the body, and returned to the fountain head in the space of about three minutes, and this theory has been confirmed by subsequent investigations. Thus, then, there is a constant flow of the blood, passing any given part of the body; and if, by taking advantage of this fact, *we can infuse into it, on its passage, the necessary electricity,* the object is accomplished without the aid of medicine or other remedies.

My Battery effectually performs this function, constantly through imperceptibly impregnating the NERVES and the BLOOD with new *electric life*.

THE BLOOD IS THE LIFE. By its impure and impoverished condition nearly all ailments are caused, and only through its purification can those diseases be cured.

Knowing these facts, I have arrived at the conclusion that, by electrifying the blood, it stimulates the entire system, so that it enables nature to throw off nearly all diseases, and causes the blood to become youthful and vigorous in its action.

The success that has hitherto attended this BEAUTIFUL LITTLE INVENTION is fully proved by *numerous Testimonials*, and the unanimous opinion of *Medical Men* throughout the United States. This Galvanic Action, though *a new doctrine to the mass*, has been long known to scientific men, who, however, have been unable to discover the means of applying it, in a MINIATURE FORM, to the body; but now the difficulty has been overcome by my Battery.

It is true that the blood is the life; and it is also true that corrupt, poisoned diseased, impoverished and vitiated blood means DEATH. I Claim, by the use of my Miniature Battery, that the blood can be so electrified as to make it as healthful and vigorous in its action as that of a *child*.

Whoever is subject to any of the following symptoms should

wear the Battery: Restless Nights, Nightmare, Palpitation of the Heart, Loss of Confidence, Dizziness, Fainting Spells, Loss of Memory, Fullness of Blood, Fits of Melancholy, Debilitated, Lack the Power of Will and Action, Disordered Condition of the Liver, Blood, Kidneys, or Urinary Organs—these troubles arose mostly from relaxation and debility, for the relief of which electricity is eminently adapted. By its application the affected organs are reached, vitalized and strengthened, the troubles arrested, and, wherever there is a basis for reaction, the functions can be restored to their normal health.

Why neglect your health and destroy your happiness, and recklessly throw aside all that makes life a pleasure? How many drag out year after year of a miserable existence, simply for the want of knowledge in procuring a remedy with efficacy and virtue, which would be adapted to their ailments? I say to those that procrastination is dangerous. It will not do, if you wish to live, to trifle with the human system. Then why delay, when an article is at hand that has science and common sense in its use: and in no possible way can it do you an injury, if you are not restored to health by its use.

Did you, when young, draw unnaturally on the fountain of life and strength, one drop of which fluid is equal to thirty drops of the heart's blood? If you were so indiscreet in youth as to allow your passions to lead you to self-abuse, and it has left you with no vital power, and carried away from you your manhood, causing you to have an aversion to society and unfitted you for business leaving your brain to run on thoughts that can be of no possible or practical use; from the above disobedience to the laws of nature, the eyes are left dim, the mind wandering, the memory lost;

with difficulty you stand erect; every step taken draws on you for an effort, which makes your daily employment a burden instead of a pleasure; there is a dimness of sight, spasmodic pains in the head, a discontented feeling without knowing the cause, and the system is left in a nervous and a general debilitated condition. For the restoration of such shattered constitutions, there is no remedy that will relieve all the ailments caused from self-abuse with such magic as Boyd's Miniature Galvanic Battery.

The Miniature Battery will cure the following diseases, which are nearly all caused from the effects of impure blood:

Rheumatism, Gout, Swollen Joints, Neuralgia, Dyspepsia, Lumbago, Aches and Pains, Pain in the Bones, Sciatica, Scrofula, Salt Rheum, Ulcers and Sores, Tumors, Boils, Carbuncles, Chills, Vertigo, Nervous and General Debility, Loss of Manhood, Impotency, Seminal Weakness, Female Complaints, Barrenness, Liver Complaint, Fever and Ague, Bright's Disease, Kidney Disease, Diabetes, Catarrh, Sore Throat, Bronchitis, Asthma, Jaundice, Pleurisy, Diphtheria, Cerebro-Spinal Meningitis, Constipation, Hysteria or Fits, Heartburn, Weak Stomach, Flatulence, Quinsy, Pustula Affections, Piles, Hypochondriasis, Deafness, Disease of the Heart, Dropsy, Gravel, Spinal Diseases, Paralysis, Weak Back, Wasting, Decay, etc., etc.

THE ELECTRA-VITA BODY BATTERY WAS ONE OF A FEW SUCH DEVICES DESIGNED FOR BOTH SEXES THAT ACTUALLY CONTAINED DRY CELL BATTERIES!

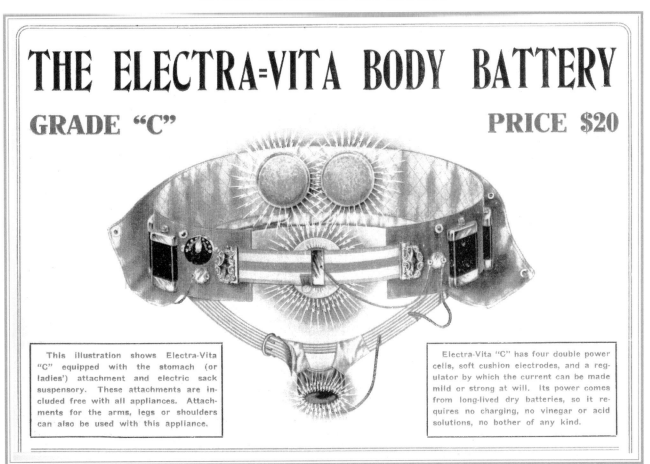

THE ELECTRA=VITA BODY BATTERY

GRADE "C"   PRICE $20

This illustration shows Electra-Vita "C" equipped with the stomach (or ladies') attachment and electric sack suspensory. These attachments are included free with all appliances. Attachments for the arms, legs or shoulders can also be used with this appliance.

Electra-Vita "C" has four double power cells, soft cushion electrodes, and a regulator by which the current can be made mild or strong at will. Its power comes from long-lived dry batteries, so it requires no charging, no vinegar or acid solutions, no bother of any kind.

Diseases that the Battery will not cure:

Yellow Fever, Cholera, Dysentery, Croup, Congestion of the Brain, Diarrhea, Sterility, Leucorrhea, Gleet, Bloody Urine, Inflammation of the Bowels, Gastralgia, Influenza, Pneumonia, Spasms, Worms, Whooping Cough, and Consumption.

DIRECTIONS FOR WEARING THE BATTERY.

Each Battery is attached to a silk cord, which should be tied around the neck, so as to allow the battery to hang as represented in the cut, and to lay on the skin. They should be worn day and night, and for at least a month after the patient is cured. Children under six years of age may wear them at night only. In extreme cases, or Chronic Rheumatism with old age combined, or the entire loss of manhood, two Batteries may be used, one to hang on the chest and the other between the shoulder blades. But in no other cases will it be necessary to electrify the blood to such a degree. When it is necessary to wear two, it can be done without the slightest inconvenience, as the battery is only the size and thickness of a silver half dollar. A Battery will last a lifetime without losing any of its power. *But in no case and under no circumstances should the same Battery be used by two different persons, as the disease from one would be conveyed to the other.*

They should be washed with warm water and soap every week. Many inquire the length of time it takes to cure certain diseases. I have known some severe chronic diseases to be cured in twenty-four hours, and others it has taken weeks and months to cure. Some persons' systems and blood are

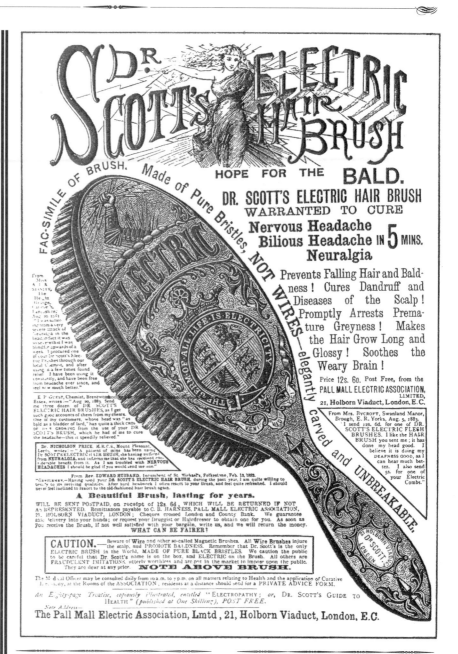

affected by electricity much quicker than others, therefore the length of time required for a cure of the same disease differs.

The Batteries can be had at nearly all druggists in large cities and will be supplied by my agents in small places, or sent from me by mail on receipt of price.

Address all communications to

J. C. BOYD
203 West 49th St., New York, N.Y.

Dr. Scott's Magnificent Electric Brushes

In the 1880s, fake electric brushes appeared. The predominant manufacturer was George A. Scott, who sold magnetism as electricity. Dr. Scott's brushes *seemed* high tech, for each brush came with a round compass made of glass and brass. When the compass was moved over a Dr. Scott's brush, its needle miraculously moved! A small rod of magnetized iron embedded in the brush casings caused the compass needle to jump. This action was the so-called electricity in Dr. Scott's electric brushes.

Dr. Scott's brushes were a classical tribute to emerging electrical technology. While the brushes were well constructed using stiff natural bristles, their hallmark was the patented design carved into the casing. At the top of the design, seemingly a paean to Zeus hurling down lightning bolts from atop Mount Olympus, an armored arm and a clenched fist held four zigzagged lighting bolts. In the circus-style poster font popular in the late nineteenth century, the brush was labeled with the word ELECTRICITY carved one-half inch high. Under this, the British Mr. Scott added a four-paneled circular crest topped by a crown as if Dr. Scott's Electric Brushes had their own heraldry. Beneath the crest was printed the motto: "VENI, VIDI, VICI," a motto seemingly appropriate for Mr.

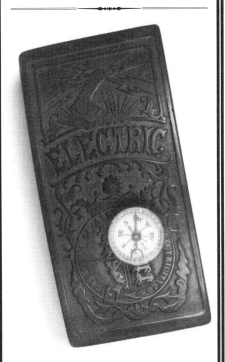

TOP VIEW OF DR. SCOTT'S ELECTRIC BRUSH
(NOTE ACCOMPANYING COMPASS)

Scott. The hair brushes' handles contained elaborate curlicues leading to a small panel noting the Dr. Scott's brand. Charming on the brush, the carvings were

outstanding when rendered as printed black and white illustrations—the major graphic advertising medium of the time. Dr. Scott's brushes were "widely advertised and sold everywhere."

One Dr. Scott's ad quotes an unnamed New York newspaper: "The first and heaviest load to cross the Brooklyn Bridge was the immense truck of Dr. Scott, carrying the average daily shipment of his Electric Brushes, Corsets, Belts &c. President Arthur remarked that he would rather be Dr. Scott than President." The Dr. Scott's truck in the accompanying illustration is so immense one wonders how the bridge withstood the load! The point of the ad was that while the Brooklyn Bridge was made of wire, while Dr. Scott's brushes were not.

The company claimed the hairbrushes would prevent premature graying, arrest hair loss, and cure baldness, dandruff, scalp diseases, headaches, and

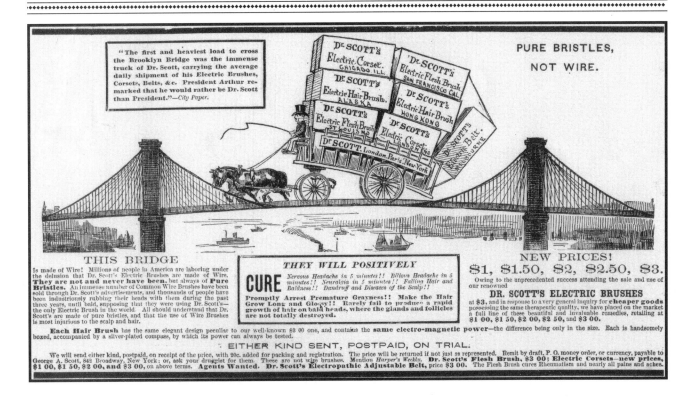

neuralgia. Claims for Dr. Scott's skin brushes were not only an improved complexion, but curing constipation, rheumatism, and backaches as well. Mr. Scott routinely warned consumers away from copies of his brushes: "Beware of Wire and other so-called Magnetic Brushes. All Wire Brushes injure the scalp, and PROMOTE BALDNESS. Remember that Dr. Scott's is the only ELECTRIC BRUSH in the World. MADE OF PURE BLACK BRISTLES. We caution the public to be careful that Dr. Scott's name is on the box, and ELECTRIC on the Brush. All others are FRAUDULENT IMITATIONS, utterly worthless, and are put in the market to impose upon the public. They are dear at any price."

The Wonder Electric Generator.

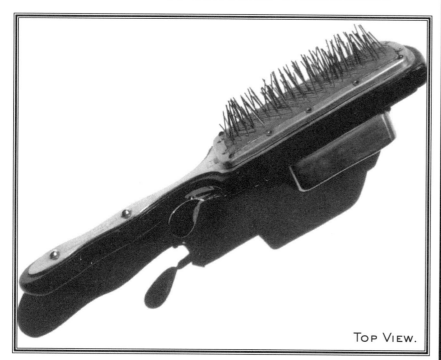

TOP VIEW.

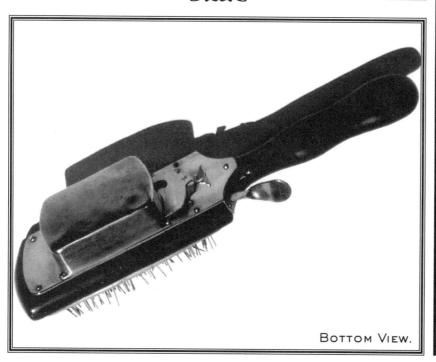

BOTTOM VIEW.

The Wonder Electric Generator may be one of the fraudulent imitations which so irritated the Dr. Scott's Pall Mall Electric Company. Its advertisement mimics the style and layout of the Dr. Scott's hairbrush ads. The ten inch handle, wood finished in black enamel, contains the marking PALL MALL ELECTRIC CO INC, PATENTED U.S.A., NEW YORK, but the device has none of the distinctive Dr. Scott's carvings on the casing. There was no room for them, for the "Wonder" endeavored to be truly electric. It contains a trigger-activated mechanical generator encased in a metal box on the back side of the brush. By rapidly depressing the trigger, the generator produces static electricity which seems not to be conducted to the wire bristles on the opposite side of the brush handle. The wire bristles sit atop a rubber pad which contains an outlet for connecting a hand-held electrode. Unfortunately, the brush produces only static electricity when used vigorously on the hair.

The Failure of the MacGregor Rejuvenator

Plenty of quack devices will supposedly make you live longer by improving your overall health. But few devices have been as ambitious as the MacGregor

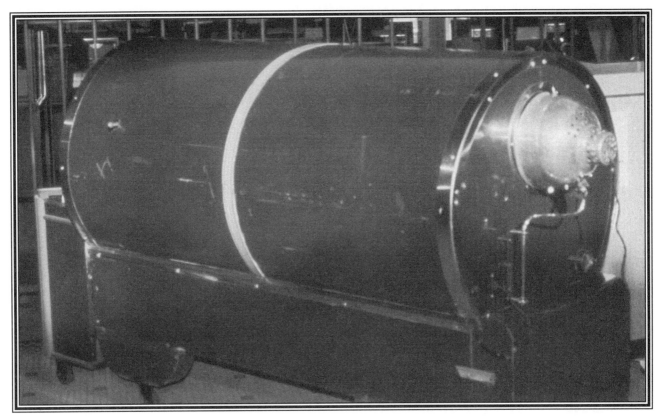

Rejuvenator. According to its inventor, this technological fountain of youth from the 1930s could actually reverse the aging process and make people younger.

Although the claims may sound too good to be true, people have been searching for the secrets to longevity since ancient times. Finding the special combination of chemicals that might make someone immortal was one of the main objectives of the early alchemists, and famous sixteenth-century Spanish explorer Juan Ponce de Leon set out to North America to find the fountain of youth (but ended up in Florida instead). This interest in longevity has continued today.

Observers often comment that the MacGregor Rejuvenator resembles an iron lung machine. This might be more than a coincidence, as the iron lung was invented in 1927, only a few years before 1932 when William. E.

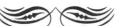

THE MACGREGOR REJUVENATOR

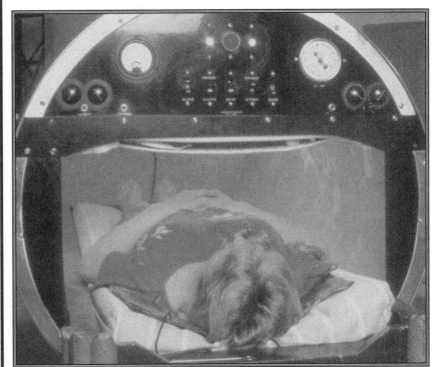

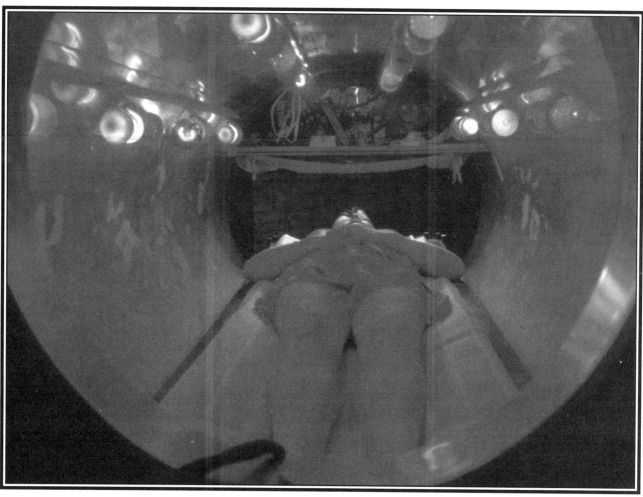

The interior of the Rejuvenator.

Mortrude Jr. of Seattle, Washington, filed a patent for the MacGregor Rejuvenator. By lying down inside the machine, with their head sticking out, patients would receive AM radio signals from the black pads under their head. Although many quack devices use only one form of energy to allegedly cure people, the MacGregor Rejuvenator used several. A timer on the outside of the machine could be set for as long as an hour as a special combination of infrared and ultraviolet lights transmitted energy to the patient and the whole tank became magnetic.

Did patients actually think the Rejuvenator made them younger? Considering that the inventor

went bankrupt and kept his five machines locked away in a warehouse for forty years, the answer would have to be, "No, not many." At an auction, Ed Fitzgerald of Wilson Creek, Washington, purchased the machines, scrapped three of them, and provided the Museum of Questionable Medical

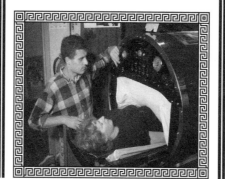

Devices in Minneapolis with the best remaining example.

Gas Grill Igniters Spark Controversy

In the mid-1990s, usually on late night cable TV, millions of consumers watched an infomercial called "Saying No To Pain," which promoted a miraculous drugless pain cure, the Stimulator. The program featured celebrity spokesman Evel Knievel, who exclaimed, "When I wake up in the morning, my wrist tends to hurt me very badly. When I put [the Stimulator] on and I click it, and use it, say, half a dozen or a dozen times on different parts of

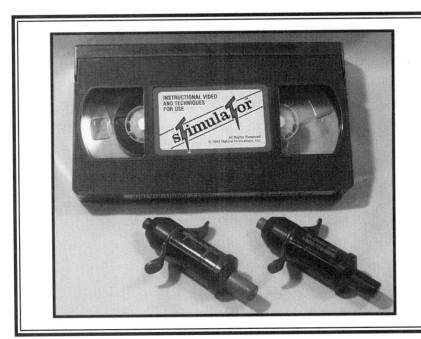

The Stimulator.

my wrist, my wrist begins to feel good. . . . [Friends] know that if I use it after all I've been through and all the things that I've tried to kill pain, that if I use it and they don't see me taking any kind of a drug for pain–everybody that knows me knows that I do not take drugs–and they just absolutely know that if I've got a product and I'm using it to help me, then it must be working for me and you can keep things that do not belong in your system out of your system." Mr. Knievel failed to add that he was being paid for his endorsement, an amount reported to have been $10,000 a week.

The Stimulator is a common gas grill igniter encased in plastic with finger holds attached. Pushing on the end button causes a plunger to hit a crystal which emits a high voltage spark. The spark is then applied to the skin. The manufacturer, Universal Management Services, Inc. of Akron, Ohio, claimed that the Stimulator cured pain, menstrual problems, arthritis and carpal tunnel syndrome, and was as or more effective than aspirin, acetomyacin, codeine, and physical therapy. The device cost about $1 to produce and sold for $88.30! About 800,000 Stimulators were sold during the 1990s.

The U.S. Food and Drug Administration issued a consumer alert on the Stimulator in 1995 and requested a preliminary injunction against the distributor. In May 1995, the FDA seized Universal Management Company, Inc.'s inventory of Stimulators, an inventory worth $1.5 million. On December 30, 1997, a federal judge enjoined Universal Management and allied businesses from distributing the Stimulator and ordered that the company make refunds available to consumers who purchased the device. This ruling was appealed in March 1998.

In the meantime, the attorney for Universal Management continued to accept orders for the Stimulator, orders that could not be filled after the inventory was seized. He diverted these funds into a personal account which eventually reached six figures. This was judged to be swindling and the attorney received a 33 month prison sentence. He was ordered to pay restitution as well.

On the appeal, the company lawyers argued that no one has been hurt by the Stimulator (except in the pocketbook?) and that other companies have peddled almost identical products. These other companies would include Magna Plus of Twinsburg, Ohio with its "Acupoint Pulse Stimulator," Bright Marketing of Burlington, Ohio, purveyors of the "Piezo D-X Quartz Crystal," and Crystaldyne Inc. of Scottsdale, Arizona which sold the "Crystaldyne Pain Reliever." By August 1999, as the 6th Circuit U.S. Court of Appeals prepared to hear oral arguments on the Stimulator appeal, the price of similar quack gas grill igniter pain cures had risen to $139.

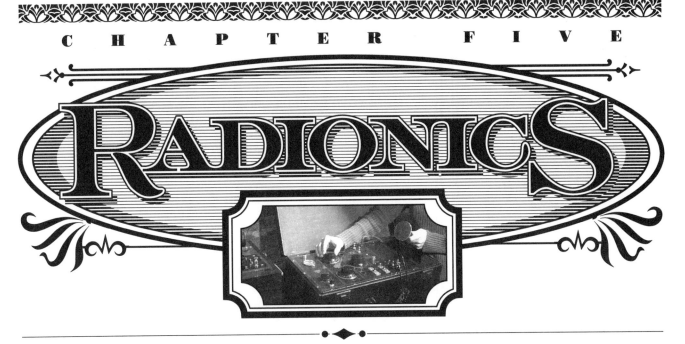

RADIONICS

ALBERT ABRAMS, RUTH DROWN, AND THE MIRACLE OF VIBRATIONS.

The Dynamizer and the Oscilloclast

BY JACK COULEHAN

in memory of Albert Abrams, an American quack

1.

Here is the machine, the dynamizer,
whose boxes, wires, and rheostats
reveal the hidden names of pain.
On the cot my assistant lies.
His scalp is connected by a wire
to this, the measurement device
in which I place some drops of blood.
Then, I finger my assistant's skin
to find the place the patient hurts.
He groans. The needle cries its name.

Poor distant people see my face
smiling from the back of magazines.
They send me shreds of paper
soaked in blood and tell their tales.
I am their savior, their last hope.
When I feed their stories, one by one,
here, into the mouth of this device,

my assistant moves, the needle turns.
YES! I write them. Come. Come soon.
For I have named your suffering.

2.

One more rheostat, another gauge.
At night in my basement shop
I work on the oscilloclast,
a new machine that oscillates disease
and restores the harmony of health.
In my mind's ear the oscilloclast
already sings. There! Can you hear
those songs, those streams, those crickets?
When I rush to fit their frequencies
to my machine, the music disappears.

The sick are selling their farms in Kansas.
They are buying their tickets in Georgia.
They are putting their houses in order.
My letters told them, Come! Come soon!
What could I do but give them hope?
The sick are pounding at my door.
I must finish the oscilloclast tonight!
One more rheostat, a final gauge
and then, My friends, the sick, come in.

Radionics, a branch of quackery which thrives today, has its roots in San Francisco, California where

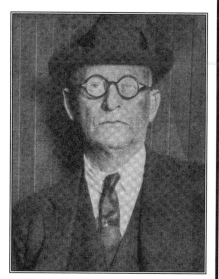

Dr. Albert Abrams

neurologist Albert Abrams devised a system for "sensing" electronic reactions in combination with radio waves to diagnose and cure disease.

Ken Raines, publisher of the *JW Research Journal*, contributed the following history of Albert Abrams and the birth of radionics:

Albert Abrams and the Electronic Reactions of Abrams (E.R.A.)

"The electronic technique has been conceived by a master mind. It is far more intricate and ironclad than medical fads of the past. It deals with a new form of energy which, we are told, cannot be detected by the physicist's most delicate instruments, but can be detected by the abdominal reflexes under the guidance of an electronic diagnostician. These reactions are said to be affected by the presence of skeptical minds. . . . It has given rise to all sorts of occultism in medicine. It has been a renaissance of the black magic of medieval times. It has given free reign to idiotic ideas . . ."

—SCIENTIFIC AMERICAN, September, 1924

Dr. Albert Abrams of San Francisco began to make some astounding medical claims in the early 1920s. His claims were so outrageous as to be viewed by many as absurd on its face. He claimed that all substances radiated electronic vibrations that could be detected and measured. All human organs, diseased and healthy, transmitted radiation or "vibrations" unique to that organ or disease. All that was needed from a patient for diagnosis was a drop of blood, a single hair, or even a handwriting sample as these would give off the unique "vibrations" of that individual. Not only were diseases ascertained by a drop of blood or handwriting, but one could determine a person's religion, golf handicap, sex, age, present location, when that person would die, and innumerable other tidbits of information.

Did Abrams discover something of significance? Was the scientific diagnosis and cure of every conceivable disease within reach? This became a huge controversy

---

"SPONDYLOTHERAPY," "ELECTRONIC REACTIONS," THE "OSCILLOCLAST," THE "ELECTROBIOSCOPE," ETC.

For some time THE JOURNAL has received inquiries of which the following recent examples are typical. This from an Ohio physician:

"Please give me some information concerning Dr. Abrams and his diagnostic and therapeutic devices known as reflexaphore and oscilloclast. If this is published please withhold my name."

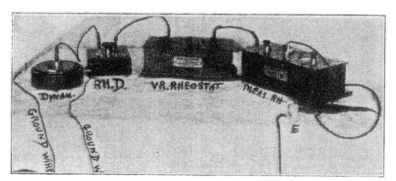

This is the apparatus used by Albert Abrams and his disciples for diagnosing the disease of John Doe from a few drops of John's blood. The specimen of blood is put in the "dynamizer" ("*Dynam.*"). The "energy" which is said to emanate from this blood ("energy" which nobody but Dr. Abrams and his disciples has ever been able to demonstrate) travels through the wire to the "rheostat dynamizer" ("*Rh. D.*"), which is said to be used "for stepping up energy." The mysterious force is then said to travel by wire to the "vibratory rate rheostat" ("*VR. Rheostat*"), which is said to admit energy "at vibratory rate of disease." From this the "energy" travels by wire to the "measuring rheostat" ("*Meas. Rh.*") for "determining energy." But it has not yet reached the end of its trip; it goes on through a wire to the electrode ("*E.*") which is applied to the healthy "subject" who has to face west and must be in a dim light! Then Abrams, and his followers, by percussing the abdomen of the "subject" purport to tell what ails John Doe and where his ailment is located.

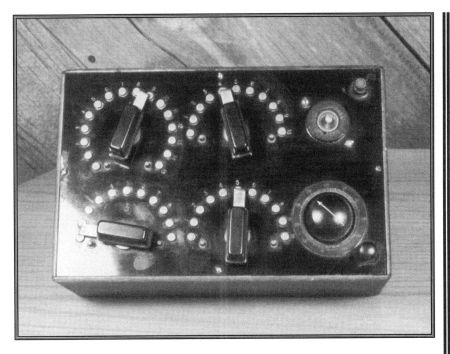

A control box that was used with various Abrams devices. Inside it has meaningless connections.

book on a medical technique he called Spondylotherapy. This volume "constituted his first definite departure from medical orthodoxy." Even in Abrams' estimation, "spondylotherapy" was his version of Chiropractic and Osteopathy which were viewed as "cults" by "orthodox" medicine at the time. For this reason Dr. Abrams began to be viewed with some suspicion and concern by his peers for promoting questionable medical practices.

In 1916, Abrams published his New Concepts in Diagnosis and Treatment book. He had been experimenting with what came to be called "the electronic reactions of Abrams" or the E.R.A. This was a complete departure from

in the early 1920s when the famous author, Upton Sinclair, wrote the article "The House of Wonders" for Pearson's Magazine in June of 1923 which promoted Dr. Abrams' theory and methods. This led to numerous articles in popular magazines both pro and con. The scientific and medical communities in the United States and Britain were forced to respond to this situation. Two scientific investigations were conducted to get to the bottom of the matter.

Who was Dr. Abrams and how did his peers in the medical community view his theory and methods? What did the scientific investigations of his claims and methods discover?

Albert Abrams was born in San Francisco in 1863. In his teen years he learned German and graduated as an MD from Heidelberg in 1882. He became Professor of Pathology at Cooper College in San Francisco in 1893 and resigned in 1898. He was also elected vice-president of the California State Medical Society in 1889 and made president of the San Francisco

Medico Chirurgic Society in 1893. By the early 1900s Abrams had become a respected expert in neurology. By all accounts, Abrams had a respectable background and promise of a distinguished career.

In 1910 Abrams published a

RADIOCLAST NEWS

Vol. III   PUBLISHED IN THE INTEREST OF BETTER HEALTH
By Radioclast Research Department, Tiffin, Ohio   No. 1

BODY ILLS ARE REVEALED IN EXPERIMENTS

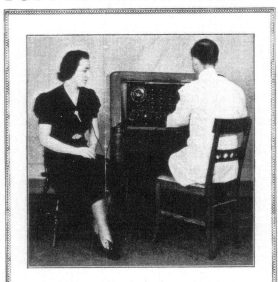

The Radioclast

New Device Measures Life Processes

NEW HAVEN, Conn., Nov. 9— Development of a device which utilizes animal electricity to reveal secrets of the body was announced today by Yale scientists.

The instrument, a vacuum tube microvoltmeter, may rival the microscope as a means of studying biological processes of life, reported the Yale authorities, who have made thousands of measurements with it.

The instrument can measure bodily electrical changes as small as five one-millionths of a volt, indicating alterations in physiological activity before they can be detected by other methods now available.

Dr. Harold S. Burr, professor of anatomy; Dr. Cecil T. Lane, of the physics department, and Dr. Leslie N. Nims, of the physiology department, developed the device.

With it they have conducted experiments on a wide variety of subjects, from fish to man, and have found that each species has a characteristic electrical pattern which

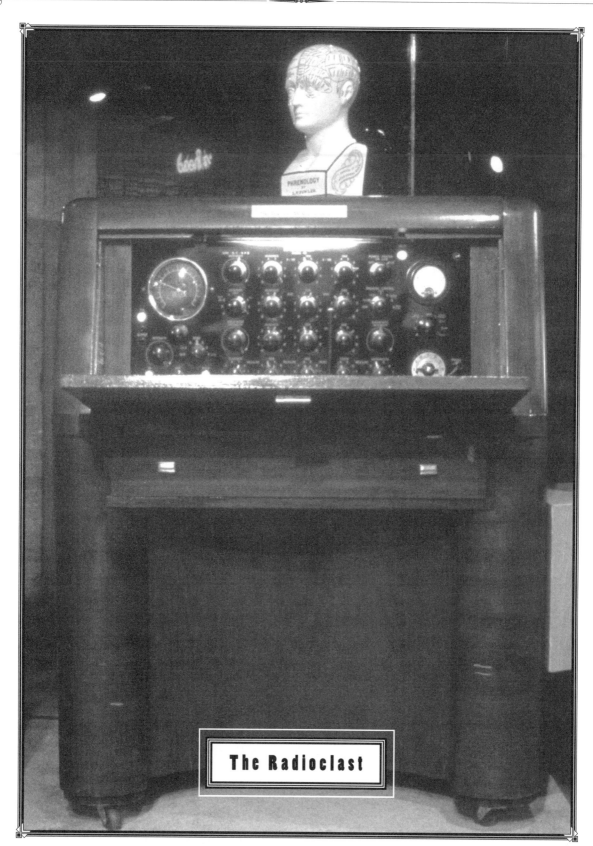

The Radioclast

"Radioclast Fraud is Nationwide!" announced the Indianapolis Better Business Bureau Bulletin in 1942. The Electronic Instrument Co. of Tiffin Ohio sold 1,400 of these contraptions for $945 each! The device contains a variety of radio parts—including a short-wave tuner—but nothing is connected in any meaningful way. The BBB flyer stated that "Modern Medical Mechanics Make Much Money Mending Many Maids and Misters, but the Mending IS MOSTLY Mental and Misleading."

conventional medicine and those in the medical community were not hesitant to call him a quack as a result.

Describing the E.R.A. can be difficult due to its complex nature and theory as well as the numerous methods and devices used. Briefly, the theory behind the E.R.A. was the human body transmitted radiation or "electronic vibrations" from the atomic level, specifically from the electrons. These electronic vibrations emanating from the electrons, if normal, would vibrate at a specific rate. If they vibrated at an abnormal rate, it would indicate the presence of disease. Each disease vibrated at a unique rate. In this theory, one could cure disease by transmitting back at the disease the same electronic vibratory rate it was transmitting. This would neutralize the abnormal vibrations and allow the electrons to return to normal vibration rates and eliminate the disease. Abrams believed that drugs worked when they had the same or similar "vibrations" as the disease they cured.

How Abrams detected and normalized these "electronic vibrations" of diseases was bizarre and complex. He would take a hair, handwriting or blood sample (sometimes a photograph) of a patient to be diagnosed. This would be placed into a device he called a Dynamizer. This was hooked up by wires to a headpiece to be worn on a healthy individual (called a reagent) who, while facing west, would "react" biologically through the central nervous system to the diseased "vibrations." These "reactions" could be detected by percussing (thumping) the abdomen of the reagent which would reveal areas of "dullness." The location of the dullness and its size would indicate the precise disease and its location in the patient.

The precise rate of vibrations were ascertained by boxes containing resistance coils which were also hooked up by wires to the reagent and Dynamizer. Dials would be turned to different "ohmage" rates once the disease was identified. This would pinpoint the exact amount and rate of the disease the patient had. Sometimes horseshoe magnets were placed over the reagent's head to "clear" him of extraneous "vibrations" to get a better "reaction."

Bob McCoy holds a Radioclast electrode to Stephanie King's forehead while she holds an electrode in the palm of her hand.

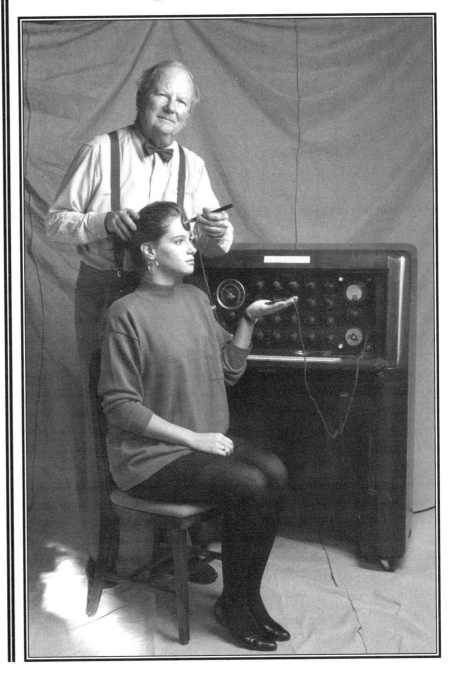

Methods used later by Abrams and his followers involved stroking the reagent's abdomen with a glass rod to obtain the "reactions."

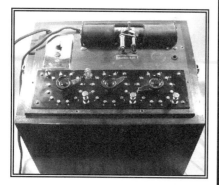

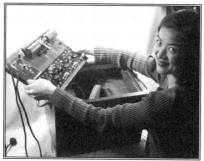

Albert Abrams' Oscilloclast had a warning label "Do Not Open This Device!" So we did. It is empty except for a piece of wood at the bottom.

Later the reagent was dispensed with altogether and the operator stroked a plate hooked up to the Dynamizer, etc. with his fingers to feel the "vibrations" from the patient's blood or handwriting.

In all this, numerous things could interfere with the vibrations as they were sensitive in more ways than one. In collecting a blood sample, the patient had to be facing west in dimmed light. No strong orange or red colored material could be present in the room. The same was true when getting the reactions from the reagent to the sample. In addition to the above, reactions could be driven away by the presence of skeptical minds or enhanced by other mental activity. For these reasons, most have compared the

E.R.A. to psychic phenomena, sympathetic magic and the occult.

Abrams had another device called an oscilloclast which he used to cure patients. This machine supposedly transmitted back at the diseased tissue the same electronic vibrations it was emitting until the patient was "clear" of the electronic reactions in the reagent. The best account of how Abrams came up with this theory and how he developed these strange methods is given in the pro-E.R.A. book, *Report on Radionics*.

The AMA and
Dr. Albert Abrams

The American Medical Association (AMA) never did take Dr. Albert Abrams' claims seriously. No formal investigation of Abrams' methods was ever undertaken by

the AMA. The AMA believed Abrams' methods and claims were ridiculous on the face of it, and that they therefore weren't worth the time and money to investigate. The AMA commented on Dr. Abrams and the E.R.A. in their two periodicals: *Journal of the American Medical Association* (JAMA), and *Hygeia* (changed to *Today's Health* in 1950), the latter being a magazine on health issues for the general public. Both were edited by Dr. Morris Fishbein during the 1920s and 1930s. Fishbein also wrote numerous articles for various popular level magazines on quackery.

JAMA began commenting on Dr. Albert Abrams and the E.R.A. in response to readers' letters, beginning with their March 25, 1922, issue (pp. 913-914). This and following articles appeared

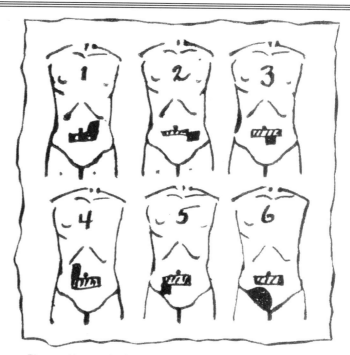

Photographic reproduction from Albert Abrams' house organ *Physico-Clinical Medicine* for September, 1922. This chart represents the areas of dulness Abrams claims to have found in determining the religion of individuals by means of the "Electronic Reactions." 1 represents the areas of dulness for a Catholic; 2, Methodist; 3, Seventh Day Adventist; 4, Theosophist; 5, Protestant; 6. Jew.

in "The Propaganda for Reform" section of the Journal that dealt with quackery. The articles mainly presented some of the clearly ridiculous claims and experiments that Dr. Abrams made with the E.R.A., such as carrying around on one's person a cut potato for curative and diagnostic purposes, his claim that numbers and vowels have a "sex," experiments with determining the outcome of a chicken's sex before it is born, determining the religion and present location of a patient from a drop of blood or handwriting sample, etc.

A couple of JAMA articles dealt with Medical Associations that made the decision to either charge MDs that used Abrams' oscilloclast with "unethical conduct" for promoting and using quackery, or expelling from their society those who used it. Some JAMA articles recounted tests by other's of E.R.A. practitioners' diagnostic ability by sending them blood samples in the mail as requested. In one case, a blood sample from a fictitious "Miss Bell" was actually a blood sample from a male guinea-pig. "Miss Bell" was diagnosed as having various ailments including a streptococcus infection of the "the left [fallopian] tube." Another article presented the results of a similar test of an E.R.A. practitioner who was sent the blood of a rooster. The "innocent" and apparently virtuous rooster was diagnosed as having a venereal disease. JAMA also noted that the California State Journal of Medicine invited Dr. Abrams to participate in a scientific test to see how accurate his E.R.A. tests were in diagnosing diseases. Abrams "flat-footedly" refused.

The AMA's popular magazine *Hygeia*, later *Today's Health*, contained numerous articles on quackery and medical "cults" it believed the public should be informed of and warned about. The *Hygeia* articles on medical fads and quackery continually referred to Abrams as a quack, even stating he may have been the greatest quack of the 20th century:

"IF SOME ONE were to set about the task of selecting the

AUTOGRAPHIC EXAMINATIONS †

Autograph	Date of Writing	Ohmage	Remarks
Dr. Samuel Johnson	Feb. 7, 1775	48	Reaction acquired syphilis (cerebro-spinal strain) and tuberculosis
Edgar A. Poe	Dec. 30, 1846	31	Cong. syphilis (cerebro-spinal) and reaction of dipsomania
H. W. Longfellow	May 14, 1855	10	Cong. syphilis
Oscar Wilde	No date		Male reaction 18/25 Female reaction 1 16/25 Acquired Syphilis (cerebro-spinal)
Samuel Pepys	July 5, 1693	60 10/25	Congenital syphilis (cerebro-spinal)
Bret Harte	No date		Jewish on father's side Cong. syphilis (cerebro-spinal)

Photographic reproduction from *Physico-Clinical Medicine* of March, 1922. Here Abrams makes a diagnosis of several well-known men, long since dead, by subjecting the autographs of the individuals to his "Electronic Reactions."

greatest medical quack in history, he would find a long list of colorful competitors. . . . In recent times, our country has produced no greater charlatan than Albert Abrams . . . the founder of the 'electronic' and 'radionic' hokum that still flourishes among many medical cults."

Many *Hygeia* articles in the 1920s and 1930s on quackery mentioned Abrams or recounted his story. As late as 1939 they printed a full length article on Abrams' life and quackery. Most of the Hygeia articles, like the JAMA articles, ridiculed Abram's bizarre experiments, instruments, and claims, such as his "Reflexa-phone" device which allowed him to diagnose and even treat patients over the phone.

Dr. Morris Fishbein ridiculed Abrams numerous outrageous claims, methods and endless gadgets. He also made it a point to mention how much money Abrams was making as the result of his "practice." He believed quackery was perpetrated for the revenue it generated. Abrams was reportedly worth two million dollars when he died in 1924. Courses in Spondylotherapy and the E.R.A. went for two hundred dollars a head with the terms being cash—in advance. His oscilloclast was leased at around two hundred dollars with a monthly five dollar charge thereafter. The lessee was required to sign a contract stating he would never open the device. These things were pointed out by Fishbein to show that to him, the whole thing was a sham operation designed to "separate sick people from their money" as the Watchtower Society later claimed about radionics.

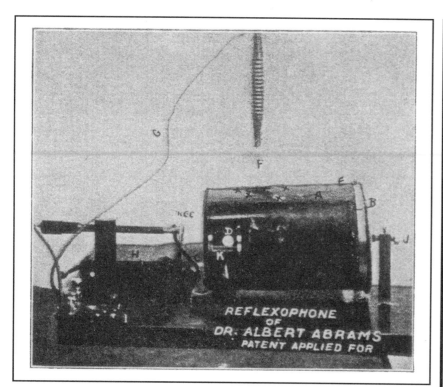

REFLEXOPHONE.

Another "patent applied for" device of Albert Abrams: the "Reflexophone." By means of this instrument Abrams claimed to be able to diagnose pathological specimens over the telephone.

Science journals such as *Nature* commented as well on the Abrams controversy. It wasn't taken any more seriously there than by the medical community.

"Orthodox" Medicine and the E.R.A.

In 1923 and 1924, the *Scientific American* magazine put together an investigation committee and investigated the "electronic reactions of Abrams." The investigation lasted about one year and cost the *Scientific American* twenty thousand dollars in 1923/1924 dollars. The *Scientific American* reported on the progress of the investigation in each monthly issue from October, 1923 to September, 1924. The adventures of Alice in Wonderland are tame in comparison of those of an investigator in the land of E.R.A.

In the second installment in the series they printed the results of their first test of an E.R.A. practitioner in New York City. The practitioner was to diagnose the diseases contained in six vials. These contained pure germ cultures from diseased patients. For example, tube #2, which simply contained Pneumococcus (a bacterium that causes pneumonia), was diagnosed as being syphilis, tuberculosis, septococcus, malaria and the flu, at which the committee decided that was enough diagnosing, which they called a "broadside." "The purity of the germ culture was questioned" by the doctor. There was no such thing as a pure germ culture according to the doctor. After a few more tests, the doctor "sought some reason for his flat failure." The *Scientific American* reported:

"He asked to look at one of the pure germ culture vials. Looking at it in full light, presumably for the first time, he discovered the red edge on the label, as well as the blue handwriting. Right then and there Dr. X found the reason for his unsuccessful diagnosis. He explained to us that red is fatal to the accuracy of the electronic reactions! The presence of that bit of red on each label was sufficient to upset the reactions completely. . . . Furthermore, there was handwriting on our labels. No doubt the electronic emissions from the writer of those labels were being carried along in the diagnosis. If so, the writer of those labels must have been in a terrible state of health—and mind, so we reflected at the time."

This was typical of the problems and obstacles the committee faced in testing E.R.A practitioners. They accommodated such complaints by taking pains to eliminate any possible electronic contaminations. For example, in

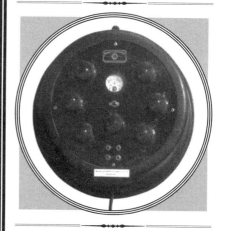

THE BLANCHARD ELECTROPATHIC SUPER RADIONIC DEVICE WAS IMPRESSIVE OUTSIDE— HODGEPODGE INSIDE.

the above case, after "Dr. X" complained about the red edged labels and the blue handwriting, the committee had new labels attached in accordance with the doctor's specs, such as typing the numbers on plain labels, etc. Further testing, as their chart indicated, resulted in "broadside upon broadside" diagnoses that were completely off the mark. Further tests with other E.R.A. practitioners using various techniques in the following months resulted in complete failures as well.

Additional strange complaints and requests of the doctor in the above case were common in the various *Scientific American* tests. Dr. X several times during the tests requested that all those present:

". . . and especially the reagent, keep their minds off the pure germ cultures. . . . It seems that even the thoughts of those present have a serious electronic effect on the reagent and the accuracy of the

diagnosis. Sensitive—super-sensitive, these reactions!"

Later, in mentioning an ongoing correspondence with Dr. Abrams in which he said he would "demonstrate" his technique but not submit to test by their committee, they wrote:

"Dr. Abrams, it will be noted, calls attention to the psychological factor. He indicates that when the E.R.A. diagnostician is working under test conditions, he is at a decided disadvantage because of his anxiety regarding the outcome of the test. From time to time we have been warned against a

---

See The Amazing Device of the Modern Age!!!
The Electro Metabograph

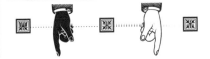

---

skeptical turn of mind, for such a state on the part of the investigator has a decidedly detrimental influence on the reactions . . ."

The committee came to the conclusion that the E.R.A. was occultic or psychic in nature. Before beginning the test with Doctor X, they said the preliminaries (subduing the light in the room, etc.) reminded them "in no little degree of a psychic seance." After tests with other doctors that included similar and even more bizarre claims and procedures ("queer" they said), they came to the conclusion that:

"The whole thing bears striking resemblance to the subjective psychic phenomena. Compare it to the Ouija board. . . . Compare it with automatic writing . . . . The E.R.A. technique works—when it does work—in just this way."

Dr. Abrams himself diagnosed his own "life expectancy" and predicted his death would

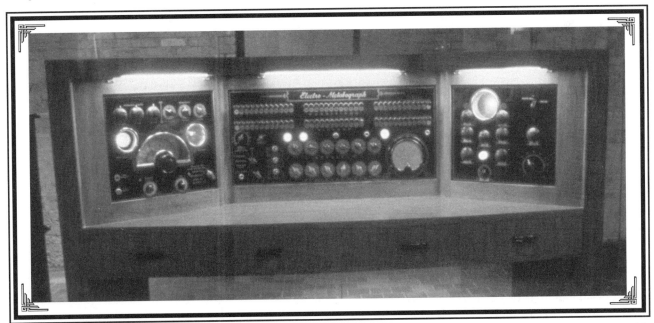

The Electro Metabograph was an impressive device made by the Art Tool & Die Co. of Detroit in 1940. The patient was connected to two ankle electrodes and seated so as to be able to view the various wave forms in the cathode-ray tube. There are 117 switches on the machine which supposedly send specific AM radio signals to the patient. For example, #13 cures jealousy, #17 impatience, and #42 nymphomania. Seized by the FDA in 1965. Notice of Judgment #7515.

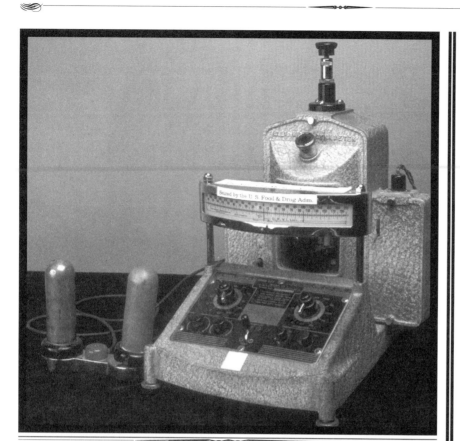

The Micro-Dynameter, a scientific looking but worthless device, was falsely promoted as curing disease. The FDA seized 1,268 in 1953. Then FDA Commissioner Lerrick called the machine "a peril to public health because it cannot correctly diagnose any disease. Thousands of patients are being hoodwinked by its use into believing they have diseases which they do not have, or failing to get proper treatment for diseases they do have."

occur in January of 1924 based on his own E.R.A. diagnosis, which was fulfilled.

After one year of tests and twenty thousand dollars spent, the *Scientific American* committee's conclusion as to the scientific basis of the E.R.A. was that it was "the height of absurdity" and "utterly worthless." Their official statement was:

"This committee finds that the claims advanced on behalf of the electronic reactions of Abrams, and of electronic practice in general, are not substantiated; and it is our belief that they have no basis in fact. In our opinion the so-called electronic treatments are without value."

In 1924, a British committee

was put together to investigate an adaptation or modification of Abrams' E.R.A. apparatus and technique by Dr. W.E. Boyd of Glasgow. This committee's investigation and mostly negative conclusions are intriguing and a little puzzling; it has given rise to debate and claims by those who endorse radionics that the E.R.A. was vindicated by this committee.

A report of the committee's findings was recorded in both *The Lancet* and the *British Medical Journal* in January of 1925. Basically, the tests of Dr. Boyd were at first complete failures. He was asked to differentiate between two different substances placed in the Dynamizer at random. His results were much less than what

OPPOSITE PAGE
From a 1922 issue of Science and Invention magazine.

would be expected by chance. A physicist was also employed for six months to determine if "any effect measurable or detectable by orthodox physical apparatus was associated with the so-called 'reactions'. No such change could be found, and this aspect of the work was ultimately abandoned."

However, after complaining about electronic interference, Dr. Boyd undertook further tests at his insulated residence in which he was able to differentiate between substances with remarkable accuracy.

Overall the committee obtained numerous negative results with other E.R.A. practitioners of the Abrams and Boyd variety when dealing with diagnosing diseases, much like the *Scientific American*. However, they obtained some success from Dr. Boyd in differentiating certain non-pathological substances such as "sulfer" and saliva.

Their four stated conclusions were as follows:

"(1) That certain substances,

The Rx Micro Tabulometer consisted of a wooden cabinet with a large ammeter, bridge circuits, lots of toggle switches, and a hand electrode. It was supposed to detect variations in skin resistance along the spinal column. Seized by the FDA 1963. Notice of Judgment 8034.

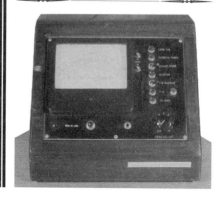

A Modern Charlatan

By A. B. TRIPP

WE HAVE HAD MANY LETTERS FROM OUR READERS REGARDING DR. ABRAM'S SUPPOSED
ELECTRONIC CURES. WE GIVE OUR OPINION BELOW.

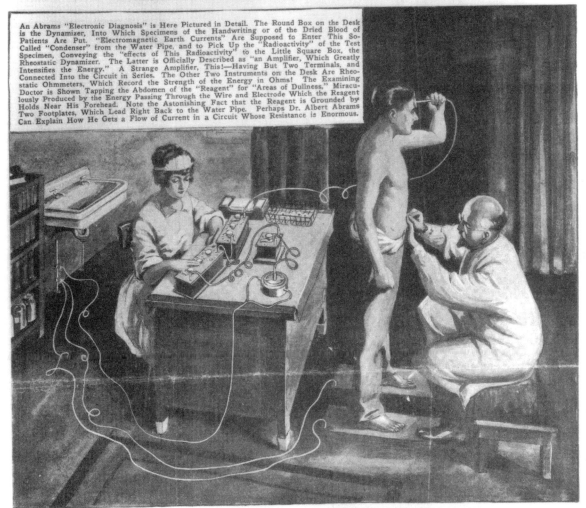

An Abrams "Electronic Diagnosis" is Here Pictured in Detail. The Round Box on the Desk is the Dynamizer, Into Which Specimens of the Handwriting or of the Dried Blood of Patients Are Put. "Electromagnetic Earth Currents" Are Supposed to Enter This So-Called "Condenser" from the Water Pipe, and to Pick Up the "Radioactivity" of the Test Specimen, Conveying the "effects of This Radioactivity" to the Little Square Box, the Rheostatic Dynamizer. The Latter is Officially Described as "an Amplifier, Which Greatly Intensifies the Energy." A Strange Amplifier, This!—Having But Two Terminals, and Connected Into the Circuit in Series. The Other Two Instruments on the Desk Are Rheostatic Ohmmeters, Which Record the Strength of the Energy in Ohms! The Examining Doctor is Shown Tapping the Abdomen of the "Reagent" for "Areas of Dullness," Miraculously Produced by the Energy Passing Through the Wire and Electrode Which the Reagent Holds Near His Forehead. Note the Astonishing Fact that the Reagent is Grounded by Two Footplates, Which Lead Right Back to the Water Pipe. Perhaps Dr. Albert Abrams Can Explain How He Gets a Flow of Current in a Circuit Whose Resistance is Enormous.

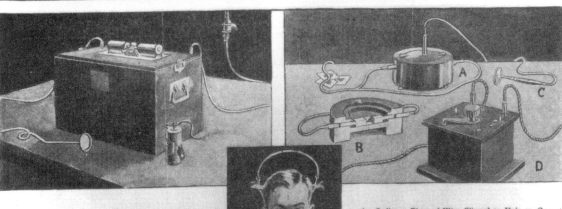

The "Oscilloclast." Above—Abrams' Cure-all Treating Machine, Pictured Beside a Worn-out Dry Cell. The Cell, Picked Up from an Ash Heap, Was So Feeble That it Would Scarcely Run a Doorbell for More Than Two or Three Seconds. Yet This Old, Burst Cell Running Its Doorbell Was a Very Hercules of Power as a Generator of Electronic Oscillations When Compared with the Glorified Electric Buzzer Towering Impressively Above It. The Only Energy That the Oscilloclast Generates is Sound, Noise. Small Center Picture Shows How Abrams "Short-circuits" the Brain. "Brain Waves May Be Conducted Through Wires," Says Dr. Abrams.

An Ordinary Piece of Wire Clipped to Hair on Opposite Sides of the Head Will "Short-circuit" These Brain Waves. (Page 108 New Concepts of Diagnosis and Treatment by Dr. Albert Abrams). Above a Close-up View of the "Diagnostic Instruments." A—"The Wonderful Little Dynamizer," Which Abrams Pretends is a "Condenser." B—The Dynamizer Cut in Two, After the Cover-Electrode Has Been Removed. Note the Two Aluminum Electrodes Inside, Upon Which the Wrapped-up Blood Specimen is Placed. C—A Brow Electrode, with Rubber Rim to Prevent Metallic Contact with the "Reagent's" Skin. D—The Abrams Rheostatic Dynamizer.

when placed in proper relation to the emanometer of Boyd, produce, beyond any reasonable doubt, changes in the abdominal wall of "the subject" of a kind which may be detected by percussion. This is tantamount to the statement that the fundamental proposition underlying, in common, the original and certain other forms of apparatus designed for the purpose of eliciting the so-called electronic reactions of Abrams, is established to a very high degree of probability.

"(2) That no evidence justifying this deduction is yet available from the work of those who practice with the apparatus as yet designed by Abrams himself.

"(3) That the phenomena appear to be extremely elusive, and highly susceptible to interference, so that in order to obtain reliable results it is necessary to take the most elaborate precautions, particularly as regards the elimination of effects due to irrelevant objects.

"(4) That it would be premature at the present time even to hazard in the most tentative manner any hypothesis as to the physical phenomena here described."

The first conclusion has of course been quoted by just about every pro-E.R.A. individual since then as confirming the E.R.A. However, this had nothing to do with the diagnosing of disease as the successful tests were done on non-pathological substances such as saliva and sulfer. As the committee said after their above conclusions:

"It is impossible to emphasize too strongly that nothing in this communication is to be taken as implying that any correlation of those changes in the abdominal wall, referred to in conclusion (1), with pathological conditions has yet been shown, or a fortiori, that any justification—physical,

Schenk's Radionic Therapy.

This machine was purchased by a woman in Minneapolis in 1931 for $365 c.o.d. from a healer, Mr. Schenk of Chicago. He promised to restore "the complete use of your legs again from my radio treatment." When she gave this machine to the museum, she stated that it was worthless and that she had rejected Schenk's offer of a visit for $500.

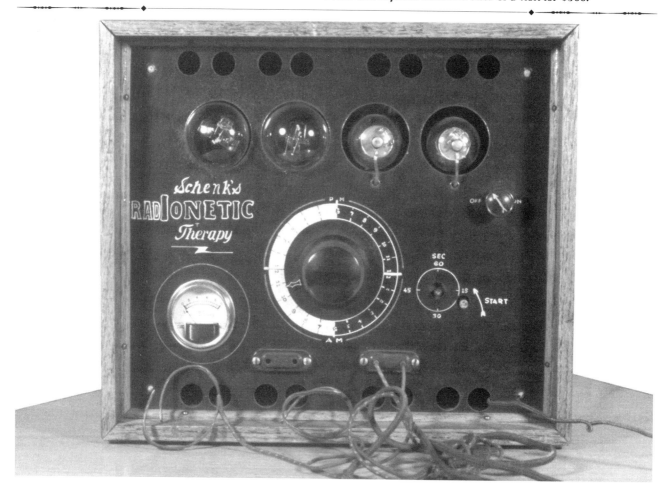

pathological, nosological, or clinical—exists for the direct use of either the Abrams or the Boyd apparatus in diagnosis or treatment."

This was further emphasized in the closing remarks of the committee's communication which has been quoted by numerous critics of the E.R.A.:

"To sum up. The conclusions arrived at in this communication leave the practicing electronist as scientifically unsound and as ethically unjustified as it was before. They give no sanction for the use of E.R.A. in the diagnosis or in the treatment of disease. Nor does there appear to be any other sanction for this kind of practice at the present time."

This communication was delivered before the Royal Society of Medicine. At the end it was put to a vote as to whether the matter should be discussed further then or at a later time. Neither was decided; the matter simply dropped for the most part and hasn't been taken up again as far as scientific investigations are concerned. Some magazines picked up the controversy during 1925 based on the Horder report, but this quickly died out.

After the *Scientific American* and Thomas Horder investigations, the E.R.A. lost most of its credibility. A few individuals, such as George De la Warr and Ruth Drown, carried on with the E.R.A.. Drown was the last major E.R.A. practitioner in America. The AMA dealt with her claims the way they did with Abrams, including recounting investigations and tests of her techniques, and found no basis for her claims. She was twice charged with fraud and died awaiting her second trial. "Radionics" and associated devices are considered fraudulent by the U.S.

Government and using it to diagnose and treat diseases is now illegal.

The Drown Technic Fails

If Albert Abrams was considered "The King of Quackery," then Ruth Drown surely was the "Queen of Quackery." The Bureau of Investigation of the AMA published the following amazing account of Mrs. Drown's exploits in the *JAMA* on February 18, 1950:

A Mrs. Ruth B. Drown of Los Angeles has claimed that she can diagnose disease and treat it with devices known variously as "Drown Radio Therapy" and "Drown Radio Vision Instruments." She

has also designated them as "Homo-Vibra Ray Instruments," which are, she reveals:

". . . based on the laws of energy and adjusted to tune into the most delicate vibrations. The Drown Radio Instruments are the most fundamentally scientific known today in the field of diagnosis, remedy selection and therapy. . . . Drown Instruments tune into the vibrations of the body for function and disease. . . . Also, the impinged nerves may be recorded, and a blood count, urinalysis, blood pressure and temperature taken on the instrument. . . . When diagnosis with the Drown Instrument is finished, the doctor has a complete and scientifically accurate blueprint of the patient's body such as can be

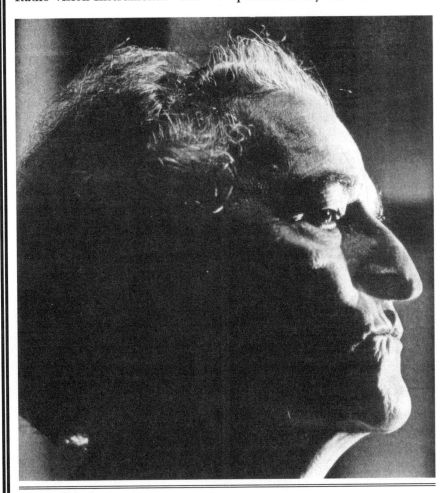

Mrs. Ruth B. Drown

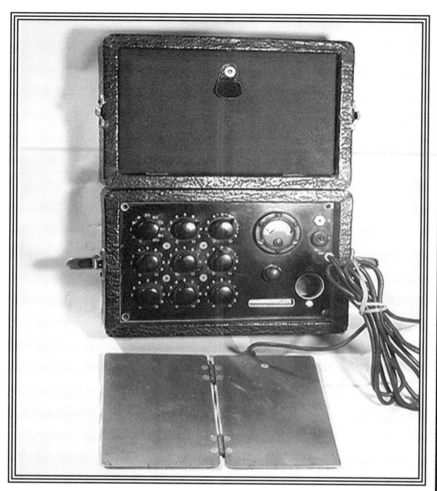

DROWN HOME RADIONICS KIT

The Model 98 sold for $500; it is a scaled down version of the standard kit.

investigation. Terms and conditions were drawn and agreed to by both parties to the protocol. The committee's report summarized observations which serve to corroborate statements previously reported in *The Journal.* On "diagnosis" the committee reported as follows:

"Diagnosis by means of the Drown diagnostic machine: It is our opinion that the machine is a sort of Ouija board in which the operator develops the audible end point by the amount of pressure applied to the stroking finger without any causal relationship to the position of three potentiometer dials. In the three patients that she attempted to diagnose, Mrs. Drown registered spectacular failures. It is our belief that her alleged successes rest solely on the noncritical attitude of her followers. Her technic is to find so much trouble in so many organs that usually she can say 'I told you so' when she registers an occasional lucky positive guess. In these particular tests, even this luck deserted her."

obtained in no other way, and many obscure conditions are uncovered which otherwise would have been impossible to locate."

Mrs. Drown has failed completely in a test entered into by her voluntarily to determine her ability to diagnose pathologic conditions by means of a drop of the patient's blood, to "photograph" soft tissue and to stop hemorrhages.

Before a committee of scientists appointed by the Dean of the Division of Biological Science of the University of Chicago, tests were conducted in December 1947 and January 1950. University officials had been persuaded by prominent Chicagoans that Mrs. Drown was entitled to such an

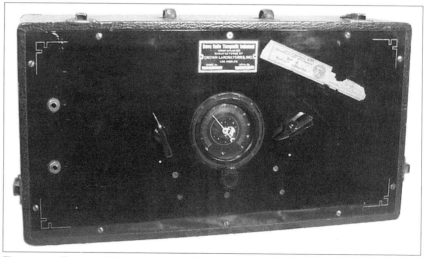

DROWN LONG-DISTANCE MACHINE

The model 300 was the device that Drown used to send healing rays to Tyrone Power and his wife after a car accident in Italy, using samples of their blood from her "library." When they recovered and returned home she sent them a more tangible message—a bill for her services!

Concerning photography of soft tissue, the committee reported:

"The alleged radio photographs: we find that the film images which have intrigued Mrs. Drown and her disciples are simple fog patterns produced by exposure of the film to white light before it has been fixed adequately. These images are significantly identical regardless of whether or not the film is placed in Mrs. Drown's machine before being submitted to the highly unorthodox processing which has been devised by her. In the numerous old films shown to us by Mrs. Drown we can see no resemblance to other anatomical structures, appliances, bacteria, etc., that Mrs. Drown professes to see. In short, it is our opinion that the so-called Drown radio photographs are mere artifacts and totally without clinical value."

As to Mrs. Drown's claimed ability to stop hemorrhage during surgical operations and at other times, the committee reported:

"Hemorrhage control: In the opinion of all observers including herself. Mrs. Drown failed completely to control or modify hemorrhage from the nicked femoral artery of an anesthetized dog."

Mrs. Drown has sold these instruments to chiropractors, osteopaths, naturopaths and some doctors of medicine. She also has sold a portable model for self treatment and has represented that practitioners may give "absent treatments" wherein the patient remains at home. A blotter containing a drop of the patient's blood is kept on file in the practitioner's office. By placement of the blotter in a slot in the machine in the "doctor's" office, the patient

The radio dial implied it could send healing rays worldwide!

is "tuned into the machine" and pathologic conditions are thus treated.

Prior to the investigation by university personnel, it was agreed that blood specimens of ten patients and ten dogs would be furnished to Mrs. Drown for "diagnosis" and she was to be furnished film for the purpose of demonstrating her technic in "soft tissue" photography. Her results on three persons were so erroneous that no attempt was made by her to undertake demonstrations on the other seven. She gave the diagnosis for a tuberculous patient as "a type IV cancer of the left breast with spread to ovaries, uterus, pancreas, gallbladder, spleen and kidney" and warned that the patient was devoid of vision in her right eye and that "the blood pressure was 107/71, the ovaries were not producing ova, and that the following structures showed reduced function: pancreas, adrenal, pituitary, uterus, right ovary, parathyroid, spleen, heart, liver, gall bladder, kidneys, lungs, stomach, spinal nerves, intestines, ears, right eye."

Her diagnosis for a patient having severe hypertension and a bleeding marginal ulcer secondary to gastroenterostomy was "coronary disease with dilated pulmonary veins, diseased heart valves and non functioning gallbladder. Blood pressure 127/80." Actually, it was 218/138 on one occasion, 230/135 on another. Mrs. Drown was not given the sex of this patient, "and she concluded that there was a normal function not only of a uterus but also of a prostate. She reported low function or non function in the following structures; pituitary, pulmonic and tricuspid valves, gallbladder, stomach, spleen, parathyroid, pancreas, kidneys."

Her diagnosis for a healthy young man with normal blood pressure was "an ischiorectal abscess, serious trouble with the prostate, probably carcinoma with spread to urethra, pelvic bones, and with loss or at any rate non function of the left testicle. The blood pressure was reported as being 166/78, and she said that the prognosis was very poor."

The ten samples of blood from laboratory animals reported on by Mrs. Drown followed the same pattern of failure. She reported on six of the ten animals, on four of which she could get no "recording," and reports on the other two were meaningless.

In the hemorrhage "control"

DROWN
HEMORRHAGE
CONTROL

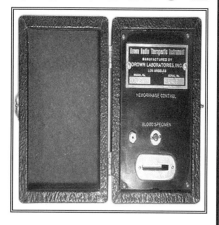

experiment, Mrs. Drown was invited to permit ligature at any time or produce a clotting with her machine. Ligature was demonstrated in the control animal. After she had permitted considerable blood to pour from the test animal, and after her friends had found the sight beyond their capacities, it was reported:

"Eventually she asked that the vessels be ligated and then suggested that instead of hemorrhage

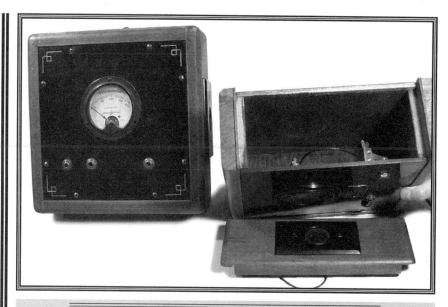

⚜HOMO-VIBRA RAY⚜

The Homo-Vibra Ray was claimed by Mrs. Drown to be the star of her line of devices. It consisted of a series of small boxes wired together. However, when the lid is removed it is empty; there is no power source.

control she now show us how she could bring the dog out of the anesthesia by means of the machine . . ."

In 1934, while trading as the Homo-Vibra Ray Company of Los Angeles, Mrs. Drown wrote to an officer of the American Medical Association in part as follows:

"The Homo-Vibra Ray has been in existence since December 15, 1929. It has been sold to a few doctors only to prove that others could use it as well as the inventor. So far it has been checked conscientiously by every known scientific method used in the healing art.

"We feel it is worthy of a fair investigation by those whose privilege it is to do so for the medical profession and we are now making a formal request of you for this investigation. Should you find this instrument to be scientific, as we know it to be, and it meets with your approval, we wish to

say to you that we would deem it a great privilege to give to the good of the cause a certain percent royalty over a set period of time on each instrument sold, feeling that this money would be utilized for the purpose of assisting humanity, even as we feel our instrument is for that purpose.

"We have not sold this instrument to any particular school of therapy because we realize it is an instrument and not a machine; therefore, being an instrument, it requires the knowledge of the operator to utilize it along with all other known methods, and without this knowledge, the instrument could not be a success.

"We demonstrated it, by request, at the Homeopathic Convention in Chicago, and also at the Eclectic Convention. These people took it upon themselves to investigate us very thoroughly, and they checked our findings with as many as three laboratories on one case.

"It has also been checked by the x-ray, the fluoroscope, and post mortem. We do not consider the Homo-Vibra Ray a panacea nor do we say that we cure people with it, but the diagnosis made with it permits the physician to have better vision of his case and to utilize to the best of his knowledge the therapy in which he is proficient. . .

"This is merely an outline of the things that the Homo-Vibra Ray is capable of determining, and a complete investigation by an open-minded investigator would prove the fact that it is definitely scientific and not hokom (sic) as so often those who do not know will attribute to it."

The reply from the Association was:

"Neither in your letter nor in your advertising matter is there given any scientific support for the claims made for the Homo-Vibra device. Nor do you give information regarding its physical constraints or the electrical hook-up. In other words, the device seems to be surrounded with the secrecy common to all nostrums."

The Bureau's files concerning Mrs. Drown reveal that she has lived in Los Angeles for many years and formerly was employed in the electrical assembly department of the Southern California Edison Company. According to information available to the Bureau of Investigation of the American Medical Association she had become "interested in radio and its possibilities as an aid to physicians in the diagnosis of disease" and attended the School of Osteopathy at Kirksville, Mo. She attended this school for about three years, but did not complete the course, although she is a member of the American Naturopathic Association. She is now a licensed osteopath and commenced her present activities in 1939, conducting a laboratory in which she continued research and developmental work, at the same time offering treatment and care to a small clinic clientele. During 1936 she devoted her efforts toward the developing of radio apparatus used in the diagnosis of human ailments and known by the name of Homo-Vibra Ray. . . .

For the past several years Mrs. Drown has also operated a "college" in Los Angeles, where she professes to teach her unique theories. In a folder called "Bulletin—The Drown College—1948-1949 it is stated that the "college" is "dedicated to the teaching and healing."

Using a Drown machine, she is reported to have given a Tribune reporter the diagnosis of "feverish infection, malaria, undulant fever, afternoon temperatures, weak glands in neck, bad ears, rheumatism, weak bladder, infected pancreas, infected lung (left lobe; right lobe OK), infected liver, possible diabetes, gas on stomach, constipation." The fee for the diagnosis was $35, according to the Tribune reporter, and the osteopath was reported to have given the patient "a sweet motherly smile" and two kinds of medicine. One was a tall bottle of yellow liquid labeled: "One teaspoonful in 1/2 glass of water before meals and or two at bed time." "That's for your feverish infection,"she explained. The other, an enormous package of bilious-green pills, was labeled "One or two at bed time." The reporter was told that these were laxatives; she commented that at that very moment she had been mildly diarrheic for two days.

Mrs. Drown also has been the subject of attention by the Federal Food and Drug Administration. An instrument which she sold to

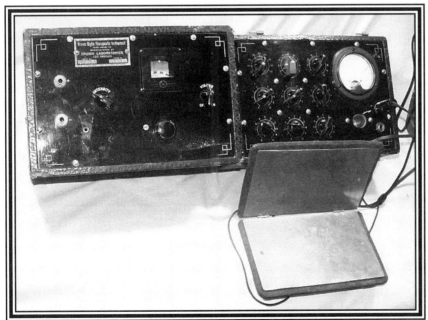

DROWN STANDARD OFFICE MODEL

When the patient's saliva was placed on the detector plate, a small dial on the upper box registered a number to indicate an illness. When the dial under the label on the left device was turned on, healing rays were supposedly sent out from an antenna.

a Chicagoan for home use was the subject of a seizure which ultimately was adjudicated by a default decree of condemnation. The charges were that literature accompanying the device contained false and misleading representations with respect to the therapeutic value of the device.

Mrs. Drown's attempt to capitalize on mechanical gadgetry has been proved for what it and similar pursuits truly are—quackery. Unfortunately, much harm can be done before prospective users realize the harm in such deceptive practices.

Spondylotherapy

Spondylotherapy, a modality of treatment espoused by Dr. Albert Abrams, is defined by

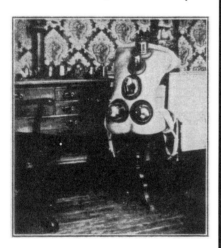

THIS IS SPONDYLOTHERAPY.

"Professor" H. N. D. Parker as "every therapeutic measure when applied to the spine curatively." This definition appears in his 1913 booklet extolling the benefits of Pneumotherapy and offering for sale pneumatic therapeutic devices which relieve human suffering and restore health by "restoring the circulation of the blood and exxential fluids of the body to

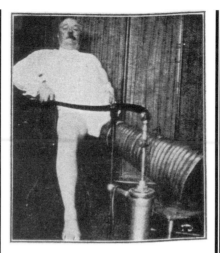

THE LEG RECEIVER IN ACTION.

the disease-weakened organs, tissue and nerve-centers."

This is accomplished by applying cups of various sizes to diseased areas, with particular attention to the spine in cases of diabetes, asthma, indigestion, hemorrhoids, incontinence and prolapse of the womb. Appliances to enclose a whole limb and indeed a cabinet for the whole body are available. Once in place a vacuum is created by a suction pump to improve circulation to the area, thus effecting a return to normal health. As an adjunct to treatment, "effectual elimination and intestinal cleansing" with Epsom salts are recommended. It is also extremely important that drafts be avoided, for "they

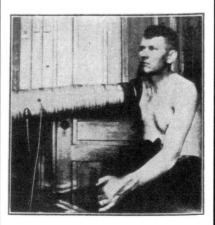

THE ARM RECEIVER IN ACTION.

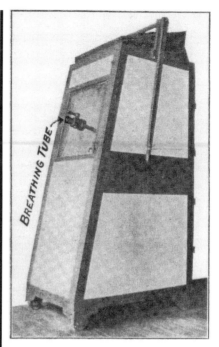

PNEUMATIC THERAPEUTIC CABINET.

who sit with their back to a draft, sit with their face to a coffin." Many of our grandmothers concur with this!

Radionics Devices

The Pathoclast is one member of a large family of 'medical' devices going back to the 1916 oscilloclast of Albert Abrams, M.D. The oscilloclast used the "Electronic Reactions of Abrams" to detect and cancel out the specific vibration rates of various diseases. As well as diseases, Abrams claimed his diagnoses revealed the religion of his patients. He did not offer conversions along with the cures; perhaps the vibrations of faith are made of sterner stuff than those of disease.

In actuality, "faith" may have quite a lot to do with the cures performed with such apparatus. The placebo effect is well-known: if a patient believes the doctor is doing something that will help, often the problem is eased. Such

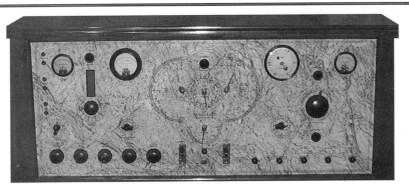

THE PATHOCLAST.

dial both numbered 1-100, plus a slot for a Food Compatible Test; the main panel with the off-on switch, a Diagnosis and Therapy Terminal, and a Diagnosis/Therapy mode switch; and the Diagnostic Pad panel where a thin paper notepad may have rested.

Magic in a Black Box!

Two Black Boxes made by George de la Warr of Oxford,

belief is aided by an impressive treatment—and whatever its actual function, this machine is impressive.

The Pathoclast, manufactured by Pathometric Laboratories of Chicago, is 22 inches long, 9 inches high, and 12 inches deep. It is constructed of wood, leather,

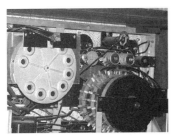

This intriguing jumble of wires and gears is the inside of the pathoclast.

plastic, bakelite, brass, other metals and glass, and contains an open storage compartment for wires, attachments, and notes on the right-hand side of the machine. This opening also held the custom personalized metal labels which included the name of the buyer. The face of the device is divided into five panels: the Pulsoidal Control Unit with one bakelite dial numbered 1-100 and a Pulsoidal Switch; the Pathodyne Diagnostic Unit containing two large bakelite dials numbered 1-100; the Aqua Potentia Unit with a Disease dial and a Potential

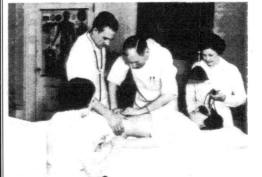
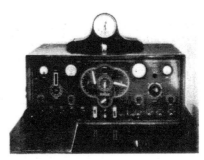

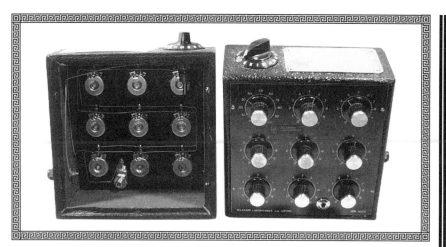

THESE GEORGE DE LA WARR MACHINES FROM OXFORD, ENGLAND, LOOK IMPRESSIVE WITH THE RUBBING PLATES AND KNOBS, BUT THERE IS NO POWER SOURCE AND THE WIRES ARE ONE CONTINUOUS CONNECTION.

England are pictured here. One is an impressive box with 9 dials, a smooth plate for rubbing, and a dial with 18 settings on the top. Removing the back of the other box reveals a meaningless string of wires. It is entertaining to twiddle the dials but it offers no medical cures.

George de la Warr was one of the pioneers in building "Black Boxes." He was a civil engineer, born in 1904 in the north of England. He resigned as assistant to the county engineer of Oxford to devote the rest of his life building "Black Boxes." These boxes work by the same "radionic" principles advocated by Dr. Albert Abrams in the 1920s and later in the 1950s by Dr. Ruth Drown. To the believer they produced amazing results in the areas of horticulture, pest control and medicine. During a demonstration of a similar device in Oxford, de la Warr claimed that he inserted a piece of ordinary photographic film into an opening in the device, and after a few moments removed a picture of his wife and himself on their wedding day . . . 30 years before! He also claimed that by just smearing a photo of a farm field with insecticide and putting it into a black box he could kill insects in that field many miles away! Interestingly, Dr. and Mrs. Crum of Indiana, the inventors of the Coetherator in 1926, made the same claim, except that their device could eradicate insects up to 70 miles away!

Calbro Magnowave Radionics

The Calbro Magnowave device is a beautiful wood cabinet housing a control panel with 26 bakelite dials which each point to a circular scale marked zero-to-ten. The panel contains a "bi-pole control" for treatment or diagnosis. The unusual feature of this device is the inclusion of various colored lights called "Screening Rays" which shine through a hole, "the Emanator," on the right side of the control panel. The oddest feature of this device is a beautifully finished and extremely heavy wood box which sits in the drawer: the box is filled with road tar!

The *Dr. Hooper Drugless Clinic News* (undated) explained how "Calbro Magnowave Radionics" used radio waves to heal:

Radionics is a truly scientific method of diagnosing and treating human ailments. It is the utilization of similar physical phenomena to that which you are using daily in your home, namely, the radio. . . . If you know the wave length or vibratory rate of a given station it is easy for you to tune in said station and determine the nature of its program. . . . Likewise, physicians who are thoroughly versed in the science of radionics know the wave length of all diseases on the radionic instrument, can tune in on them at will and definitely determine the nature of diseased processes in the body.

A radionic examination or diagnosis is made by "tuning in" your body with the master instrument; not by asking you to relate your symptoms. . . . Two wires connect you with the instrument which takes the energy from your body the same as an antenna or aetial is used to bring the vibrations from the air into your radio.

The diagnostician "tunes in" on a host of diseases to ascertain if they are present in your body, their degree of advancement and exact location. All other diagnostic methods of proven merit are used, in conjunction with radionics, to make the findings conclusive.

The radionic treatment is given with the patient lying on a couch. As in the examination, you feel nothing; the treatment being so soothing that many patients fall into a restful sleep.

Two metal plates are placed above and below the diseased part of the body and a vibratory wave of electrical energy is passed through this infected tissue. This vibratory wave is a trifle stronger than the wave emanating from the given infection thus making it impossible for the infection to survive.

Any ailment of an invective

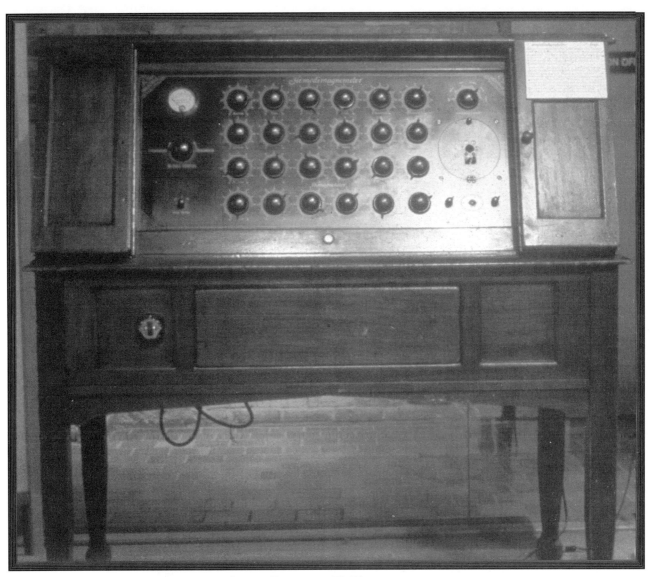

The Calbro Magnowave

This is the predecessor to the Electro Metabograph. It was obviously designed to impress patients.

origin can be successfully treated with Radionics. This means about ninety five per cent of human ills. We will cite a few which have responded favorably to this method:

ARTHRITIS
ASTHMA
APPENDICITIS
ANEMIA
BRONCHITIS
BRIGHT'S DISEASE
CATARRH
CONSTIPATION

CYSTITIS
DIABETES
FLU
GALLSTONES
GALL BLADDER TROUBLE
GOITRE
KIDNEY TROUBLE
NEURITIS
RHEUMATISM
STOMACH TROUBLE
SINUS TROUBLE
ULCERS

Where specifically indicated we employ many other forms of treatment adjunctively to radionics, such as artificial fever, colon irrigations, corrective diet, hygiene, diathermy, ultra violet rays, corrective exercise, etc.

In short, the body has the power within itself to heal; our work is directed toward removing the obstacles in nature's way in order that she may re-establish normalcy.

The Gallert Machine: Radionics Plus Astrology

Mark Gallert combined radionics with astrology and in the 1950s sold his Deluxe Model, a radionics device, for $545. The Gallert machine is about two feet square and uses no alternating current. The device, made out of five painted boards and backed with a thin sheet of plywood, contains fifty four dials. In 1952, Mr. Gallert was visited in San Francisco by an undercover investigator from the California Department of Public Health. The investigator was diagnosed with cancer of the liver, a tumor pressing on the heart, syphilis, and lympho-granuloma. Mr. Gallert was promptly arrested and charged with false advertising, misbranding, practicing medicine without a license, and petty theft. He pleaded guilty and was sentenced to two years probation after his physician testified that his health would suffer from incarceration.

The Harmonizer

The Harmonizer is actually an old-fashioned AM vacuum tube radio encased in a 1960's amplifier case. An amp meter,

The Gallert Machine

Mark Gallert of San Francisco claimed to cure cancer, syphilis, and all other diseases with this machine. He pleaded guilty when charged with fraud after practicing for only 2½ months.

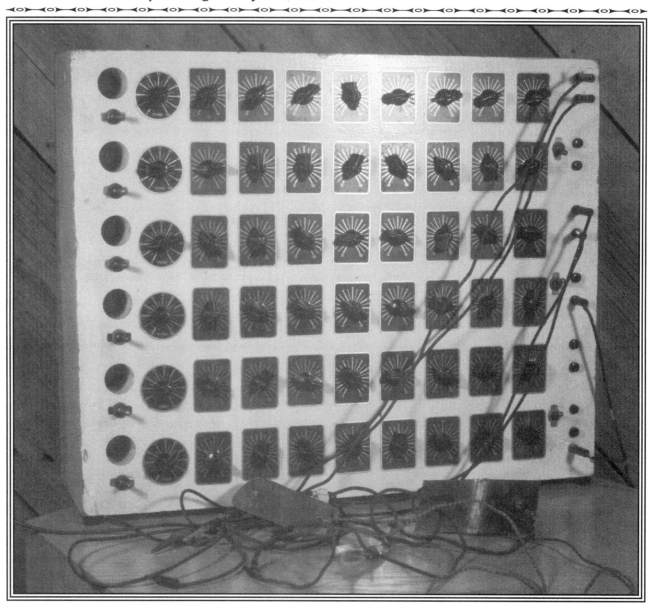

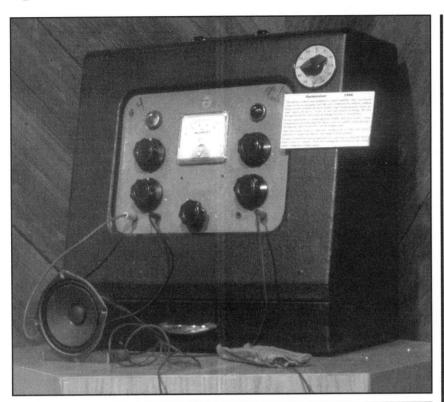

The Harmonizer

The Harmonizer has a radio speaker—indicating that it can both broadcast the ballgame as well as cure cancer!

mounted on the face of the Harmonizer, is connected to the radio volume control. The radio cannot be heard, for there are no speakers. The "patient" is linked to the device by holding a corduroy cotton pad filled with bits of copper wire which are connected to a lead wire. This wire then plugs into a dead connection on the front of the device. When the operator turns on the radio and tunes in a local AM radio station, the needle in the amp meter jumps back and forth, reflecting the volume of the broadcast, and the patient is led to believe that a cure or treatment is taking place.

The T. Galen Hieronymus Machine, 1993

This device is based on the so-called discoveries of Albert

Abrams. Its makers claim that treatment of the Electronic Reactions of Abrams "through this machine, is helping man and beast world-wide."

This device, one of two in the museum seized by Minnesota's Attorney General in 1993, came with instructions for treating humans and animals with radio waves. Pictures, saliva, blood, or

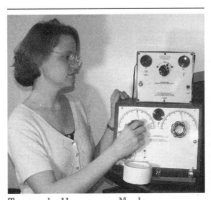

Testing the Hieronymus Machine.

Q tips were put into the various wells in the machine. The patient was not required to be present; a little blood or saliva made diagnosis possible. Besides the standard radionic schemes for making "cures," amazingly there were also such instructions as how to control the weather with the machine.

Would-be weather experimenters are warned that they must register with the National Oceanic and Atmospheric Administration in Boulder, Colorado before beginning any weather changing projects. Having done this they may then proceed, setting the dials to cause such events as rain, either in general or in specific locations, heavy snow or prevention of heavy snow, driving the Jet stream north or other ambitious manipulations of the weather. A disclaimer notes that these are experiments and there is no guarantee of success in every instance. Selling price: $1,500.

The Auto Sweep Resonator Model 526A Sweep III

This device was also seized by Minnesota's Attorney General. Its instructions include a long salute to the great American genius Albert Abrams, which should raise doubts as to the merits of the machine!

This "radionic" device will not only cure all known diseases, but you can also kill insects in a farm field. 1) Obtain photographs of the field that is infested. 2) Place a picture of the field, a bottle of insecticide, plus a dead insect in a plastic bag in a well of the machine. 3) Turn on the power switch to the Resonator. 4) Leave the Resonator on and "sweep" for several hours, repeating the process until the desired results are obtained.

It also has incredible power as a Subliminal Broadcaster: 1) Purchase an affirmation subliminal audio tape that promotes healing at a health food store. 2) Plug the tape recorder into the Resonator and put the antenna up. 3) Put a photograph of the person to be treated into the well and press play on your own recorder. A special feature of the device is that it will convert input energy to digital pulse output automatically. Your subliminal message is broadcast straight to the brain of the person in the photograph to heal him, after first

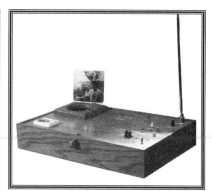

The Auto Sweep Resonator Model 526A Sweep III

When examined at the Mayo Clinic Lab, the verdict was that this device was a jumble of wires, dials, and switches with no scientific basis.

locating and diagnosing him with the AM radio antenna. The Resonator allegedly works on the principle that causes a tuning fork to vibrate in unison with an adjacent tuning fork that is already vibrating.

The so called vibration rate of matter is the underlying principle of radionics. Illnesses cause specific vibration rates which can be treated by the similar vibration rate of radio waves. This device was reported by the Attorney General's office to sell for $1,500.

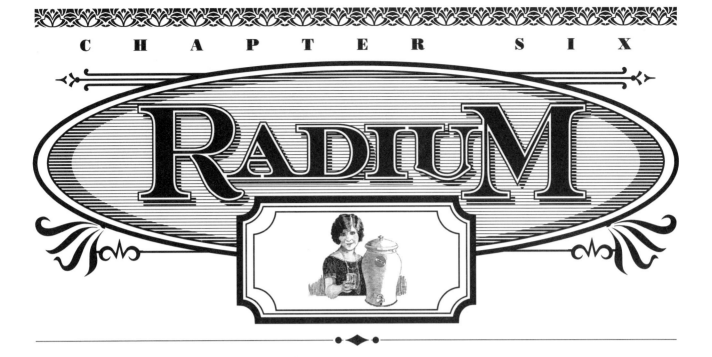

RADIUM

GOOD FOR WHAT AILS YOU.

As the 20th century began, radium was regarded as almost supernatural because of its radioactive, transformative, and healing powers. It glowed in the dark! And soon, so did clock faces. If a little radium could cure cancer, what would a lot do? Radium began appearing everywhere! In bath salts, cold creams, mouth washes, ointments, face powders, healing pads, eye washes, belts, crocks, coins, and bags.

Doctors used it, too. The 1925 standard for radium emanator generators set by the Council on Pharmacy and Chemistry was 2,000 millicuries or more in a 24 hour period. Some of the early AMA criticism of radium quackery was not that products were radioactive, but that the quackery contained too little

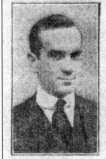

EVERYBODY KNOWS "AL JOLSON"

The Highbrow of Hilarity. He Says:

"I have used your 'Radio-X' Pad for my throat and it has worked wonders. I am singing better than ever.
"Yours very truly,
"AL JOLSON."

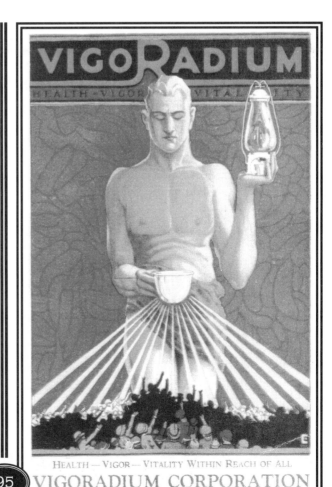

HEALTH — VIGOR — VITALITY WITHIN REACH OF ALL
VIGORADIUM CORPORATION

95

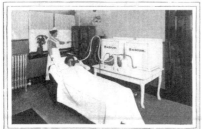

Inhaling radium at John Harvey Kellog's Battle Creek Sanitarium.

radioactivity to be effective! Some doctors also prescribed radium water, gave radium injections, or applied radium topically. John Harvey Kellogg's Battle Creek Sanitarium set aside a room where patients could "inhale" radium. For the consumer, the line between legitimate medicine and quackery was blurred in a new technology many failed to understand. In the U.S., radium was unregulated during the early part of the 20th century despite passage of the 1906 Pure Food and Drug Act, for radium was classified as a natural element, not a drug.

Fortunately for the general public, radium was expensive and most of the quack products which claimed to contain radium had no radioactive ingredients. A 1930 analysis of radium products by the U.S. Food, Drug and Insecticide Administration, then in the U.S. Department of Agriculture, found that 95% were not radioactive. Even so, some hundreds of thousands of items were sold which were radioactive. Of these, the most popular were crocks and jars for making radioactive water at home.

OPPOSITE: One of many brochures over the years touting the imagined medical benefits of sitting in a uranium mine.

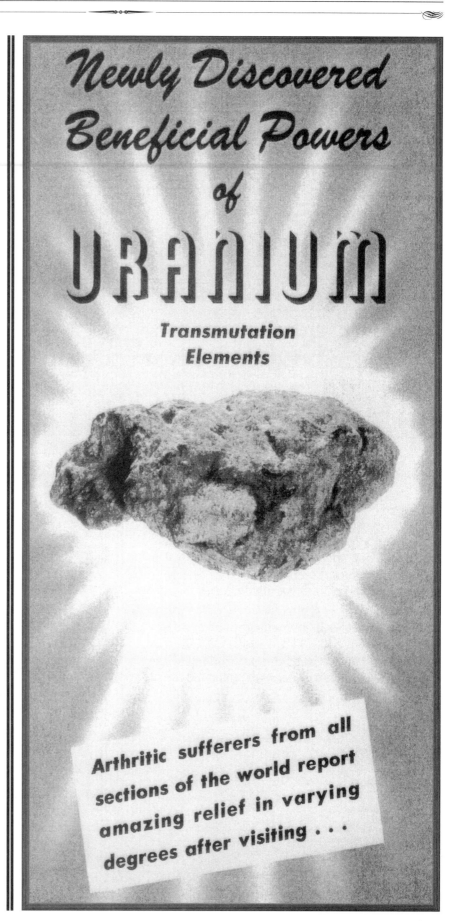

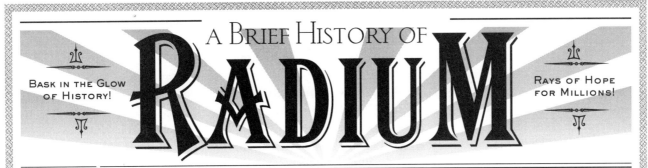

A Brief History of RADIUM

BASK IN THE GLOW OF HISTORY!

RAYS OF HOPE FOR MILLIONS!

During the winter of 1895, two exciting scientific discoveries were made. On November 8, 1895, German physicist William Conrad Roentgen was working in his lab with a cathode ray tube surrounded by black paper. While moving the tube, he noticed that a screen containing barium platinocynid began to fluoresce. He put his hand between the tube and the paper and was able to see the outline of his bones. Unsure of the nature of his discovery, Professor Roentgen called it "X-rays." His discovery would allow physicians to see inside the human body.

LIVE LONG AND PHOSPHER

Professor Antoine Henri Becquerel of France was a third generation physicist, carrying on the work of his father, Alexandre Becquerel, who had studied light and phosphorescence. When Professor Becquerel learned of the discovery of X-rays, he set out to discover if phosphorescent substances might also produce the new rays. He exposed potassium uranyl sulfate, a uranium salt, to sunlight which made it phosphorescent, and then applied it to a photographic plate covered with black paper. The plate, when developed, displayed the image of uranium crystals.

Initially, Professor Becquerel surmised that the uranium absorbed the sun's energy and transmitted it to the plate. But during a couple of cloudy days in late February 1896, he wrapped the uranium salts and stored them in a drawer with a new photographic plate. When he opened the drawer, the photographic plate was fogged. Professor Becquerel recognized that the radium salts were emitting their own rays. He soon proved that the rays were linked to uranium and they were known as Becquerel or uranic rays. These rays would also allow physicians to see inside the body. Henri Becquerel had discovered radioactivity.

Physicist Marie Curie nee Sklodowska was a student in Paris when she chose the accurate measurement of rays emitted from uranium as the topic for her doctoral thesis. She duplicated Becquerel's work and then started studying different grades of uranium. One sample gave off more radiation than would have been expected from uranium. Mme. Curie hypothesized that this was because of an unknown element even more powerful than uranium. She was joined in her work by her husband, Pierre Curie, and in 1898, they discovered the element polonium (named for Mme. Curie's native Poland) and, in collaboration with chemist Gustave Bèmont, radium. In 1903, the Curies and Dr. Becquerel shared the Nobel Prize in physics for their discoveries.

PIERRE CURIE: GIVING HIS LIFE FOR SCIENCEE

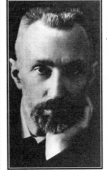

Pierre Curie decided to test radium on humans with himself as the subject. He bound radium salts to his arm for 10 hours and the resulting burn and wound took almost two months to heal. A permanent scar remained.

Curie died in an accident in 1906. However, years before his death he showed symptoms of radiation poisoning including weight loss, trembling hands and legs, constant pain, and chronic fatigue.

Physicist Ernest Rutherford and chemist Frederick Soddy at McGill University in Montreal published the theory of radioactive transformation of elements in 1901 which explained why the Curies found polonium and radium in uranium ore. Uranium is constantly decomposing, going through seven stages until it becomes lead. Radium is the fifth stage before polonium, and its daughter is the gas radon. By this time, Pierre Curie was collaborating with medical doctors studying medical applications for radium.

The major medical application they discovered was the treatment of cancerous tumors with small amounts of radium or radon. Radium destroys human cells and cancer cells are more vulnerable than healthy cells. Needles or tubes were inserted or applied to affected organs. Seeds, or small capsules, containing radon were inserted during surgery and left in place as the half life of radon is four days. Treating cancer with radium or radon became known as the "Curie treatment."

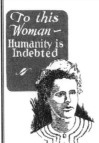

The Radium Ore Revigator

The Revigator is typical of the radium water devices popular in the U.S. during the early decades of the twentieth century. Patented in 1912, it may be the earliest such device made in the U.S. Between 1912 and 1930, there were three models of Radium Ore Revigators. The first was a six quart pottery crock in earth tone. In the mid-1920s, the shape remained the same but the glaze was changed to green/blue. The final model, circa 1929, was white-porcelain, held two gallons of water, and sold for $29.50.

Revigator interiors were porous, for the crocks were lined with radioactive ore which emitted radon. The radioactivity of water stored in the crocks was a few hundred to a few hundred thousand picocuries per liter. The concentration of radium-226

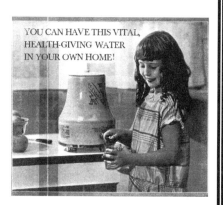

YOU CAN HAVE THIS VITAL, HEALTH-GIVING WATER IN YOUR OWN HOME!

in water left in a Revigator overnight was about five times as strong as the maximum recommended for well water today.

The radioactive water dispensers were legitimized, in part, by famous health spas and springs. As the radium craze spread through Europe and the U.S., spa operators had their water tested and many found radioactivity. The curative powers of the waters, then, was ascribed to "radium

emanation." World War I intervened and wealthy Americans could no longer visit European spas like Carlsbad, Baden-Baden, and Wiesbaden.

A 1914 newspaper article quoted U.S. Surgeon General

RADIOACTIVE JOURNALISM: This article was used by the manufacturer of the Revigator to promote the sale of radioactive water.

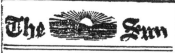

The Sun

MONDAY, SEPTEMBER 7, 1914.

RADIUM BATHS MAY SUPPLANT FOREIGN SPAS

Americans Needn't Worry Over Taking the Cure, Says Surgeon-General Blue.

WASHINGTON, Sept. 6.—Radium rays emanating through the medium of ordinary American spring water may take the place of the famous European spas which have been closed to American patients by the war in Europe. This opinion, expressed here to-day by Surgeon-General Rupert Blue, head of the United States Public Health Service, suggests another use for this rare element.

Commenting on the closing of the German and other spas, upon which so many Americans feel themselves absolutely dependent, Dr. Blue said:

"There is really no occasion for uneasiness about the closing of the baths abroad. In the first place we have springs in this country that possess amazing curative properties. In the case of patients suffering from ailments that respond to treatment by radium it will be a simple matter to charge pure water with radium and use it for drinking, inhaling or bathing purposes."

The spas to which Dr. Blue has reference and upon which persons of means in this country have been relying are at Carlsbad, Baden-Baden, Nauheim, Gastein, Wiesbaden and Pistyan. They are very popular with American victims of rheumatism and gout. Entrance to the famous watering places, however, has been cut off by the war and it is unlikely that they will be reopened until peace is restored to Europe.

The fame of these springs is centuries old, but it is of comparatively recent date that their curative properties have been found to depend upon radium emanations. The discovery of radium by Mme. Curie and the subsequent demonstration of its wonderful physical properties gave rise to the theory that what had been known as the "spirit of the springs" might claim this almost supernatural substance as its origin.

Careful investigation changed this theory into a fact and led to the perfection of mechanism whereby one billionth of a milligram of radium emanation can be recognized and measured.

Because of these facts it is pointed out here by Government scientists, and in view of the situation in Europe it is possible that artificial baths in the United States will supplant the European spas.

Rupert Blue on this event: "There is really no occasion for uneasiness about the closing of the baths abroad. In the first place we have springs in this county that possess amazing curative properties. In the case of patients suffering from ailments that respond to treatment by radium it will be a simple matter to charge pure water with radium and use it for drinking, inhaling or bathing purposes."

The purveyors of radium water cures were also promoted in the popular press. In the 1915 article "Radium Facts," the *Saturday Evening Post* reported:

"American research work has indicated that when radium water is taken as a medicine it works its way through the entire body, and proceeds to accomplish effects quite different from those of the application of a little tube of radium imbedded in a cancerous growth. The particular value of the radium scattered through the body is yet subject to a great amount of study; but it now seems to rouse all the cells of the body to greater activity—a sort of tonic for them all. In no one disease is this internal use of radium entitled to the word cure, but in a score of diseases—such as rheumatism, gout, anæmia, and neuralgia—the increased cell activity is often helpful.

"A report just issued by the Radium Institute of London on similar experimental work shows that radium water has given surprisingly good results in many cases of the terrible disease of arthritis deformans . . .

"The latest research has indicated that much stronger doses of this radium-absorbing water are advisable than had at first been expected . . . Heavy doses

continued on page 102

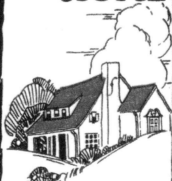
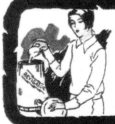
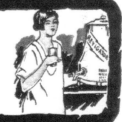

A GALLERY OF
RADIUM WATER DISPENSERS
FOR YOUR PERSONAL PERUSAL.

The RADIUM VITALIZER

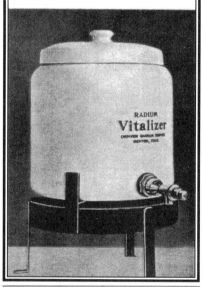

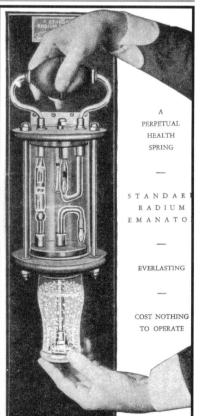

A
PERPETUAL
HEALTH
SPRING

—

STANDARD
RADIUM
EMANATO

—

EVERLASTING

—

COST NOTHING
TO OPERATE

FOR BANKS, OFFICES AND BUSINESS
INSTITUTIONS

Further information on request

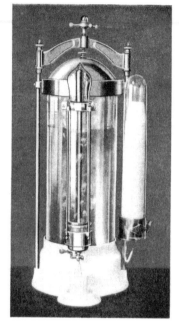

VIGORADIUM
"Truly Graces Business Places"

"For Your Health's Sake"

"Lifetime"
RADIUM WATER JAR

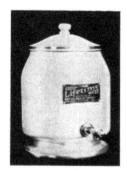

**THREE BEAUTIFUL FINISHES
IN PURE ALUMINUM**

—

**INDESTRUCTIBLE
ORNAMENTAL**

—

**INVALUABLE IN HEALTH
MAINTENANCE**

Distributed throughout the
UNITED STATES, MEXICO AND CANADA
by accredited representatives.

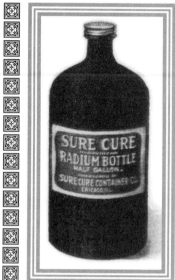

SURE CURE RADIUM BOTTLE

THE
Radioak
α β γ

U. S. TRADE MARK REG.

GENERATOR
for *RADIANT* Health.

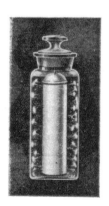

RADIUM CHARGED
WATER

Lasts a Life Time   *First Cost Is All*

RADIOAK DISTRIBUTORS
Suite 306-7, Physicians' Bldg.,
1225 Washington St.
Phone Lakeside 2127   Oakland, Calif.

RADIOAK LABORATORIES
678 Twenty-second Street
Oakland, California, U. S. A.
Telephone Oakland 1694

A GALLERY OF
RADIUM WATER DISPENSERS
FOR YOUR PERSONAL PERUSAL.

Health Fountain

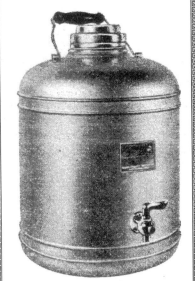

(Patent Pending)

PRICE $35.00

OUR SLOGAN

"A HEALTH FOUNTAIN IN EACH AND EVERY HOME"

MANUFACTURED BY

RADIUM-HEALTH

CORPORATION

WOOSTER, OHIO

U. S. A.

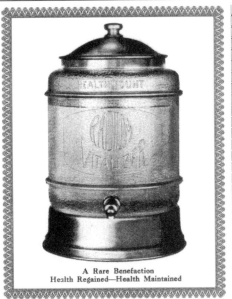

A Rare Benefaction
Health Regained—Health Maintained

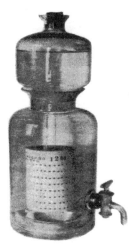

MANUFACTURED BY

DENVER RADIUM SERVICE

DENVER, COLORADO

RADIUM APPARATUS.

DOSAGE.

(1,000 to 10,000 Mache Units) per day.

Continuous activity at full measured strength guaranteed for a minimum of ten years.

NOTICE.

WE SUPPLY OUR APPARATUS ONLY UPON RECEIPT OF COMPLETE DIAGNOSIS MADE BY A QUALIFIED PHYSICIAN ON OUR DIAGNOSIS BLANK, AND RECOMMEND THAT THE TREATMENT BE TAKEN ONLY UNDER THE PHYSICIAN'S SUPERVISION.

PRICE LIST.

STRENGTH APPARATUS MACHÉ UNITS PER DAY.	
1,000	$85.00
2,500	165.00
5,000	265.00
10,000	550.00

TERMS.

NET CASH—NEW YORK FUNDS.

Clean receipt from express company constitutes delivery. The apparatus will be carefully packed for shipment and all claims for damage must be made upon the carrier. Damaged parts will be replaced at proportionate cost of apparatus. Full instructions for putting apparatus in operation will be sent with each shipment.

INTERNATIONAL RADIUM CORPORATION

220-224 West Forty Second Street,

New York, N. Y., U. S. A.

CABLE ADDRESS—"ACTIVATOR, NEWYORK."

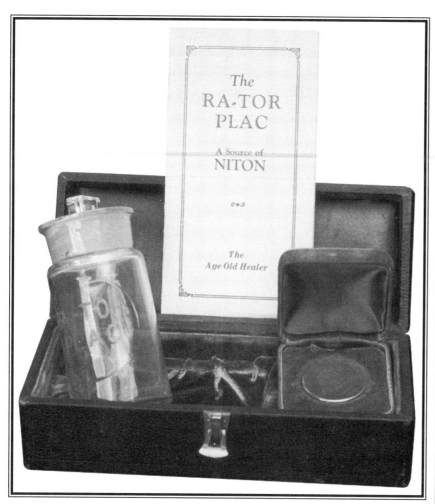

The Ra-tor Plac.

One of a number of radium water cures, the Ra-tor Plac is the "hottest" item in the museum's collection. Its rays were used to make radioactive water.

of strongly impregnated water have not yet been found to be harmful, though the limit of a prudent dose has been fixed."

This was the information available to the public, which still tended to confuse X-rays and "radium emanation," when the Revigator entered the market-place. Over the next 15 years, the Radium Revigator Ore Company would have dozens of competitors. Even so, by 1927, the company claimed to have sold hundreds of thousands of devices. The radium water fad lasted until the early 1930s when one of the Revigator's competitors, W. J. A. Bailey of East Orange, New Jersey, was a little too successful: he sold so much pre-mixed radium water that his "cure" killed a prestigious patient.

W.J.A. Bailey

William John Aloysius Bailey was born in Boston on May 25, 1884. Like the famous Kansas quack, Doc Brinkley, Mr. Bailey lost his father at a young age and grew up in poverty. A bright young man, Mr. Bailey gained entrance to the prestigious Boston Public Grammar School where he graduated 12th in his class. He entered Harvard in 1903; finances forced him to drop out of college after two years of study. Despite his dropout status, he later claimed to have not only a bachelor's degree from Harvard, but a doctorate from the University of Vienna as well.

W.J.A. Bailey's talent as a con man, and he truly was a great con man, surfaced in 1915. With two associates, he operated the Carnegie Engineering Corporation—a corporate name that falsely implied a relationship with the Carnegie Steel Corporation. Carnegie Engineering sold automobiles for $600 by mail order with a requirement of a $50 advance deposit. Mr. Bailey and his associates accepted 1,500 advance deposits. Their Kalamazoo Michigan factory, an abandoned sawmill, was incapable of producing cars. On September 15, 1915, the Postmaster General issued a fraud order against Carnegie Engineering Corporation and that December, Mr. Bailey was convicted of swindling and sentenced to 30 days in jail.

Mr. Bailey managed to stay out of trouble until 1918 when he

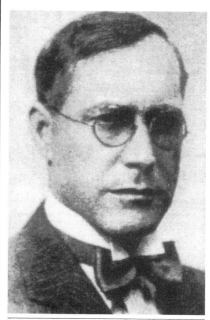

William Bailey.

The Radium Ore Revigator An Aid to Better Health

THE Radium Ore REVIGATOR is designed primarily for homes and offices to revitalize or revigorate drinking water. The REVIGATOR accomplishes this by restoring radio-activity or Natural Niton, an element lost from most drinking water by standing in reservoirs and bottles.

The REVIGATOR, by restoring this lost health element, provides the best drinking water possible for the daily use of the home. The health value of this water in the home is shown by the remarkable results obtained by the sick and afflicted, among whom its use has become very general. The value of radio-activity or radium emanation is so well established from a health standpoint that we publish the following statistical data of over 10,000 cases reported by various authorities as treated with radio-active emanation in various strengths. (This does not include such common conditions as constipation, indigestion, stomach disorders, various skin diseases, and general run-down feeling, as in practically every case of this nature marked benefits are reported).

	Cases Treated	Reported "Cured"	Reported "Benefited"	Reported "Not benefited"
Anemia	111	71	40	0
Asthma	37	..	31	6
Stiff Joints	52	30	21	1
Hardening of Arteries and High Blood Pressure	399	70	316	13
Arthritis	2371	1134	785	452
Apoplexy	81	....	70	11
Bronchitis	200	104	58	38
Inflammation of Bladder	21	11	....	10
Diabetes	395	162	147	86
Eczema	59	22	15	22
Condition of weakness after Influenza and other diseases	479	328	79	72
Inflammation of Stomach and Bowels	41	8	26	7
Inflammation of Sinus	221	110	101	10
Gout	608	128	418	62
Laryngitis	12	....	11	1
Lumbago	221	112	86	23
Inflammation of Uterus	312	45	167	100
Inflammation of Spinal Cord	14	....	11	3
Sick headaches	28	9	17	2
Inflammation of Heart Muscles	181	....	168	13
Bright's Disease	242	....	200	42
Neuralgia and Neuritis	372	153	181	38
Nervous Prostration	387	225	145	17
Peritonitis	34	22	11	1
Polyarthritis	638	316	249	73
Pyorrhoea	98	55	43	0
Skin Diseases	33	4	22	7
Rheumatism	1487	703	634	150
Hay Fever	58	39	8	11
Sciatica	483	292	130	61
Synovitis	77	39	21	17
Locomotor Ataxia	45	2	27	16
Old Age with symptoms of disease	214	....	188	26
TOTALS	10011	4194	4426	1391

RADIUM ORE REVIGATOR CO.
Pacific Coast Branch
260 California St., San Francisco

RADIUM
—A LIST OF CURES.

Radium water cures were promoted for the treatment of: Abnormal blood pressure, Acute bronchitis, Acute gout, Acute sinusitis, Anemia, Ankylosis, Apoplexy, Arterio-sclerosis, Arthritis, Auto-intoxication, Bright's Disease, Bronchial asthma, Chronic bronchitis, Chronic cystitis, Chronic metritis, Conditions of weakness after influenza and other diseases, Constipation, Diabetes, Eczema, Eye Trouble, Gastroenteritis, Glycosuria, Gout, Hay fever, Headaches, High blood pressure, Inflammation of the Bladder, Inflammation of the Heart, Inflammation of Sinus, Inflammation of Spinal Cord, Inflammation of Stomach and Bowels, Inflammation of the Uterus, Laryngitis, Locomotor ataxia, Lumbago, Myocarditis, Nephritis, Nervous prostration, Neuralgia, Neuritis, Neurasthenia, Old age without symptoms of disease, Old age with symptoms of disease, Ozena, Parametritis, Peritonitis, Polyarthritis, Pneumonia, Poluria, Post-operative deformities, Psoriasis, Pyorrhea alveolaris, Rejuvenation, Rheumatism, Sciatica, Scleroderma, Sinusitis, Skin disease, Stiff Joints, Stomach Trouble, Synovitis, Tabes Dorsalis, Typhoid, Weak Kidneys, and Weight Loss.

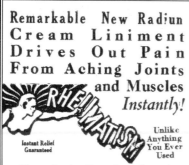

Remarkable New Radium Cream Liniment Drives Out Pain From Aching Joints and Muscles *Instantly!*

Unlike Anything You Ever Used

Instant Relief Guaranteed

Thousands of sufferers from rheumatism, neuritis, neuralgia, lumbago, sciatica and gout are daily obtaining almost unheard of benefits from LINARIUM, the new radium liniment.

No matter how bad your case may be nor how many things you have tried, this radium method is guaranteed to show astonishing results where everything else has failed, even in advanced, stubborn and seemingly hopeless cases.

The moment you apply LINARIUM it penetrates down to the very seat of the trouble, driving out inflammation and giving soothing, comforting relief almost instantly. Possessing a healing power unlike anything else known, the radium content of LINARIUM acts in a definite and marvelous way to relieve congestion, quickly stimulate the aching tissues and renew their normal suppleness and activity. Stainless, greaseless. No rubbing or friction necessary—simply apply and LINARIUM ACTS.

One man writes he would not be without LINARIUM if it cost even ten times as much.

Another says: "To apply LINARIUM is like getting the healing rays of the Sun directly on the spot that pains."

A lady writes: "I find LINARIUM far superior to any direct application I ever used for the quick relief of pain—Helped me almost immediately and brought ease and activity of the muscles."

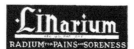

Linarium
RADIUM for PAINS and SORENESS

---

was fined $200 for selling Las-I-Go—an impotence cure containing strychnine for Superb Manhood. With Las-I-Go, Mr. Bailey discovered that sex sells, and as the Roaring Twenties began, he combined sex with the national fascination about radium.

His first radium concern was Associated Radium Chemists, Inc. of New York City. Associated Chemists promoted several radium cures, including Dax for coughs, Clax for the flu, and Linarium, a radioactive liniment. The corporation's major product was Arium, a radioactive aphrodisiac in tablet form. Arium advertising promised

---

to bring "renewed happiness and youthful thrill into the lives of married people whose attraction to each other had weakened and waned…" The company appeared to be pro-consumer for it offered a $5,000 guarantee! The guarantee simply warranted that radium was used "in the preparation of" Associated Radium Chemists' products. The U.S. Department of Agriculture judged the claims

---

FOUR EXAMPLES of outrageous radium ads. The Pure Food & Drug Act of 1906 outlawed patent medicines with poisons, but ignored radium because it was "natural."

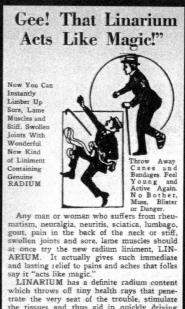

Gee! That Linarium Acts Like Magic!"

Now You Can Instantly Limber Up Sore, Lame Muscles and Stiff, Swollen Joints With Wonderful New Kind of Liniment Containing Genuine RADIUM

Throw Away Canes and Bandages. Feel Young and Active Again. No Bother, Muss, Blister or Danger.

Any man or woman who suffers from rheumatism, neuralgia, neuritis, sciatica, lumbago, gout, pain in the back of the neck or stiff, swollen joints and sore, lame muscles should at once try the new radium liniment, LINARIUM. It actually gives such immediate and lasting relief to pains and aches that folks say it "acts like magic."

LINARIUM has a definite radium content which throws off tiny health rays that penetrate the very seat of the trouble, stimulate the tissues and thus aid in quickly driving away inflamed conditions.

The use of LINARIUM as an external application for instant relief of pain is especially valuable while you are taking ARIUM internally. The combined radium action produces marvelously successful and entirely lasting results. Countless letters of praise are on file from both physicians and laymen. Satisfactory Results Guaranteed or Money Back. Fill in Coupon below NOW and have LINARIUM on hand for the first twinge of pain.

SPECIAL OFFER COUPON
Associated Radium Chemists, Inc.,
461 Eighth Ave., New York, N. Y.
Gentlemen:—Send me four $1.10 Packages of LINARIUM at special price of only $3.00 ( ). Or, one package for $1.00 ( ).
I will pay postman on delivery plus few cents postage ....( ). Or,
I enclose $.............................( ).
Name ....
Street ....
Town .... State ....

For Sure Results Have FAITH

You CAN Be Strong, Well and Full of "Pep"

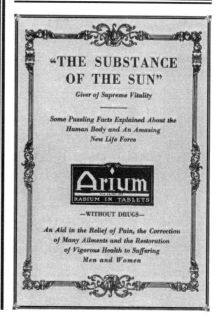

Take ARIUM KNOWING that it is going to help you. Have FAITH that pains are GOING — that new VITALITY is BUILDING itself within you—in your Blood, Glands, Organs, Nerves, Tissues and every fibre of your body. FAITH depends upon *reasoning* and here are the grounds for it. In the circular "Amazing Testimony of Physicians and Users," you have read of the *startling results* ARIUM has produced for others in such a great variety of stubborn ailments, weakened conditions and lack of "SEX FORCE." These statements are voluntarily made. It is just as certain, in our opinion, that this marvelous radium action should be equally beneficial to you.

Do not be anxious about what ARIUM is doing, continually scanning yourself every moment for signs of improvement. *Farmers do not turn over the dirt every morning to see if the seed is growing. Once sown a progressive action takes place until the green blade appears.* ARIUM works from day to day to banish every alarming symptom. It has been explained to you that the radium action is a *progressive* one. It is for this reason that each succeeding box of ARIUM makes more apparent in the way you *act, look and feel*, the completely successful and lasting results you desire.

"THE SUBSTANCE OF THE SUN"

Giver of Supreme Vitality

Some Puzzling Facts Explained About the Human Body and An Amazing New Life Force

Arium
RADIUM IN TABLETS

—WITHOUT DRUGS—

An Aid in the Relief of Pain, the Correction of Many Ailments and the Restoration of Vigorous Health to Suffering Men and Women

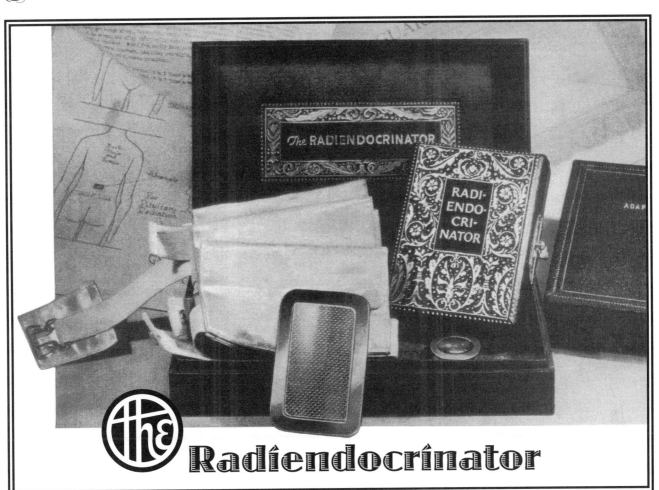

The Radiendocrinator

for Arium to be false and fraudulent and the product was ordered destroyed.

After Arium was pulled off the market, Mr. Bailey sold Thorone, which was advertised as "250 times more active than radium." With Thorone, Mr. Bailey graduated to "cure-alls" as Thorone was promoted for all glandular, metabolism, and faulty chemistry conditions. However, Thorone was marketed primarily as a cure for impotence.

In the late 1920s, Mr. Bailey entered into partnership with Ward Leathers and founded American Endocrine Laboratories in New York City. This firm was also associated with two other quacks, Dr. Herman H. Rubin and Dr. C. Everett Field. American Endo-

crine Laboratories manufactured the elegant and upscale Radiendocrinator, a device akin to the fountain of youth according to Mr. Bailey.

In a 1924 address to the Division of Medicinal Products of the American Chemical Society, "Dr." Bailey argued: "I am satisfied, from definite clinical experience with the radiendocrinator that a method of [endocrine] ionization is now available whereby we can definitely, practically without exception, retard the progress of senescence and give a new lease of relatively normal functioning power to those whose sun of life is slowly sinking into the purple shadows of that longest night . . . .

"The wrinkled face, the drawn skin, the dull eye, the listless gait,

the faulty memory, the aching body, the destructive effects of sterility, all spell imperfect endocrine performance. So definite are the external evidences as indicators of the endocrines' functioning that we have worked out a chart which enables a very accurate diagnosis of endocrine disfunctioning to be arrived at, although this endocrine 'picture' be separated by an ocean or a continent from the patient."

The product itself was simple: two pads, two inches tall by three inches wide and three-eighths of an inch thick, were attached to the body by a belt called an "adaptor." The pads were "charged with pure radium, carefully and perfectly screened to avoid every possible alpha ray (burning rays),

"Scientific Rejuvenation" Demonstrated

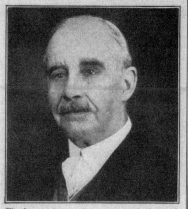

The lower picture shows a man of advanced years—unfit for further usefulness—sinking toward the end. The specialist's diagnosis showed high blood pressure, arteriosclerosis, severe kidney complication, stomach dysfunction, rheumatism of muscles and joints, prostatitis, nerve exhaustion, mental senility, impotency. Years were spent in search of health and lost energies in Europe and America without result.

The upper picture shows the same man after a couple of months of gamma ray treatment for rejuvenation—now a strong, upstanding, successful New York business man at the high-point of his life's energies. He now passes for a man thirty years younger than his actual age.

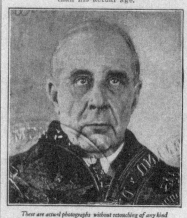

These are actual photographs without retouching of any kind

A FLYER SHOWING BEFORE AND AFTER PICTURES OF HOW THE RADIENDOCRINATOR WORKS. THE REVERSE SIDE ASKS YOUNG AND OLD TO SEND A CARD TO FIND OUT HOW GAMMA-RAYS WILL MAKE ONE YOUNGER.

and then the gamma ray is amplified by the use of mesotharium and actinium, elements rarer and in some cases much more expensive than pure radium."

The Radiendocrinator pads were worn over the thyroid, adrenals or ovaries, pituitary and prostate glands. Treatments of ten-to-thirty minutes were some-times recommended as often as three or four times a day, and overnight treatment of the "gonads" was suggested. The pads were advertised to work by causing ionization of the endocrine system, thereby increasing hormone production. Or, for the lower-tech audience, the pads were effective at "lighting up dark recesses of the body." The result, according to American Endocrine Laboratories, was rejuvenation with results guaranteed in 30 days! The AMA Bureau of Investigation called the Radiendocrinator "high-priced Hokum" appealing "particularly to wealthy neurotics interested in 'sexual rejuvenation'."

The belt or adaptor, constructed of white satin and silk elastic, contained a pocket to hold a Radiendocrinator pad. Metal parts of the belt were "heavily gold-plated in order to avoid corrosion, for in the presence of these powerful rays practically any metal corrodes rapidly." The Radiendocrinator was sold with an instruction manual and a "Radiendocrine Chart"—a diagnostic tool which could be used by doctor or patient!

The most interesting accessory in the Radiendocrinator kit was The Ray Chest, the box storing the radioactive pads. The Chest was described in detail in a 1929 advertisement:

"It is invisibly lined with lead, the most ray-resistive element known. Lead is used to impede the flow of penetrating rays constantly emitting from the instruments.

"The Chest is covered with African Morocco leather (navy blue), engrossed [sic] outside and inside. It is lined with fine French velvet (navy blue). All metal parts of both the chest and instruments are gold-covered to avoid corrosion.

"One of the secondary objects of the protective chest is to avoid the destruction by the escaping rays of all unexposed photo or negative of paper which comes within fifty feet of the instruments, regardless of intervening walls or objects."

Despite its alleged propensity for destroying film and corroding metal, the Radiendocrinator was advertised as harmless. It may have been: during the 1930s, postal authorities had the device tested and found it had "a gamma radiation equivalent to 0.21 milligrams of radium in radioactive equilibrium" or about "1/250th of the dose experts considered effective for medical purposes."

The Radiendocrinator originally sold for $1,000. Not long after the 1929 stock market crash, the price fell to $500. In the early 1930s, as radium cures came under attack, the price was again reduced to $150. Postal authorities estimated the manufacturing cost of the product at $28. American Endocrine Laboratories realized $200,000 in sales with $50,000 earned in one year. The company shut down in the early 1930s rather than face fraud charges from the postal authorities.

By the late 1920s, W. J. A. Bailey had gained enough success and savvy to use sophisticated marketing techniques. Registered physicians throughout the U.S. received a direct mail promotion for Radithor and doctors were promised a 17% commission on Radithor sales, a practiced exposed and denounced by the AMA Investigative Bureau. At least one associate with bona fide medical credentials published a supportive article in a mainstream medical journal; post-publication inquiries were then routed to

Radium's Gamma Rays Sought as Fountain of Youth

London's "Discovery," However, that Rejuvenating Gas Can Be Captured and Put in Tiny Phials Is Not News to U. S., Says Dr. William J. A. Bailey, Expert in Radioactivity.

By Margery Rex

"Gimme a gamma" is the cry of prematurely old humanity in search of rejuvenation. Emory Buckner can never padlock Ponce de Leon's jazz fountain of youth, at least not as long as radium maintains its own private white light district.

Alpha, Beta and Gamma, sound like a hotel wrecking fraternity dance. But when they serve as the Christian names of various forms of radium rays, the sorority of youth-seekers know the schoolgirl complexion is being paged and will readily answer. Each of the sorority will demand science's spotlight as well as the male thing of beauty who would be a boy forever.

Middlesex Hospital, London, gives out the "news" that an important discovery has been made which "will simplify the whole technique of treating disease by radium." The London institution says radium gas called "radon" can be captured, put in little glass bottles the size of a Boston or lima, but not string, bean and sent anywhere on receipt of your name, address and ten cents in stamps—or something like that.

NO LONGER NEWS.

But is this "news?" Not at all, declares Dr. William J. A. Bailey, known as consultant to the medical profession on radioactivity and endocrinology. Says Dr. Bailey:

"Twenty-two years ago that would have been news but not to-day."

At his office and laboratory, No. 323 Riverside Drive, Dr. Bailey showed us little radium "seeds" which proved to be much smaller than the "beans" described in cable despatches

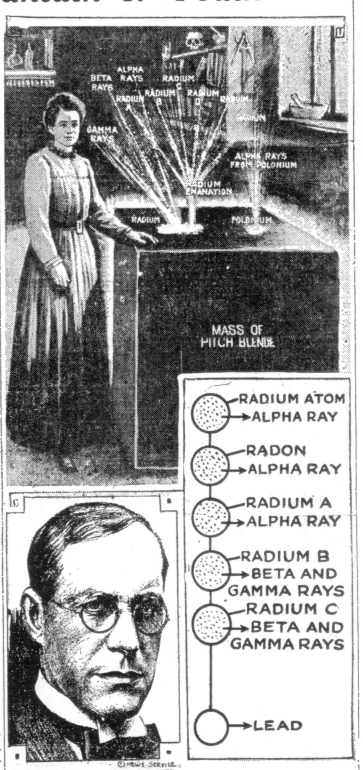

MASS OF PITCH BLENDE

RADIUM ATOM → ALPHA RAY

RADON → ALPHA RAY

RADIUM A → ALPHA RAY

RADIUM B → BETA AND GAMMA RAYS

RADIUM C → BETA AND GAMMA RAYS

→ LEAD

DR. WILLIAM J. A. BAILEY. RADIUM AND ITS RAYS.

Bailey's company. After the article appeared, an enraged physician complained to the AMA:

"I wrote J. Coleman Scal, M.D., of New York, in re to his article on the Treatment of Diseased Tonsils by means of Radium. I was referred to Radium Emanation Corp. of New York, from whom I have received literature. Promptly, I received literature from Bailey Radium Laboratories of East Orange, N.J., as to the value of Radithor. I smelled a 'rat,' put two & two together & have found its 'nest.' All of the rats are of the same breed, & connected, let me tell you. Muir, Bailey, and Dr. Scal must be in [cahoots] . . . What the hell the Editors of the Journal of Otolaryngology mean by letting one of that clique put one over on them, I don't know . . ."

In 1925, W. J. A. Bailey founded Bailey Radium Laboratories in East Orange, New Jersey. Bailey Radium Laboratories produced Radithor, Mr. Bailey's best-known and most notorious quack radium cure. Radithor was premixed radium water packaged in a squat ugly brown bottle stopped with a cork. The nostrum sold for a $1 a bottle with a case of 30 bottles, a one month supply, considered a minimum order. Production costs were estimated to have been 25¢ a bottle which made Radithor a very profitable product.

In 1989, scientist Roger Macklis M.D. discovered five bottles of Radithor at a medical antiques shop. He bought one bottle, tested it, and published his findings in "The Great Radium Scandal" (*Scientific American*, August 1993):

"Because my laboratory research centers on treating cancer with biologically targeted radioactive compounds, I knew it was possible to make water temporarily radioactive by incubating it with radium. The radium gives off radon, a radioactive gas whose half-life is short. I assumed that the maker of the patent medicine had resorted to this very inexpensive process and that Radithor's residual activity had decayed to insignificance long ago.

These three bottles of Radithor were given to the museum a few years ago. They are empty but still register a moderate signal on a Geiger counter.

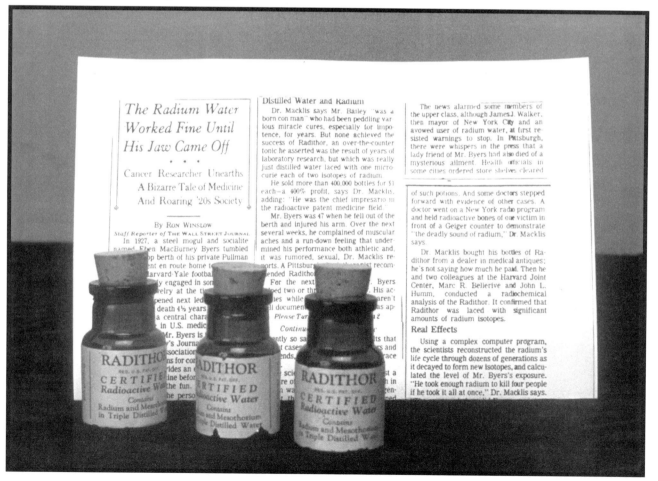

"I was wrong. Tests performed by my colleagues John L. Humm and Marc R. Bellrine in our gamma-ray spectroscopy unit at the Dana-Farber Cancer Institute in Boston revealed that almost 70 years after it had been produced, the nearly empty bottle [of Radithor] was dangerously radioactive. We estimated that the original bottle must have contained approximately one microcurie each of radium 226 and radium 228."

Radithor was alleged to cure 160 diseases and conditions though, in the Bailey tradition, sexual rejuvenation was touted.

W.J.A. Bailey mocked up a full page story-cum-advertisement about Radithor, "Science to Cure the Living Dead," and distributed it to newspapers hoping they would run the story as straight news. Some did. The "Living Dead" was a euphemism for the mentally ill; the story implied that Radithor would cure mental illness and empty the

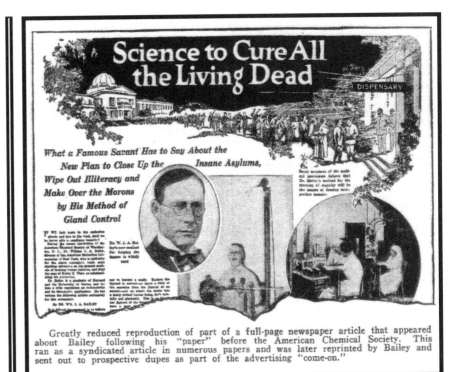

Greatly reduced reproduction of part of a full-page newspaper article that appeared about Bailey following his "paper" before the American Chemical Society. This ran as a syndicated article in numerous papers and was later reprinted by Bailey and sent out to prospective dupes as part of the advertising "come-on."

insane asylums.

Mr. Bailey's marketing strategies worked. Legitimate doctors did recommend Bailey products. Between 1925 and 1930, Bailey Radium Laboratories sold 400,000 bottles of Radithor. Ironically, it was the success of Radithor that ushered in the end of the "Era of Mild Radium Cures" though, tragically, death served as the catalyst.

The victim was Eben M. Byers, a steel tycoon from Pittsburgh, Pennsylvania, and a character who could have walked off the pages of *The Great Gatsby*. He was rich and handsome. An avid athlete, Mr. Byers once held the title of U.S. Amateur Golf Champion. He owned homes in New York, Pittsburgh, Rhode Island, and South Carolina, and maintained horse racing stables in the U.S. and Great Britain. Unmarried, he had quite a reputation as a ladies' man. An injury received during a train ride caused lingering pain in his arm and his physician prescribed Radithor. Byers could afford it.

Eben Byers was so enthusiastic about Radithor that he sent cases of the nostrum as gifts to his friends

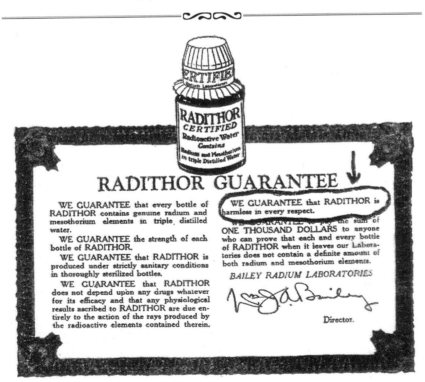

RADITHOR GUARANTEE

WE GUARANTEE that every bottle of RADITHOR contains genuine radium and mesothorium elements in triple distilled water.

WE GUARANTEE the strength of each bottle of RADITHOR.

WE GUARANTEE that RADITHOR is produced under strictly sanitary conditions in thoroughly sterilized bottles.

WE GUARANTEE that RADITHOR does not depend upon any drugs whatever for its efficacy and that any physiological results ascribed to RADITHOR are due entirely to the action of the rays produced by the radioactive elements contained therein.

WE GUARANTEE that RADITHOR is harmless in every respect.

WE GUARANTEE to the sum of ONE THOUSAND DOLLARS to anyone who can prove that each and every bottle of RADITHOR when it leaves our Laboratories does not contain a definite amount of both radium and mesothorium elements.

BAILEY RADIUM LABORATORIES

Director.

and paramours. He drank about 1,400 bottles between 1927 and 1930, and then became extremely ill.

Initially, he experienced aches and pains and these were misdiagnosed as sinusitis. His teeth began to fall out. Specialists were called in and recognized that Mr. Byers was dying from radium poisoning. Most of his upper and lower jaw were surgically removed and Byers' weight dropped to under 100 pounds.

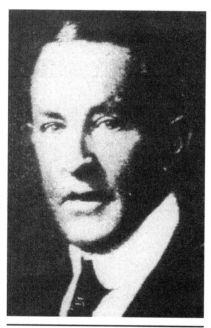

Eben Byers.

Holes began to appear in his skull. Desperately ill, he found the strength to meet with government investigators at his home a few months before he died on March 31, 1931.

Bailey Radium Laboratories had been under investigation by the U.S. Federal Trade Commission since 1928, just months after Eben Byers started his love affair with Radithor. But it was two years before a false advertising complaint was filed and it took until December 1931 to complete

the investigation and obtain a cease-and-desist order. At this point, Mr. Byers had three months left to live. After his death and its cause were headlined on the front page of the *New York Times,* government and the medical profession increased their efforts to warn consumers away from the dangerous radium nostrums.

W.J.A. Bailey, of course, denied that Radithor had killed Eben Byers. "I have drunk more radium water than any man alive," Mr. Bailey said, "and I never have suffered any ill effects."

As Radithor was being investigated, Bailey, ever the entrepreneur, founded three more companies promoting three more radioactive products. The first was the Bio-Ray, which looked something like a paperweight. It was called "a miniature sun" and claimed to provide a continuous supply of gamma rays. The Bio-Ray

was followed by a water nostrum, the Theronator, a two-ounce vessel said to create radioactive water using thoron. For his last hurrah, Mr. Bailey returned to the sexual rejuvenation theme with the Adrenoray, a belt containing five radioactive disks which "cured" impotence and the usual long list of diseases. The companies promoting these products appear to have gone out of business during the early 1930s as the economy soured and consumers turned away from radium nostrums.

W.J.A. Bailey died of bladder cancer in Tyngsborough, Massachusetts on May 16, 1949.

Home Products of Denver, Colorado

Most radium quacks–including W.J.A. Bailey and his cronies–were relatively subtle in claiming rejuvenation or sexual rejuvenation would result from their radioactive products. At least they used euphemisms and testimonials to discuss sex. This was not the case with the Home Products Company of Denver, Colorado, which was forthrightly frank about the sexual nature of its products in its 1930 booklet, "Glands and Radium." Home Products Company promoted a strategy of combining tablets made from animal glands with items containing radium salts in order to help "weak discouraged men bubble over with joyous vitality."

The gland tablets were purportedly made from animal glands "removed from the still-warm body of the animal selected" to ensure that the gland was "active and fresh." The glands were dried over five to six days and ground into a powder. The powder became Nu-Man Gland Tablets "for fatigued, prematurely aged men," or Vagatone Tablets for women. The Nu-Man Gland Tablets were advertised to "each contain 4 grains of the active, sperm-secreting cells of the boar's testicle" and "two other gland substances for activating corresponding human glands that are so vitally concerned in man's sexual well-being and general vitality." The promised results were "restored glandular activity, sex-impulse and power; build-up of pep, personal magnetism and action; and raised resistance to colds."

The ad fails to say what animal was used to produce the women's Vagatone Tablets, which allegedly contained five different gland substances—including ovarian glands— and which promised to remedy "sexual indifference," menopausal symptoms, and dysmenorrhea. While the gland tablets might be used alone, even greater results

An order form for Home Products' tablets. Note the price reduction—as the tablets' popularity waned, the prices continued to fall.

were promised when they were used in tandem with Vita Radium Suppositories (for men) or Women's Special Suppositories.

Vita Radium Suppositories were to be inserted in the rectum so the radium would be absorbed by the colon and intestinal walls.

The company stated the harmless radium would be gone in three days. In addition to "restoring sex power," claims for the suppositories were ameliorating prostate problems, ending frequent urination, and curing piles and rectal sores. The radioactive

MEN IF YOU ARE NOT PHYSICALLY FIT

Let This Marvelous Combination of

Glands And Radium

MAKE YOU THRILL AGAIN WITH JOYOUS VITALITY!

YOU WANT MANLY STRENGTH!

NO MATTER whether you are old or young in years, if you are weak, you want STRENGTH! If you are feeling "down and out," you want of course to become PEPPY and ACTIVE again! If you are physically unfit for the duties and pleasures of a REAL MAN, you must long for a return of your normal, natural powers that fill life with joy, charm and happiness!

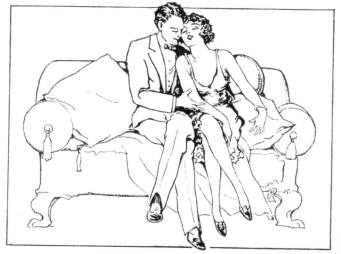

The very consciousness of your unfitness for marriage is enough to make you despondent. To know that you are sexually inefficient, outside the pale of certain joys, is well warranted to give you the "blues," make you cross, irritable and discolor your outlook upon life. Such knowledge may be seriously interfering with your daily work, making it almost impossible for you to CONCENTRATE ADEQUATELY upon what you are trying to do. Certainly, if your vitality is low, you haven't the pep, courage, the incentive, to push your work and make a success of it. Rather, you go at it as drudgery and in a listless, half-hearted fashion.

Can there be anything more humiliating to a man's pride, can anything make him more dejected in spirit, than to find himself the subject of INDIFFERENCE from his wife, knowing that it is due to his own PHYSICAL DEFICIENCY? A man whose vigor is failing him, loses his attraction and cannot command the love, respect and admiration that he craves and that is due him as a husband. Oftentimes he is no more than just tolerated.

Not only this, but your physical incompetency may be depriving another of the strong, virile love she craves and causing domestic discord, discontent and unhappiness. And, after all, is not SEXUAL HARMONY the very foundation of the finer, nobler qualities of peace, love and devotion in the home?

Likely as not you know of men 70 years of age, or thereabouts, who look and act young—gay, sprightly men they are, who walk with brisk, firm step, head and shoulders erect, face aglow with health—men who can enter into the sports and pleasures of youth and who are fully the equal, if not the superior, of many a man much younger in years.

How you must look with envy upon the COURAGEOUS, AGGRESSIVE SELF-CONFIDENT man, the man abounding in vigor and strength, the man who is the "life of the party," the man who is admired and RESPECTED by the opposite sex, and who is SUPREMELY ABLE to measure up to any pleasurable opportunity.

Yes, if you have a spark of manhood in you—and you doubtless have—you want to "come back." You must long for a return of your SEX FORCE so you can again partake of the SWEET JOYS of life and REALLY LIVE AGAIN!

And the question is, HOW?

YOUR FOUNTAIN OF VITALITY

SCIENTISTS assert that the ductless glands are the DYNAMOS of the human body, and that when they run low, we experience a premature decline of our vital forces. You know that when the dynamos in the power plant are not generating enough power, the electric lights are dim and low. Just so it is when the marvelous ductless glands grow weak, the various vital processes within the human body SLOW UP, FAIL and "burn low."

Of all the ductless glands, probably the glands most essential to bodily and mental efficiency and happiness of the individual are the SEX GLANDS—the testes in the male, and the ovaries in the female. It seems that the whole life of the individual revolves around these glands, and that his or her health and well-being are more dependent upon the proper activity of these glands than on any of the others.

They pour into the blood stream a vital fluid which spreads happiness and a feeling of well-being and plentitude of life throughout our bodies. The period of their greatest activity corresponds to the greatest expansion of all our faculties. It is the moment when our brains are "on fire," so to speak—when we are overflowing with energy and are incited to the most daring actions.

A noted physician also states that, "the preservation of the sexual glands in advanced old age proves also the important fact that though the actual age be there, the symptoms of it may not be very pronounced if the sexual glands are in good order. Of course, the condition of the other ductless glands is of importance, for old age must be regarded as the consequence of the degeneration of the different ductless glands, not of any particular gland alone."

WHEN THE GLANDS FAIL

When the various ductless glands grow weak and fail to secrete a sufficient quantity of their marvelous vitalizing secretions into the body, it is then that a man loses his ardor of affection, becomes deficient in qualities of vigorous manhood, and undergoes a change in his physical, moral and mental makeup, which his family and friends are quick to notice.

Especially is this true when the sex glands become exhausted, shrink and atrophy. When Manly Courage, Ambition and Vigor are lacking, the individual sadly realizes that he is not the "man he once was" and is no longer a fit mate. He lacks the peculiar appeal that once was his, and he feels that life has become almost a mockery—a vain and empty thing to him instead of a life of glorious pleasure, enjoyment and happiness as it should be. No wonder he loses his sense of humor and is morose and melancholy —no longer the jolly, peppy fellow he used to be. He feels he is almost alone in the world because of his inability to take part in social pleasures, and that everyone is trying to shun him. His disposition changes gradually—there isn't anything that really pleases, but much that displeases. Trivial things get on the nerves—it becomes difficult for the family and friends of the weakened man to get along with him harmoniously.

Your Glorious Opportunity Is Before You!

Women's Special Suppositories, inserted vaginally, were supposed to stimulate nerve-currents, revive sluggish tissue, increase tone, and stimulate vaginal secretions. They were also recommended for inflammation, ulcers, discharges, infections, other afflictions of the vaginal area, heavy menstrual flow, and uterine hemorrhages. In the presence of "sex apathy," women were exhorted to use both the gland tablets and radium salt suppositories because "the woman is a better mother when her sex organs are toned up."

Home Products Company had two additional products for men. The most unusual nostrum made by the company was Soothol Radium Bougies to counteract prematurity (and congestion and irritation from self-abuse). The company argued that premature ejaculation might be caused by "excessive indulgence, venereal infection and bad habits" resulting in inflammation. The bougies, an eighth inch in diameter and six

VITA RADIUM SUPPOSITORIES

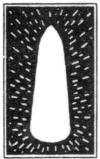

Actual Size of Suppository

OUR VITA RADIUM SUPPOSITORIES (HIGH STRENGTH) are one of the outstanding triumphs of Radium Science. These Suppositories are guaranteed to contain REAL RADIUM—in the exact amount for most beneficial effect. They are inserted per rectum, one each night, this being one of the several practical and successful ways of introducing Radium into the system.

After insertion, the Suppository quickly dissolves and the Radium is absorbed by the walls of the colon; then, within a few minutes, it enters the blood stream and traverses the entire body. Every tissue, every organ of the body is bombarded by its health-giving electric atoms. Thus the use of these Suppositories has an effect on the human body like recharging has on an electric battery.

And remember, Radium taken into the system remains for months, continuing its curative, restorative work. Thus, the effects are NOT merely temporary.

VITA RADIUM SUPPOSITORIES are guaranteed to be non-injurious—they are perfectly safe for anyone to use. Their action is due solely to the Radium contained therein.

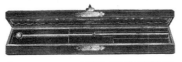

A VELVET LINED RADUIM APPLICATOR BOX.

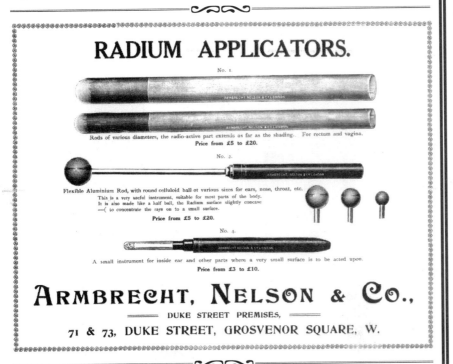

inches long, were to be inserted in the urethra so as to treat "the deep urinary canal." A thirty day treatment period was recommended.

They also produced a radium belt: the Testone Radium Energizer and Suspensory (alleged to contain 20 micrograms radium), which promised "new energy for weak sagging men." This diaper-like contraption was supposed to radiate the testicles! "It is much like the 'trickle' charger used to recharge wet cells of storage batteries. As radium will not lose over half its strength in one thousand years, it is evident that with reasonable care the Testone Appliance should be good for a lifetime."

Home Products Company was operated by Dr. Davis (an osteopath) and Marko Gacina. Mr. Gacina peddled Haelan, a stomach nostrum containing alcohol, water, sarsaparilla root, and burdock root, throughout the Pacific coast states from 1908 until 1922 when he arrived in Denver. He teamed up with Dr. Davis and they repackaged Haelan as Heilol, a mail order tuberculosis cure. The postal authorities banned Heilol in 1924, so the pair formed Home Products Company. Home Products Company's rejuvenation cures were judged to be fraudulent and the company was barred from using the U.S. mail on August 25, 1931.

Radium wasn't the only source of rays which captured the fancy of the American public in the industrial age. As you'll see in the next chapter, some folks looked for cures in the benign rays we call colored light.

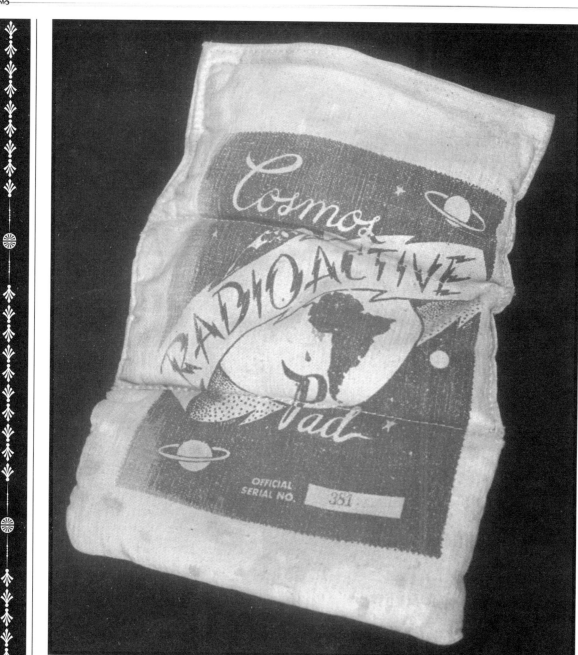

The Cosmos Radioactive Bag is heavy and radioactive. It was promoted by a man supposedly named Cosmos and was sold to relieve the pain of arthritic joints. Oddly, the reverse side says, "Do not eat the contents of this bag."

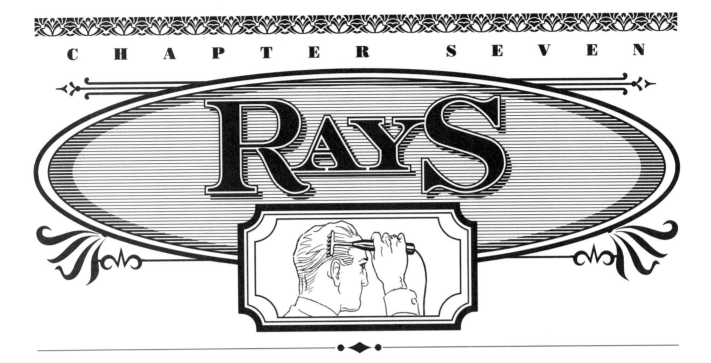

LET THE SUN SHINE IN.

Throughout history, people from a variety of cultures have believed in "healing rays"—beginning with the therapeutic benefits of sunshine. The earliest devices which sought to harness the healing power of rays were amulets made of metal, gemstones, and other materials believed to have the power to ward off illness or attract a cure. These amulets were thought to be magic or a way to get the attention of the gods. In modern America, quack medical devices which emitted "healing rays" also relied upon faith and magic. By the turn of the twentieth century, electricity made new "healing ray" quack devices possible: colored glass combined with light bulbs, violet ray generators, ozone generators, and misapplied X-rays. Ironically, at the end of the twentieth century, the latest "healing ray" device in the collection of the Museum of Questionable Medical Devices is a "therapeutic necklace," which in reality is nothing more than a yellow plastic amulet.

One of the earliest colored light cures in the U.S. was the Blue Glass Craze in the 1870s, a story

JUST AS LIGHT is the recognized source of all vegetable, animal, and human life, so it is—in the specific use of the seven spectral colors—the greatest assistant to nature. The Chromaray claimed to treat all known diseases, from appendicitis to veneral disease. (1937)

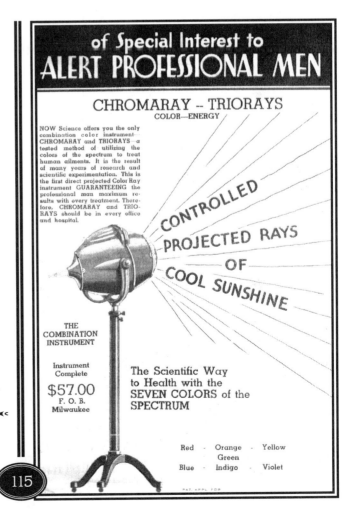

of Special Interest to
ALERT PROFESSIONAL MEN

CHROMARAY -- TRIORAYS
COLOR—ENERGY

NOW Science offers you the only combination color instrument—CHROMARAY and TRIORAYS—a tested method of utilizing the colors of the spectrum to treat human ailments. It is the result of many years of research and scientific experimentation. This is the first direct projected Color Ray instrument GUARANTEEING the professional man maximum results with every treatment. Therefore, CHROMARAY and TRIORAYS should be in every office and hospital.

CONTROLLED PROJECTED RAYS OF COOL SUNSHINE

THE
COMBINATION
INSTRUMENT

Instrument
Complete

$57.00
F. O. B.
Milwaukee

The Scientific Way
to Health with the
SEVEN COLORS of the
SPECTRUM

Red	Orange	Yellow
---	Green	---
Blue	Indigo	Violet

well-told by medical historian Dr. James J. Walsh in his 1924 book, *Cures That Fail*:

A glass-making firm by an egregious blunder of a clerk made much more blue glass than they could find any sale for. It was a drug on the market. They offered a salesman a substantial bonus if he would dispose of it. He had a scientific friend of whom he asked what new use might be discovered for blue glass. The scientist had a sense of humor and he said: "Well, the blue end of the spectrum is where the actinic rays are which act upon photographic plates; they ought to also to stimulate tissues and cure disease." So the salesman got the idea of advertising the blue glass as good for all sorts of pains and aches. One of the well-known old generals of the Civil War wrote in to ask about the value of blue glass for the chronic pains and aches of his old wounds and the salesman assured him that it would certainly do him good, and inspired entirely by a patriotic motive, of course, offered to supply the old general with the blue glass necessary for him to try it. The old general bared his wounds and let the blue light shine on them for several hours of the day and very soon to his agreeable surprise they were much better.

At the moment the general was one of the best known survivors of the Civil War officers, a leader in the Grand Army of the Republic—the American Legion of that day. Any news with regard to the old general was of national import, so the item was flashed through the country. Every newspaper published an account of it. It was the easiest bit of national advertising ever accomplished. And that was before the days of national advertising as we know it. For one thing, there were several hundred thousand men North and South whose old wounds, healed in the pre-antiseptic days, when laudable pus was considered a valuable indication of the healing power of tissues and therefore with much scarring and destruction of substance, inflicted on them especially in rainy weather, discomforts similar to those of the old general. They took up the new cure with avidity so that it is easy to understand that it was not long before blue glass was much in demand. The factory disposed not only of

Elco Combination Health Generator No. 12

Generates Medical Electricity, Vibration, Violet Ray and Ozone.
Write for Descriptive Literature.

The Elco Combination Health Generator No. 12 was typical of such devices and was clearly designed to appeal to all the senses—the sight of the coil's electrical spark; the smell of ozone; the crackling and buzzing sound of a serious, powerful machine; and the brilliance of the gas-filled tubes—so that patients would feel their visit to the doctor was worth the fee.

its surplus blue glass stock, but had to manufacture an immense amount more. And other glass foundries throughout the country had to take up the manufacture of blue glass and the demand for it could scarcely be supplied.

I remember an uncle of mine who sat under the blue glass for an hour and more every day and was perfectly sure that nothing in the world had ever done him so much good as the "blue glass cure." Pains in his back and shoulders that had been bothering him for years and were always worse in rainy weather, disappeared, as if by magic. He persuaded a brother of his, an old soldier who had been much exposed to rain and dampness during the war and then subsequently in a series of western adventures, to try the glass and he also was very much benefited by it. I remember seeing the glass many years afterwards in a garret of the old homestead and being reminded then of what I had heard about it as a boy. Evidently, the cure did not last, for both uncles continued to complain of rheumatic pains and aches of various kinds that were "cured" by many other things after the blue glass was given up. . . . Of course after a time the fad for blue glass dropped out and now is almost completely forgotten. Blue glass is of no special value for the relief of pains and aches, but for a time it looked as though it were one of the heaven-sent dispensation of relief for the old soldiers whose wounds and exposure during the war had rendered them the subject of so many discomforts.

Plain colored glass cures made a comeback in the 1920s and 1930s when a thick circle of colored

glass was enclosed in a handle similar to the design of a hand mirror. The devices were cure-alls claiming to treat dozens of common medical complaints, including aches and pains. The most notable was the Von Schilling Surgical Ray, a thick lens of green

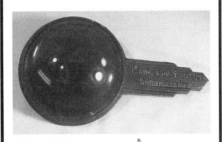

THE VON SCHILLING
SURGICAL RAY

glass set in an Art Deco-style cast iron handle. The hand-held glass cure-alls never knew the popularity of the Blue Glass Craze; such popularity would follow the higher tech colored glass cures which used electric light.

Dr. George Starr White and the Rithmo-Lite Generator

Dr. George Starr White might be the Renaissance Man among the great American quacks for he engaged in all major forms of quackery with some success. He graduated from the New York Homeopathic Medical College in 1908, accumulated four additional degrees from a California chiropractic college, and an LL.D. and a Ph.D. from bogus diploma institutes. By 1915, Dr. White was a traveling salesman working for Albert Abrams, conducting Spondylotherapy seminars throughout the western United States.

About this time, Mr. White also got into the testimonial racket. He appeared on the literature of

"Oxylene," an ozone device sold by Neel-Armstrong Company of Ohio. He endorsed "Radiumacti" of California, a fake radium cure; the "Electrothermal dilator" for prostate trouble manufactured in Steubenville, Ohio; and the "Traction Couch," made in Duluth, Minnesota. Dr. White was a networker who belonged to 39 medical or quasi-medical organizations, and these memberships made his endorsement all the more impressive. Dr. White's testimonial earnings are unknown, but another doctor during this period reported being offered $750 to write an endorsement letter for a quack concern.

During 1918-19, there was a severe flu epidemic in the United States and, in response, Dr. White produced and sold an influenza nostrum for $30 a gallon. After the epidemic, Dr. White became a gadget quack. His Filteray Pad, a patented heating pad, was recommended for 150 conditions including hair loss, lumps in the breast, tuberculosis, and tumors.

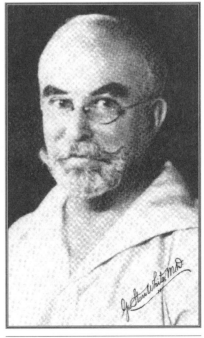

Dr. George Starr White

He borrowed an idea from a former client and manufactured the Valens Bio-Dynamic Prostatic Normalizer (for prostate and rectal problems, $35) and Valens Bio-Dynamic Pelvic Normalizer (a sexual "normalizer" for women, $45). The two sexual devices were said to contain magnets imbedded in plastic and so were promoted as magnetic cures.

Dr. White rounded out his products with two light cures: the Rithmo-Lite Generator and the Rithmo-Chrome. He encouraged the use of his products in combination so the patient sat on the Filteray heating pad in front of the Rithmo Chrome achieving "rhythmic recurrence [of colors] to harmonize with any individual" while breathing the fumes of his Oxygen Vapor.

As with the ancient amulets, colored light cures needed an element of magic to be believable. George Starr White's "magic" was Bio-Dynamic-Chromatic (B-D-C) Diagnosis, a fresh pseudo-scientific diagnostic technique remarkably like Albert Abrams' E.R.A. The patient faced east or west while the doctor percussed the abdomen until a dull spot was located. Then the patient faced north or south and again his abdomen was percussed while being bathed in different colored lights. Ruby plus blue signified gonorrhea and, again like Abrams, Dr. White found a lot of syphilis. Rithmo-Chrome Therapy was advertised as "treatment by means of rhythm, complementary colors, and the magnetic forces of the earth."

The Rithmo-Lite Generator was described by Dr. White as a powerful machine devised "for fading in and fading out light from one or more fifteen-hundred watt

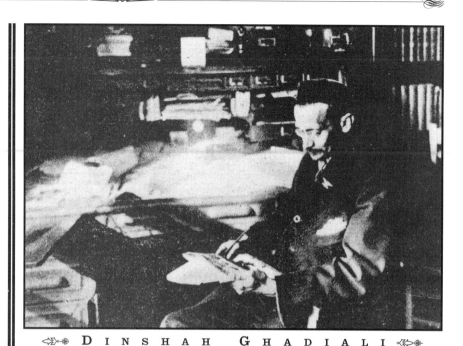

◁≍≍≍◈ D I N S H A H   G H A D I A L I ◈≍≍≍▷

lamps at one time "to provide rhythmic harmonization of the person being treated."

In his 1936 autobiography, Dr. White wrote "I built my first outfit for giving rithm to powerful lites, as well as color, in treating human ills, in 1908. Making the outfits practical required a great deal of experimenting. . . . I have learned that to get the greatest benefit from the use of powerful lamps, the radiation must be given in rithm to suit each patient. In other words the Lite of Color radiations must be given in such a manner as to bring the patient 'up to par.' I do this by having the patient inhale when the lite or color comes on, and exhale while the same goes off. Experience has taut me that the ratio between the inspiration and expiration of the average helthy person is as four is to five. That is to say: If the patient consumes four seconds to exhale, I have develpt a machine that automatically makes and breaks the electric current to the big lamps in just this ratio [spelling original]."

The secret to the Rithmo-Lite Generator was lights flashing at the rate of normal respiration!

Dinshah Ghadiali and the Spectro-Chrome

Following in the footsteps of Dr. George Starr White was Dinshah Ghadiali, who spent over 35 years peddling his colored glass cure, Spectro-Chrome Therapy. The Spectro-Chrome came in several models. The smallest model sold for $30 in the 1930s and consisted of a hood, a lamp bracket, 15 feet of cord, an attachment plug, and color slides. A larger model was a box, made out of aluminum or plywood, which contained a 1,000 watt light bulb so hot that the box also included a fan for cooling. The box, placed atop a stand, had a front window covered with slides of colored squares—glass in the aluminum model and plastic in the plywood model. The Spectro-Chromes used standard alternating current.

Treatments were given by lay healers or at home. The patient sat nude in front of the Spectro-Chrome during the right moment of the lunar phase, generally the new moon or full moon, and was bathed in different colored lights for various conditions. In "The Latest Effort of the Healing Art," Dr. Cramp of the AMA Investigative Bureau exposed this branch of quackery:

Now comes into the field Colonel Dinshah P. Ghadiali, exponent of "Spectro-Chrome Therapy" and founder of the "Spectro-Chrome Institute." Ghadiali has an appalling list of titles. The leading one, for his present purpose at least, is that of "M.D." So far as the records of the American Medical Association show, and they are the most complete extant and based on official data, no man by the name of Dinshah P. Ghadiali has ever been graduated by any reputable medical college nor licensed to practice medicine in any state in the Union. . . . He tells us that "among other honors" he holds the following degrees: "Doctor of Chiropractic," Doctor of Philosophy," "Doctor of Legal Law" (sic!).

He is

- Fellow and Ex-Vice-President, Allied Medical Associations of America
- Member and Ex-Vice-President, National Association of Drugless Practitioners
- President, All Cults Medical Association
- President, American Association of Spectro-Chrome Therapists
- President, American Anti-Vivisection Society
- Member Anti-Vaccination League of London
- Member American Association of Orificial Surgeons

During the war Ghadiali seems to have received a commission in the New York Police Reserve. Most of his advertising bears a picture of him in full regalia.

What is Spectro-Chrome Therapy?

Here is the thesis developed and commercialized by Ghadiali: Every element exhibits a preponderance of one or more of the seven prismatic colors; 97 per

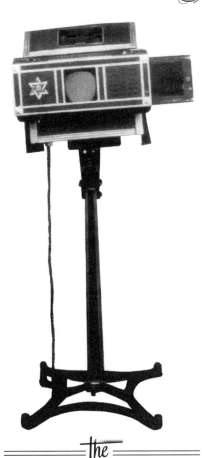

the SPECTRO-CHROME

cent of our body is composed of the four elements, oxygen, hydrogen, nitrogen and carbon; the preponderating color wave of these four elements are blue, red, green and yellow, respectively; the human body is responsive to these four "color wave potencies." In health our four colors are properly balanced; when they get out of balance we are diseased; ergo, to cure disease administer the lacking colors or reduce the colors that have become too brilliant.

Part of Ghadiali's paraphernalia is a chart describing the "Spectro-Chrome Therapeutic System." From this we learn that Green light is a pituitary stimulant, a germicide and a muscle tissue builder. Yellow light is a digestant, an anthelmintic and a nerve builder. Red is a liver

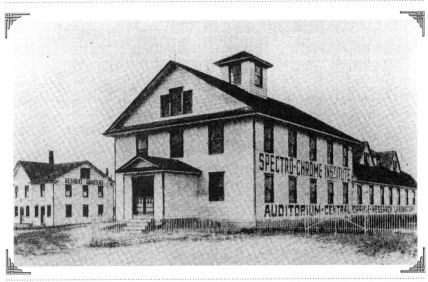

THE WORLD-RENOWNED SPECTRO-CHROME INSTITUTE, IN MALAGA, NEW JERSEY.

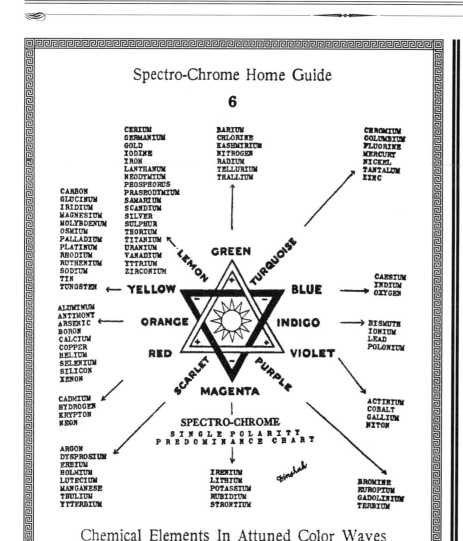

Spectro-Chrome Home Guide

6

CERIUM
GERMANIUM
GOLD
IODINE
IRON
LANTHANUM
NEODYMIUM
PHOSPHORUS
PRASEODYMIUM
SAMARIUM
SCANDIUM
SILVER
SULPHUR
THORIUM
TITANIUM
URANIUM
VANADIUM
YTTRIUM
ZIRCONIUM

BARIUM
CHLORINE
KASHMIRIUM
NITROGEN
RADIUM
TELLURIUM
THALLIUM

CHROMIUM
COLUMBIUM
FLUORINE
MERCURY
NICKEL
TANTALUM
ZINC

CARBON
GLUCINUM
IRIDIUM
MAGNESIUM
MOLYBDENUM
OSMIUM
PALLADIUM
PLATINUM
RHODIUM
RUTHENIUM
SODIUM
TIN
TUNGSTEN

LEMON GREEN TURQUOISE

YELLOW BLUE

CAESIUM
INDIUM
OXYGEN

ALUMINUM
ANTIMONY
ARSENIC
BORON
CALCIUM
COPPER
HELIUM
SELENIUM
SILICON
XENON

ORANGE INDIGO

BISMUTH
IONIUM
LEAD
POLONIUM

RED VIOLET

CADMIUM
HYDROGEN
KRYPTON
NEON

SCARLET PURPLE

MAGENTA

ACTINIUM
COBALT
GALLIUM
NITON

SPECTRO-CHROME
SINGLE POLARITY
PREDOMINANCE CHART

ARGON
DYSPROSIUM
ERBIUM
HOLMIUM
LUTECIUM
MANGANESE
THULIUM
YTTERBIUM

IRENIUM
LITHIUM
POTASSIUM
RUBIDIUM
STRONTIUM

BROMINE
EUROPIUM
GADOLINIUM
TERBIUM

Chemical Elements In Attuned Color Waves

energizer, a caustic and a hemoglobin builder. Violet is a cardiac depressant; Blue is a vitality builder; Indigo is a hemostatic; Turquoise, a tonic; Lemon, a bone builder; Orange, an emetic; Scarlet, a genital excitant; Magenta, a suprarenal stimulant, and Purple an anti-malarial . . .

The disciple is told that the "attuned color waves" should be applied to the bare skin as clothing will intercept them. In giving the "systemic treatment" which from the testimonials, seem an important feature, the "color wave" is applied to the entire nude body, both front and back. For local treatment, the "color wave" is applied to the area that is designated by the number given in the chart.

The later history of Dinshah P. Ghadiali is interesting. In May 1925 newspapers reported that Ghadiali was arrested after a pistol battle in Portland, Ore., charged by the federal authorities with violation of the Mann Act in having transported a 19-year-old girl from that city to Malaga, N.J., and back for immoral purposes. He was indicted on six counts and was found guilty on all of them. At the time of the trial the Portland Oregonian reported that the girl in question was engaged as a secretary by Ghadiali while he was delivering so-called lectures in Portland on Spectro-Chrome Therapy. The paper went on to state: "Illicit relations, the girl testified, started while at Wildwood, N.J., on a vacation and continued until she was taken from his control at the Portland hotel upon her return to this city in April of this year. Two illegal operations were said to have been performed while the young woman was at Malaga.

On Dec. 4, 1925, Ghadiali was sentenced to five years' imprisonment in the Atlanta penitentiary. During his incarceration there was an outbreak among the prisoners in the penitentiary, and because of Ghadiali's services at that time, his sentence was commuted and he was released March 1, 1929. Since his release he has gone back to his Spectro-Chrome quackery and has claimed in his advertising that he was pardoned by the President. He wasn't. The Department of Justice at Washington D.C., under date of Oct. 18, 1934, reported that "while Dinshah P. Ghadiali was released from the Atlanta penitentiary by commutation of sentence, granted by the President, he has never, in fact, been pardoned for the offense of which he was convicted."

In 1931 Ghadiali was arrested in Cleveland, Ohio, and found guilty in the local court and fined $25 and costs. But he still finds an ample supply of dupes and issues elaborate colored advertising booklets. He sells a "Spectro-Chrome Cabinet" for home use, ranging in price from $75 to $150, and a very elaborate contraption that he calls the Graduate Spectro-Chrome for professional use, which sells for $750. The latter reminds one of some of the marvelous gadgets illustrated by cartoonist Goldberg and appears to be a cross between a stereopticon and an automobile heater.

By 1940, Dinshah Ghadiali had made over a million dollars selling the Spectro-Chrome. The U. S. Food and Drug Administration seized a Spectro-Chrome device in 1944, the first step in a three year process which resulted in Mr. Ghadiali's conviction on twelve counts for which he received a sentence of five years probation and a $24,000 fine. One probationary condition was that he no longer sell Spectro-Chromes. This decision was appealed to no avail and Mr. Ghadiali served his five years probation. He returned to the Spectro-Chrome business in 1953 when he founded the Visible Spectrum Institute. In 1959, a permanent injunction was issued against Mr. Ghadiali and sale of the Spectro-Chrome. Dinshah Ghadiali died in Malaga, New Jersey, home of the Spectro-Chrome, in 1966. In 1995, his son Darius Dinshah published

Let There Be Light, an updated version of the Spectro-Chrome manual currently for sale from the non-profit Dinshah Health Society, also of Malaga, New Jersey, which is trying to revive spectrochrometry.

The Ether-eal Rays of Dr. Heil Crum

The Coetherator, patented in 1936 by Heil Eugene Crum and his wife, Anna May Crum, is a wooden box, 26" x 8" x 7" with two interior compartments. The main compartment contains a track on which a small lamp house and light bulb are moved manually via a knob on the front of the box. Behind the lamp house is a strip with small circles, each containing celluloid color patches. By moving the knob side-to-side, the light bulb illuminates the various patches and the colored light shines through circles in the front face of the cabinet. The practitioner moved the knob until

locating the desired color. Then, a matching strip of celluloid was inserted through a slot in the top of the box into a small square wire basket affixed to the back of the compartment. This compartment was also used to hold unnamed chemicals if the practitioner so desired.

The second compartment held the workings of a 25-hour clock "which is preferably electrically operated." The standard model appears to have used a clock set which was moved manually. The purpose of the clock was to turn off the light in the larger compartment.

Sometime before 1927, Heil Crum attended the College of Drugless Physicians, a diploma mill, for a year and emerged with degrees of Doctor of Naturopathy, Doctor of Electro-Therapeutics, Doctor of Chiropractic, and Doctor of Herbal Materia Medica. Under the Medical Practice Act of 1927, Indiana required licensing of certain medical practitioners.

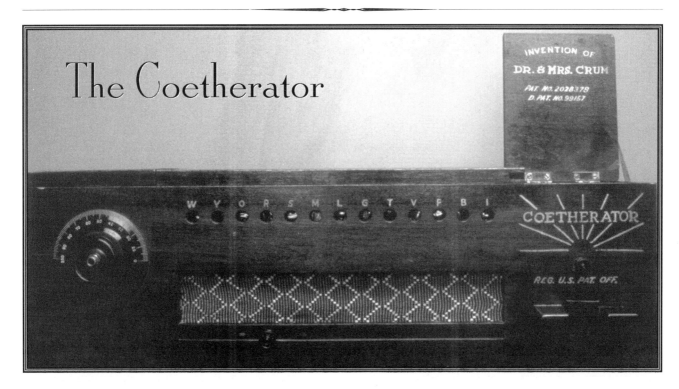

Mr. Crum believed his licenses for chiropractic, naturopathy, and electrotherapy would be deemed legal without examination under the Act's grandfather clause, and he established a practice in Indianapolis.

The 1936 patent documents call the Coetherator the "etheric vibrator, " a device supposed to "treat human ailments by the vibration rate of ether." The Crums alleged that ether is readily present in the atmosphere. Further, the vibration rates of ether waves *affecting the eye* change with color. This variation in ether movement, said the Crums, "enables the practitioner to treat disease by varying the vibration rate as accomplished by the use of colored screens."

The State of Indiana promptly disagreed with Dr. Crum's new treatment method and moved to revoke his licenses. A trial was held in Marion and Dr. Crum lost. He appealed to the state supreme court. In the case, Heil Eugene Crum v. State Board of Medical Registration and Examination, the Indiana Supreme Court found the following:

The charge was, in effect, that the appellant used a device of no possible therapeutic value under any recognized system of treatment, and that he knowingly made false and fraudulent claims with respect to it for his own profit and to the injury of others. No licensee of this state may rightfully claim that privilege . . .

In 1936, he obtained a United States patent on the machine with which we are presently concerned. The granting of a patent does not imply that the subject there of will accomplish what is claimed for it or that it has any merit. In view of the overwhelming evidence that the appellant's contraption had no value in the treatment of diseases, it is reasonable to infer that his purpose in obtaining letters of patent was to impress his patients with the thought that the device has some measure of governmental approval . . .

The machine was a small wood box with a number of holes in the front, over which various colors of thin paper were pasted. On the inside was an ordinary light bulb with a cord for making contact with electricity. The bulb could be moved about so that light would penetrate the various paper-covered holes. The box also contained a quantity of disconnected wire, such as is commonly used for radio aerials, and a glass tube filled with ordinary hydrant water. There was a pedal and a dial on the outside of the box, neither of which had any connection with the interior.

The usual method for treating human ailments was to have the patient moisten a slip of paper with saliva and deposit it through a slot on the top of the box, although it was claimed by the appellant that the same results could be obtained by similar use of the patient's photograph or a specimen of his handwriting. After this was done, the appellant rubbed the pedal with his thumb and talked to the machine, repeating the popular names of diseases and organs of the body. Among the diseases which the appellant claimed to be able to treat and relieve, and in some instances cure, by this method were cancer, blindness, arthritis, nervous disorders, hemorrhoids, abscesses, kidney ailments, stomach disorders, leakage of the heart, skin ailments, ovarian trouble, varicose veins, and tumors. He asserted that he could lengthen or shorten a patient's legs; cause amputated fingers to grow back into place; and fill cavities in teeth, not with a foreign substance but by restoring them to their original condition. He said that it was not necessary for patients to be present or to visit his office, but that he could broadcast treatments to them wherever they might be located.

The appellant's practice was not limited to the treatment of human ills. He also claimed to be able to administer "Financial treatments," by means of which money could be put into the hands of his patients; that he could fertilize fields to a distance of 70 miles; kill dandelions over any particular area; and treat golf greens as far from Indianapolis as Decatur, Illinois, so that clover would turn brown and dry up and give the grass a chance to grow.

The mention of the extravagant claims made by the appellant is sufficient to suggest their untruthfulness and brand them as designedly fraudulent . . . The above summary of the evidence, taken from the appellant's own brief, was sufficient, in our judgment, to justify the above trial court in finding him guilty of gross immorality . . ."

Gross immorality was grounds for license revocation and so, on November 3, 1941, Dr. Crum lost his licenses to practice medicine in Indiana.

Violet Rays

Violet Ray generators are the most common quack medical device found in the United States antique market today. These devices began as cure-alls during the nineteen-teens, reached the

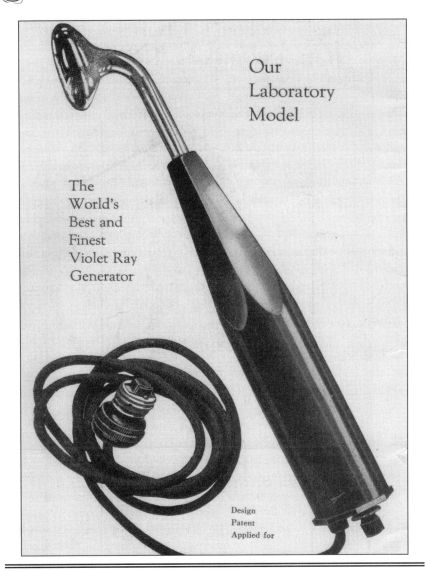

Our
Laboratory
Model

The
World's
Best and
Finest
Violet Ray
Generator

Design
Patent
Applied for

THE SHELTON VIOLET RAY

Induction Coils, Vacuum Discharge Tubes, Diathermy Machines, and related high voltage devices and contraptions. Following is Behary's history of violet ray generators:

"Violet Ray" and High Frequency Devices

Two distinctly different versions of "High Frequency Currents" were discovered in the 1880s by two individuals. First by Nikola Tesla in the United States, and second by d'Arsonval in Paris. Nikola Tesla experimented with alternating currents of extremely high frequency and voltage, with relatively low current. D'Arsonval experimented with high frequency currents of relatively lower voltages and higher amperage. Both Tesla and d'Arsonval currents are noted for their physiological effects on the human body.

Tesla (who incidentally referred to the earlier faradic coils and magneto-electric machines as more-or-less fraudulent quackery) reported the stimulating and vitalizing action of these currents in

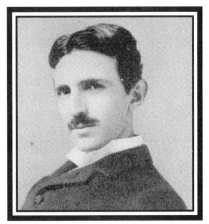

Nikola Tesla.

the cases of several of his assistants, and upon his own organism—implying further that they would possibly become the "healing art of the future." In the December

height of their popularity during the 1920s and 1930s, and continued as a cosmetology tool into the 1990s. The device consists of an "appliance," the handle, with a glass electrode inserted at the top. Dozens of electrodes were manufactured in shapes and sizes to fit every nook and cranny of the human body. The most common glass electrodes were either shaped like a mushroom for removing warts, pimples, blackheads and freckles, or like a rake to stimulate the scalp and make hair grow. The most knowledgeable collector of violet ray generators in the United States may be Jeff Behary, from Loxahatchee, Florida. Behary began taking apart and reassembling violet ray generators when he was 15 years old. Aside from collecting devices, he also repairs machines and builds reproductions. Recently, he has started to remanufacture glass electrodes. His online website, "The Turn of the Century Electro-therapy Museum (http://www. lvstrings. com/quack.htm)," contains a wealth of information on Violet Ray machines, Faradic Batteries, Magneto-Electric Machines, Carbon Arc Lamps, Tesla Coils,

****
THE THOMPSON PLASTER
ELECTRICAL CABINET
****

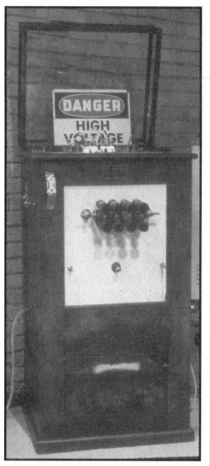

The Thompson Plaster Electrical Cabinet, circa 1880, contains a large motor and air compressor. The violet ray attachment is "quack."

1891 issue of *The Electrical Engineer*, he wrote:

"I trust that the brief communication will not be interpreted as an effort on my part to put myself on record as a 'patent medicine man', for a serious worker cannot despise anything more than the misuse and abuse of electricity which we have frequent occasion to witness . . . without vouching for all the results, which must, of course, be determined by experience and observation, I can at least warrant the fact that heating would occur by the use of this method of subjecting the body to bombardment by alternating currents of high potential and frequency such as I have long worked with."

Tesla was a brilliant showman and inventor—with thousands of patents leading to his name. He is credited with the invention of remote control devices, the wireless transmission of electricity and wireless lighting, alternating current motors and generators, polyphase systems, radio, and countless others. He was rarely photographed without million volt streamers and sparks dozens of feet long surrounding him.

In 1896, Kinraide developed a primitive but interesting machine of the Tesla type for radiography, introducing high frequency currents to the medical field and commercial market. It was inexpensive, consumed little electricity, and was lightweight: the exact opposite of everything else in the field for powering X-ray tubes. The currents however were not well suited for therapeutic use because of several technical flaws in design that needed further investigation. With the help of Mr. Howard Jackson, Kinraide developed a new high frequency coil of improved design. This coil proved less satisfactory for radiography, but worked quite well for use of high frequency currents therapeutically.

As high frequency electricity was a relatively new concept when used therapeutically, physicians generally published their results. As varied and unique as the treatments themselves were, the actual instruments used to deliver these currents to the body were quite numerous as well. The most famous and familiar was the vacuum electrode, invented by Dr. Frederick Finch Strong. In 1897, Strong discovered that while working with condenser discharges from leaden jars, a vacuum tube evacuated to the geissler degree would prevent direct sparks from burning or searing the skin. Strong published his findings and went on to design dozens of tubes made for the application of high frequency currents to specific body parts. He also further developed various modalities of currents

Early advertisement for the Roentgen Ray Current.

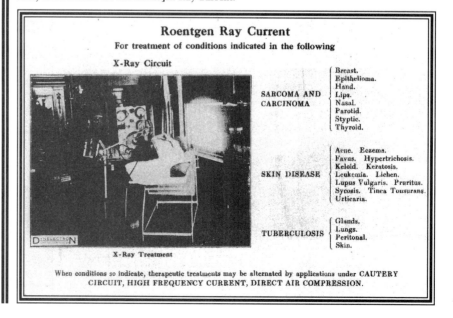

Roentgen Ray Current
For treatment of conditions indicated in the following
X-Ray Circuit

SARCOMA AND CARCINOMA	Breast. Epithelioma. Hand. Lips. Nasal. Parotid. Styptic. Thyroid.
SKIN DISEASE	Acne. Eczema. Favus. Hypertrichosis. Keloid. Keratosis. Leukemia. Lichen. Lupus Vulgaris. Pruritus. Sycosis. Tinea Tousurans. Urticaria.
TUBERCULOSIS	Glands. Lungs. Peritonal. Skin.

X-Ray Treatment

When conditions so indicate, therapeutic treatments may be alternated by applications under CAUTERY CIRCUIT, HIGH FREQUENCY CURRENT, DIRECT AIR COMPRESSION.

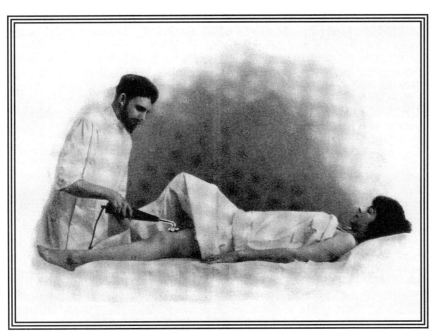

Healer treating a patient with a high-frequency violet ray device.

that could be derived from Tesla type apparatus. The door was opening to a world of opportunity in this new and exciting field of electricity.

Soon literally dozens of coils were developed and experimented with across the country and in Europe, each slightly different in design and electrical output including Oudin Resonators, Guilleminot Spirals, and Piffard's Hyperstatic Transformer. Serious experimentation was done with these coils on patients, and truthful results were published in various texts across the country. For example, Dr. Sinclair Tousey in his 1915 *Medical Electricity, Röntgen Rays, and Radium* offered this advice for treating Postobstetric Hemorrhoids: "Bilinkin treated 6 cases, eight to nineteen applications, 4 were cured . . . bad results in exceptional cases are an increase in swelling, considerable pain, and some hemorrhage . . . when this takes place this line of treatment had better be abandoned."

Many of these early high

frequency apparatuses were large and bulky, and very costly. But when nothing else was available they proved to be invaluable in the treatment of many conditions. Many modern devices for surgery, electrotherapy, and diathermy were based on these early apparatuses. The weight of the machines and amount of electricity needed to run them limited their usefulness. Many patients required home visits—and many homes either did not have alternating current, or did not have a large enough supply of electricity to operate the machines correctly.

Portable Violet Ray Devices

Around 1910 several portable high frequency devices showed up on the now-booming electrotherapy market. One such device was manufactured by Remco. It was sold for cauterizing small growths and moles, and came with a glass vacuum condenser electrode for the spark treatment of moles and small epitheliomata and for the

vacuum electrode treatment of neuralgia. It had a large advantage of running on small amounts of electricity, either direct or alternating current, and being lightweight, could hang freely from an electric light socket. This was one of the first portable high frequency apparatus. Despite its generally limited use, it was one of the first of the now-common "Violet Ray" devices.

Several companies such as AS Aloe, HG Fischer, Campbell, and Frank S. Betz decided to make similar lightweight apparatuses (under 35 pounds) that could offer high frequency currents, and other electrical functions as well. Soon platinum coagulation tools, cold cauterizing surgical tools, diagnostics lamps, ultraviolet mercury vapor lamps, special high frequency X-ray tubes, and glass vacuum electrodes could all be operated by one unit that was the size of a small suitcase.

With more and more portable apparatuses showing up on the market, several companies decided to market these devices to the public for home use. Many people were embarrassed to approach doctors about female problems or problems of a sexual nature

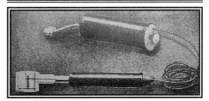

and resorted to buying "home treatment" apparatuses that claimed to fix these problems in the privacy of the home. With the production of high frequency devices for home use, the now-familiar term "Violet Ray Generators" came into use.

Booklets which came with these home devices often had ridiculous claims that lacked the authority and truth of the previous high frequency machines. Eastern Laboratories' *The Marvel Violet Ray* instructions included:

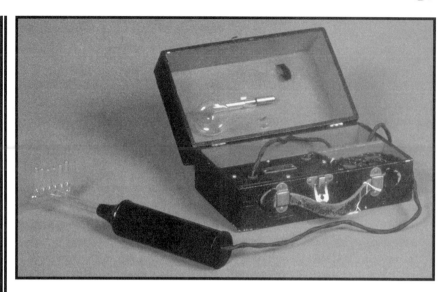

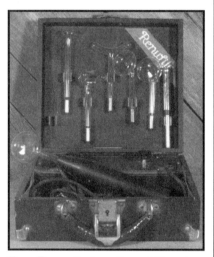

THIS PAGE displays three different violet ray generators from the Renu Life Corporation. It also shows the wide variety of glass and metal inserts available. The device on the lower right also came with a vibrator.

"Freckles: Cover the surface with gauze . . . Use daily for 4-6 minutes with a medium current. Results are apt to be slow, therefore be patient.

"Obesity: . . . fat will decrease and redistribute."

The thought of one device claiming to cure everything did not go over well in the medical profession. Dr. Tousey wrote:

"Violet-Ray Treatment: — This is a term which has been used very carelessly, as there is really no such treatment. It has

usually been applied when a vacuum electrode is used, without regard to whether the current was a high-frequency or simply a high voltage one, either being sufficient to cause the violet color to appear in the electrode.

"Ultra-Violet Treatments: . . . as the ultraviolet ray will not penetrate the thinnest piece of mica or celluloid, the results which have been obtained when using the vacuum electrode are due to the form of current applied, and

not so much to the ultra-violet rays, which are given off from the sparks forming outside of the electrode."

Eventually, several cases appeared in front of U.S. Courts over the years concerning the claims given to the Violet Ray machines.

By the 1930s most (but not all) of the companies manufacturing Violet Rays decided to drop the "cure-all" claims, and resorted to selling them as beauty products,

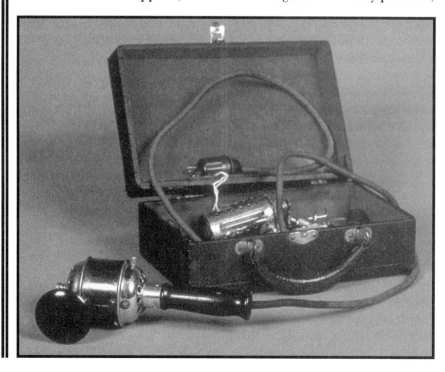

as some companies still do to this day. Companies such as Renulife attacked the quackery claims as they arose (from Renulife Violet Ray instruction manual, 1919): "There is no quackery or uncertainty about high frequency current. It is not claimed to be a 'cure-all.' Its effects are systematic as well as local, and therefore it treats fundamentally."

As to the actual construction of the machines, they are early forms of Tesla "Disruptive Discharge Coils," not to be confused with modern-day "Tesla Coils"

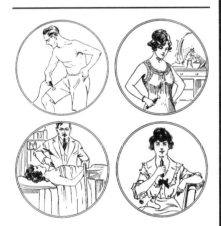

FOUR views showing proper application of Master Violet Ray devices.

which are of different design both physically and electrically. The outputs however are quite similar.

Different Violet Ray models can be run for longer periods of time than others due to better insulation of the resonator ("spark") coil to prevent inefficiency and overheating. Overheated coils produce weak sparks and can eventually burn out. Design characteristics were often the selling point of machines. Two-part machines were made to sell at high costs, because they can run for extended periods of time without needing the frequent "cooling off" periods that the one-piece units require.

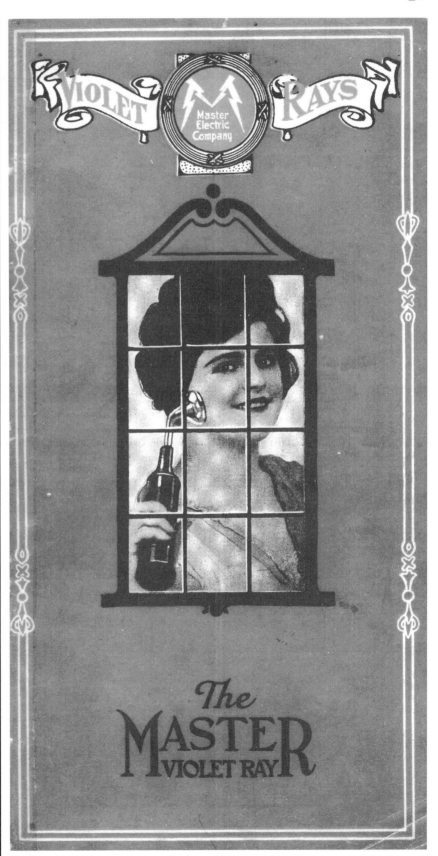

VIOLET RAYS

Master Electric Company

The MASTER VIOLET RAY

The Master Violet Rays are an example of many such devices that made a wide range of health and beauty claims. The FDA Ordered most of them seized in the 1950s, "because they were not capable of fulfilling the promises of benefit made for them." FDA Notice of Judgment 4168, June 1953.

The oscillator circuit consists of an electromagnetic interrupter that is used to rapidly charge a condenser to a high voltage and then discharge it through the primary of the disruptive discharge coil. This electromagnetic interrupter and condenser are essentially the same for all Violet Ray manufacturers.

Vacuum Electrodes

The one impossible goal for any collector is finding every single glass electrode made for these machines. Shelton Laboratories sold over 63 different electrodes. To complicate matters, many manufacturers sold tubes with different vacuums or contents. Standard vacuum electrodes are made of annealed Pyrex glass, with the exception of specialty tubes. Tubes made to produce X-rays were generally soda-lime glass, whereas tubes made specifically to transmit ultra-violet light were made of quartz. Because of the rarity of neon, argon, helium, etc., early tubes simply were partially vacuumed. A low pressure vacuum

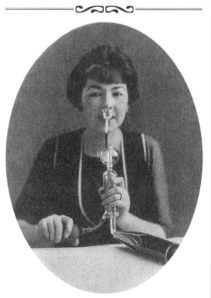

Optional Shelton ozone electrode.

resulted in a reddish to violet discharge, whereas a high vacuum would appear more of a white color. Neon filled tubes glow red-orange. Different vacuums and different gases conduct the sparks in different ways. Some physicians preferred tubes filled with salt water to conduct the electricity— these tubes were quite powerful, and never burned out. Obviously they did not light up in any way, but proved quite useful to conduct the electricity. Metal electrodes were also used. Cauterizing electrodes were made with platinum wire sealed into the glass, and were used to sear the skin with caustic sparks.

Tube shaped "Saturator" metal electrodes were sold for indirect treatments. The patient firmly gripped the metal electrode while the doctor turned the current on. The doctor could hold a glass electrode in his or her hand and draw sparks out of the patient using this method. Alternatively, the doctor may have held the metal electrode and conducted the electricity through his own body to a vacuum tube in his other hand and then to the patient for very mild treatments.

The metal electrodes should be noted as somewhat dangerous.

Should there be a mechanical fault with the tungsten interrupter contacts, there is a chance that the metal electrode would be charged to 120 volts from the wall circuit.

Today, Violet Ray machines are still manufactured for both industrial leak detection and as beauty products for the treatment of various skin conditions. Despite the trials and quackery claims of the Violet Ray machines for medical purposes, their scientific uses

Directions for Operation

From the Shelton Violet Ray manual, circa 1920s

1. Insert the Glass Applicator into the handle of machine.

2. Attach the plug to the lamp socket.

3. Turn the current on: first electric light switch; second, knob switch on the machine.

4. Turn the adjusting knob switch to the right or left also to increase or to diminish the Violet Ray discharge. Also give extra turn when finished to insure electric current is broken.

5. In orificial treatments, the electrode should be first inserted into the orifice without inserting it in the instrument. Then place Electrode No. 6 in the instrument. Hold this metal electrode against the metal cap of the electrode the current carries. This simple method will prevent the electrode from moving while inserted. Use lubricant on all orificial electrodes. (For physicians).

6. In the indirect treatment, the party to be treated should hold the instrument, with the metal Electrode No. 6 attached in hand. The current should then be turned on and some second party, with either hand, fingertips or another applicator, draw the current to the desired spot of the patient's body. The method can be used for body massage, facial massage and scalp treatment. No. 1 Applicator may be used in place of No. 6 although it is not so strong, and desired result is not so easily obtained.

7. Do not attempt to repair instrument, if the necessity arises, but write to the factory, advising of your difficulties, and we will inform you what to do.

8. *Do not use our* instrument in connection with any *tonic containing alcohol on the hair.*

9. Any treatment should be started with a mild current and gradually increased to the required strength.

10. When a treatment is completed, do not forget to turn off the current at the switch, or to be on the safe side, *remove plug from the electric light socket.* Damage arising from carelessness is not covered in our guarantee.

11. The standard winding for this instrument is 110 Volts. If voltage is higher or lower than 15 per cent, special windings or series resistances must be used to obtain best results. We will supply all necessary information upon request.

12. Take care of the connecting cords. They should be kept dry and free from knots and twists and must be repaired when signs of wear are apparent.

13. Should you break the glass Electrode off in the machine accidentally, simply take a pair of long-nose plyers and pull out the broken part.

ELECTRODES

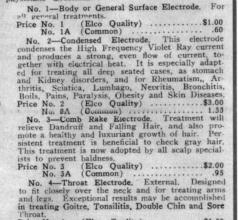

Elco Violet Ray Electrodes are made of special glass, blown by highly skilled experts. Each electrode must pass a special rigid laboratory test, to insure it being perfect in every detail. Inasmuch as electrodes are made of glass, we cannot guarantee them against breakage. Internal Electrodes should not be used except under physicians' directions.

No. 1—Body or General Surface Electrode. For all general treatments.
Price No. 1 (Elco Quality) $1.00
No. 1A (Common) .... .60

No. 2—Condensed Electrode. This electrode condenses the High Frequency Violet Ray current and produces a strong, even flow of current, together with electrical heat. It is especially adapted for treating all deep seated cases, as stomach and Kidney disorders, and for Rheumatism,, Arthritis, Sciatica, Lumbago, Neuritis, Bronchitis, Boils, Pains, Paralysis, Obesity and Skin Diseases.
Price No. 2 (Elco Quality) $3.00
No. 2A (Common) 1.55

No. 3—Comb Rake Electrode. Treatment will relieve Dandruff and Falling Hair, and also promote a healthy and luxuriant growth of hair. Persistent treatment is beneficial to check gray hair. This treatment is now adopted by all scalp specialists to prevent baldness.
Price No. 3 (Elco Quality) $2.00
No. 3A (Common) .... .95

No. 4—Throat Electrode. External. Designed to fit closely over the neck and for treating arms and legs. Exceptional results may be accomplished in treating Goitre, Tonsilitis, Double Chin and Sore Throat.
Price No. 4 (Elco Quality) $1.50
No. 4A (Common) .... .50

No. 5—Sensitive and Eye Electrode. This electrode is especially suited for delicate treatment of the Eye, Face, Forehead and around the Ear, Breast, etc. It is also suitable for treating Pimples, Blackheads, Wrinkles, Eczema, Facial Neuralgia, Inflammated Sinus condition and regular Facial treatments. Its shape permits it to fit snugly over the eye. With eye lid closed, treatments can be taken for weak eyes, stimulating Optic nerves, and for general eye troubles.
Price No. 5 (Elco Quality) $1.00
No. 5A (Common) .... .45

No. 6—Spinal Electrode. Is designed to fit both sides of vertebrae so that treatments may be applied to the nerve centers of the spine. (See chart.) "The Spinal Nerve Centers."
Price No. 6 (Elco Quality) $1.50
No. 6A (Common) .... .50

No. 7—Double Eye Electrode. For treating both eyes at the same time. Price $2.00

No. 8—Cataphoric Electrode. Made with an indentation so cotton saturated with liquids that do not contain alcohol can be used. Price $3.50

No. 10—Tongue or Spatula Electrode. For mouth or tongue treatment, and for crevices of the face or body. Price $1.00

No. 11—Ear Electrode (Insulated). For treating Deafness, especially Catarrhal Deafness, ringing in the ear, earache and chronic middle ear infections. Price $2.25

No. 12—Metal Saturator Electrode. This electrode is especially valuable in treating Anemia, Nervousness, Insomnia (sleeplessness), High Blood Pressure and for constitutional effects.
Price No. 12 (Elco Quality) $1.00
No. 12A (Common) .... .45

No. 14—Urethral Electrode. (Plain.)
Price $1.00

No. 15—Vaginal Electrode. (Plain.)
Price $1.00

PLAIN ELECTRODES

as Tesla Coils are quite numerous . . . and have remained one of the most popular and familiar "quack medical devices."

Rays and Ozone

Ozone generators made wonderful "healing ray" cures: their light was fluorescent, their sound was a static-like hum, and they gave off a gas—a gas said to purify and clean. These devices, another group of cure-alls, experienced a surge of popularity after World War II.

The U.S. Food and Drug Administration seized seven shipments of Radiant Ozone Generators, distributed by J. C. Gage and the Ozone Clinic of Kansas City, Missouri, in 1948

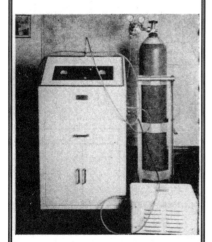

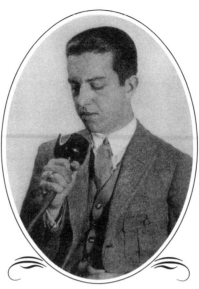

This method of Ozone treatment is built into Shelton's Outfits Nos. 205 and 206. This style, therefore, permits a greater volume of Ozone and is easily operated.

and 1949. The charge was "misbranding" and Mr. Gage denied the charge. The case went to trial on November 14, 1949, and on November 18th the case was sent to the jury. District Judge Duncan's charge to the jury, partly quoted here, was included in the Notice of Judgment:

"The intent with which H. C. Gage, the claimant, acted in making the shipments is not a question for your consideration in this case. The government is not required to prove a wrongful intent or an awareness of wrongdoing. It is not necessary for you to find that J. D. Gage intended to make false or misleading statements in the labeling. The question of whether Mr. Gage acted in good faith is not material in this case. It is sufficient for a finding for the Government that the statements complained of, or any one of them, be false or misleading regardless of whether Mr. Gate was aware that any false or misleading statement in labeling on the reader's mind is the same whether the

representations were made in good faith or not.

"It is the responsibility of the person who used the channels of interstate commerce for the distribution of devices to be assured that the labeling of the devices contain no false or misleading statement or representation. The statute places the burden of acting, at their own risk, upon person who ship devices. It does not place the risk on the public, who are largely helpless in this regard."

The jury deliberated less than three hours and found for the Government on all seven counts. Judgment of condemnation was entered and the devices and advertising were turned over to the FDA.

One of the prettiest devices at the Museum of Questionable Medical Devices is the Color-Therm, circa 1948-1952, a powerful ozone generator. The device features a wooden base holding six U-shaped curved tubes plus a hand applicator, and a wand consisting of one straight and two u-shaped curved tubes. The Color-Therm displays multi-colored lights similar to neon. The machine generates so much ozone that the seller instructed that "a suction fan should be installed in the room in which the Color-Therm operates so as to draw the ozone out of the room and thereby

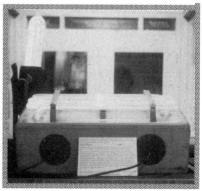

The Color-Therm.

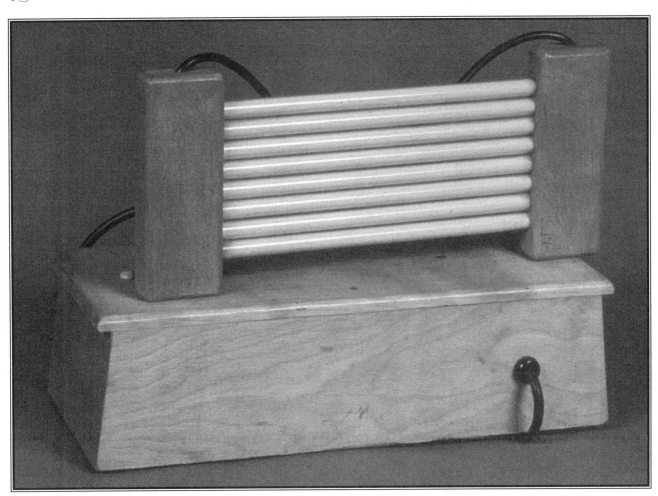

⊕ The Ozonator. ⊕

This device from 1953 provided an electrical discharge from tubes when activated, and was described by the Manufacturer as "Ozone, God's Gift to Humanity." It was misbranded with false and misleading statements, and claimed that it was effective in treating all kinds of ailments and diseases, including: asthma, all respiratory diseases, cardiovascular and renal disease. It also supposedly made one more active physically, psychologically, and sexually. The attachment of tubes on the top can be picked up and scanned over the affected parts of the body.

prevent breathing an excess amount." Treatments of 10-30 minutes were recommended one or more times a day.

The manufacturer falsely claimed that the Color-Therm was "similar to Short Wave [for] it creates an electric field thereby producing heat." The device was alleged to treat sprains, strains, tendon injuries, sinusitis, inflammatory pelvic conditions, iritis, pleurisy, osteo-arthritis, bursitis, and muscle pain. To this list, the

seller offered a final caveat: "There is no such thing as a cure for any condition that I may mention. It is only to assist and up to the doctors desecretion [sic]." Eight devices were seized by the U.S. Food and Drug Administration in 1951 and on December 31, 1952, the devices were condemned by the Northern District Court of Oklahoma and ordered dismantled.

The Vigoray (ca. 1948) was manufactured in Seattle, Washington. Its literature sought

to reassure consumers that concentrated ozone was not dangerous, citing laboratory tests with ozone generators running in a room 50 x 40 feet (about half the size of a city lot).

X-rays

In the late 1940s and early 1950s, the shoe-fitting X-ray unit was a common shoe store sales promotion device and nearly all stores had one. It was estimated

---

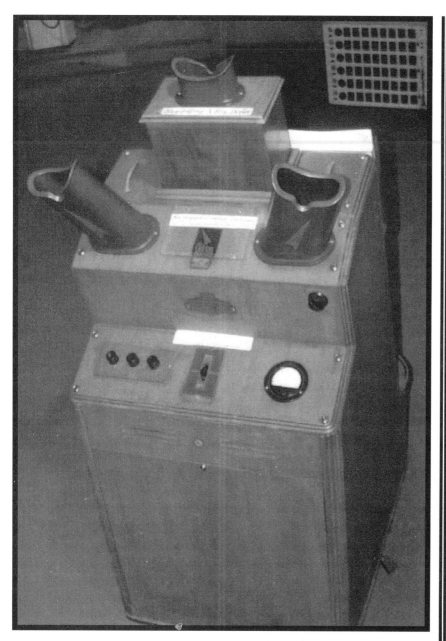

THE ADRIAN SHOE-FITTING X-RAY MACHINE.

three viewing ports at the top of the cabinet, where the customer, the salesperson, and a third person (your mother?) could view the image at the same time.

The radiation hazards associated with shoe fitting X-ray units were recognized as early as 1950. The machines were often out of adjustment and were so poorly constructed that radiation leaked into the surrounding area. By 1970, shoe fitting X-ray units had been banned in 33 states and strict regulation in the remaining 17 states made their operation impractical. Believe it or not, this particular shoe-fitting X-ray unit was found in 1981 in a department store in Madison, West Virginia. It was still being used in the store's shoe department! When it was pointed out to the store managers that it was against West Virginia law to operate a shoe-fitting X-ray unit, they donated it to the U.S. Food and Drug Administration.

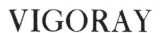
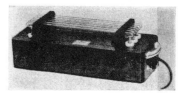
that there were 10,000 of these devices in use. The shoe-fitting X-ray unit pictured above was produced by the dominant company in the field, the Adrian X-ray Company of Milwaukee WI, now defunct. Brooks Stevens, a noted industrial designer whose works included the Milwaukee Road Olympian and an Oscar Meyer Wienermobile, designed this machine.

The primary component of a shoe-fitting X-ray unit was the fluoroscope, which consisted essentially of an X-ray tube mounted near the floor and wholly or partially enclosed in a shielded box and a fluorescent screen. The X-rays penetrated the shoes and feet and then struck the fluorescent light. This resulted in an image of the feet within the shoes. The fluorescent image was reflected to

Invisible Rays:
The Solarama Bedboard

The Solarama Bedboard is a quack medical device most of us could make at home. Cut two squares of laminated wall paneling, insert an asbestos pad in the middle, and enclose with aluminum trim. Drill a hole through the center of one edge of the aluminum trim. Run a cord attached to a plug from this hole—be sure to cap off the wire ends inside the device. Beyond this, there is no internal wiring. The final step is the hardest to accomplish: finish the device with a clear coating of Vital Solutions paint. Regrettably, the paint is no longer available.

This device, according to the World of Solarama, Ltd. and Solarama distributors from Daytona to Detroit to San Bernadino, treated headache, bursitis, and paralysis; cured cancer; served as an anesthetic; promoted "electrosleep"; controled blood pressure; and regenerated heart muscle, body organs, and missing limbs! This device sold for $150 in the mid-1970s and the company claimed to have sold over 150,000!

This worthless device proved so popular that knock-offs appeared on the market. The Solarama manufacturer issued a warning that purchasers should not be fooled by imitations, but should insist on the genuine Solarama Board! Quacks do not take kindly to their turf being invaded.

Solar Energizer,
Modern Day Amulet

Our modern day amulet claims to exchange solar power for human energy. It also claims to reduce tension, improve sleep, and reduce pain. The only way it can achieve

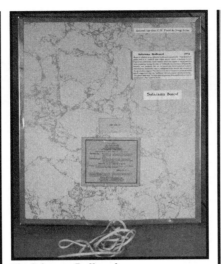

The Solarama Bedboard.

these is by relying on the wearer's faith, for the solar technology in this device is fatally flawed. The Solar Energizer therapeutic necklace was patented in 1979, before most people were familiar with solar power (solar-powered calculators had yet to become a common device). Today, the technology remains relatively uncommon, but most people know that photovoltaic cells (solar cells) generate electricity. Passive solar power, of course, collects heat.

The pendant includes a series of small connected wires encased in acrylic which are supposed to represent a solar cell. The wire configuration is reminiscent of a computer chip in appearance. The patent papers and product literature, despite their technical drawings, fail to explain how electricity might be converted to human energy.

The alleged electricity is supposed to be transferred from the pendant to the necklace chains and absorbed directly by the skin. Of course, the wearer feels nothing for there is nothing to be felt. The Solar Energizer was judged to be misbranded in 1991, but has reappeared in the marketplace today via the internet. The current selling price is $24.99.

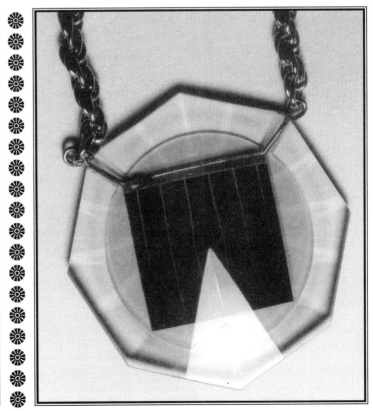

THE SOLAR ENERGIZER.

PSYCHOLOGY

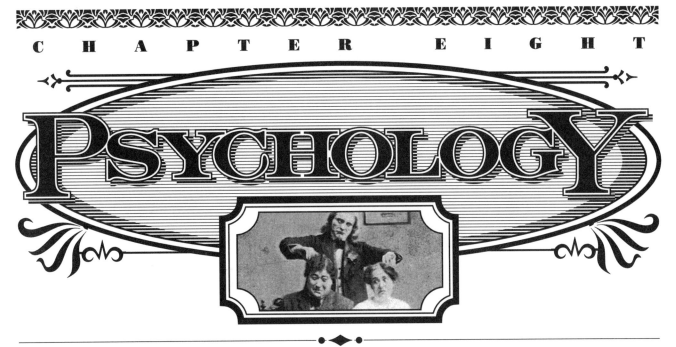

USE YOUR HEAD–
THE BUMPY HISTORY OF PHRENOLOGY.

Although many questionable scientific ideas were intended to improve the physical health of the body, a few have focused largely on the mind. Phrenology, a popular "pseudoscience" throughout the nineteenth century, is a prime example of this, as the phrenologists felt the head shape of their patients to gauge their "moral constitution"–and then prescribed a dose of practical advice on top of it.

Phrenology had its beginnings in the 1790s, when Austrian physician Franz Joseph Gall developed an intricate system to pinpoint the precise regions of the brain that influenced specific intellectual abilities, talents, and personality traits (called "mental faculties" or "organs of the brain"). Gall developed this system after making head observations of numerous individuals and concluding that people whose heads were prominent in certain areas tended to share certain characteristics. For example, after observing that people with great linguistic ability tended to have large, protruding eyes, Gall reasoned that the faculty for "Language" sat in an area of the brain found behind the eyes. Noticing that thieves tended to have large prominences directly above the ears, Gall concluded that the part of the brain that controlled "Acquisitiveness" (interest in wealth) was located there.

Gall and his student Johann Spurzheim located about 30 faculties in all, which measured traits rang-

ing from "Secretiveness" to "Mirthfulness." According to their theory, the larger the bump in each area meant that the larger the brain was in that area and the more potential someone had. Many of the categories had vocational applications. For example, having a large

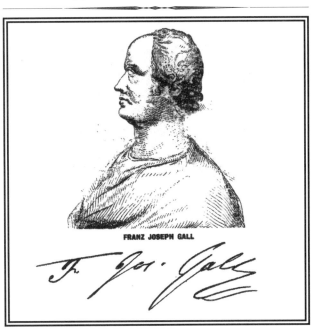

DR. FRANZ JOSEPH GALL

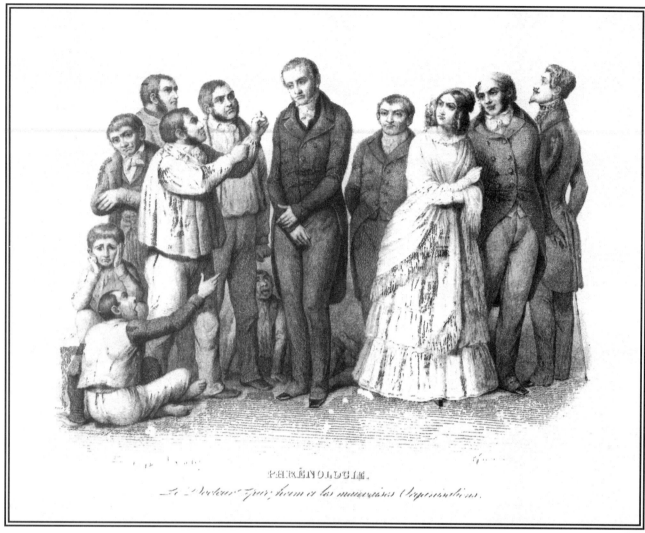

PHRÉNOLOGIE.

A lithograph showing Dr. Spurzheim seemingly flanked by depictions of character traits. The lithograph was created by Dr. Spurzheim's son.

organ of "Tune" meant you were a born musician. A large organ of "Calculation" meant you were naturally good at math. Some of the faculties measured the ability to deal with other people, from strangers to children to spouses. Finally, some faculties of the brain dealt with physical and mental health as well. Here are some examples:

• "Vitativeness" measured physical endurance. People with small bumps in this area supposedly were prone to illnesses.

• Too much "Alimentiveness" (desire for nourishment) could

lead to obesity. Too little might lead to malnutrition.

• A very large organ of "Bibativeness" (love of liquids) could lead to alcoholism.

• Too much "Cautiousness" might give you needless stress and anxiety.

• Without enough "Hope," people tend to become melancholic (or chronically depressed).

• Too much "Spirituality" (sometimes called "Wonder" or "Faith") might cause you to hallucinate or suffer from delusions.

Many physicians questioned the validity of phrenology from its

onset, and lectures on phrenology were banned in Vienna in 1802, as many people worried that the idea that brain shape reflected personality sounded too "deterministic"—as though people had no free will. Others complained that phrenology indicated that human beings weren't equal, as different people received significantly higher intellectual or emotional scores than others.

But critics did not prevent Gall's ideas from spreading to other parts of Europe during the early nineteenth century. For one thing, many of phrenology's strongest

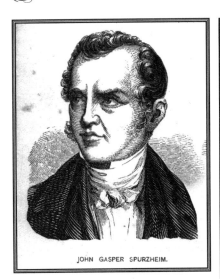

JOHN GASPER SPURZHEIM.

Dr. Johann Spurzheim

supporters were not trained scientists, but converts who thought that phrenological descriptions of their own personalities sounded accurate. A prime example of this is Edinburgh lawyer-turned-phrenologist George Combe, who introduced sizable numbers of intellectuals to the principles of head-reading during his popular U.S. lecture tour of 1838–1840. This was a time when there was broad public interest in sciences that involved basic observations and that had straightforward applications in daily life.

The Fowler Brothers

Phrenology really took off in the United States because of the company that brothers Orson and Lorenzo Fowler founded in 1835, only a few years after the deaths of Gall and Spurzheim. Headquartered in New York City, the Fowler company became the heart of phrenology in nineteenth-century America, and the leading publisher of phrenology books. Ordinary Americans easily grasped the basics of phrenology, and tourists flocked to the Fowlers' well-publicized

"phrenological cabinet," which included anatomical drawings, cranial reproductions of famous people, and numerous skulls of humans and animals.

At the Fowler company, visitors could pay for a detailed "phrenological examination" to learn about their dispositions and receive advice concerning their careers, relationships, and well-being. An exam might take an hour or so, as the phrenologist felt the various sections of a customer's head and recorded a number for each region. The higher the number, the more potential someone had. "Know thyself" was the Fowlers' motto. In addition to learning more about themselves, some people

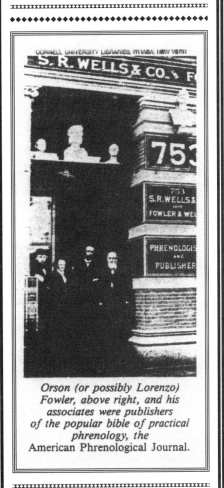

Orson (or possibly Lorenzo)
Fowler, above right, and his
associates were publishers
of the popular bible of practical
phrenology, the
American Phrenological Journal.

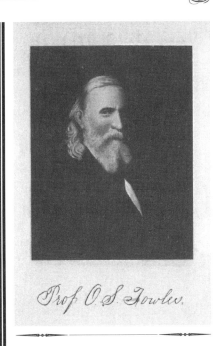

Prof. O. S. Fowler.

may have enjoyed the intimacy of phrenology as well. After all, phrenologists made physical contact with the face and head while providing customers with detailed personal information—which may or may not have been accurate.

The Fowler brothers, and other self-taught students of head shapes, confidently promoted phrenology as a "science"—perhaps the most rigorous or beneficial of all sciences. Yet as a group they did not refer to themselves as "scientists," often using the term "practical phrenologists" instead.

Although Nathan Allen, the first editor of the Philadelphia-based American Phrenological Journal, had attended medical school, he was the exception not the rule among phrenologists. Orson Fowler, for example, had been studying to become a minister when he decided to practice phrenology instead. A number of prominent Americans became strong supporters of phrenology,

continued on page 140

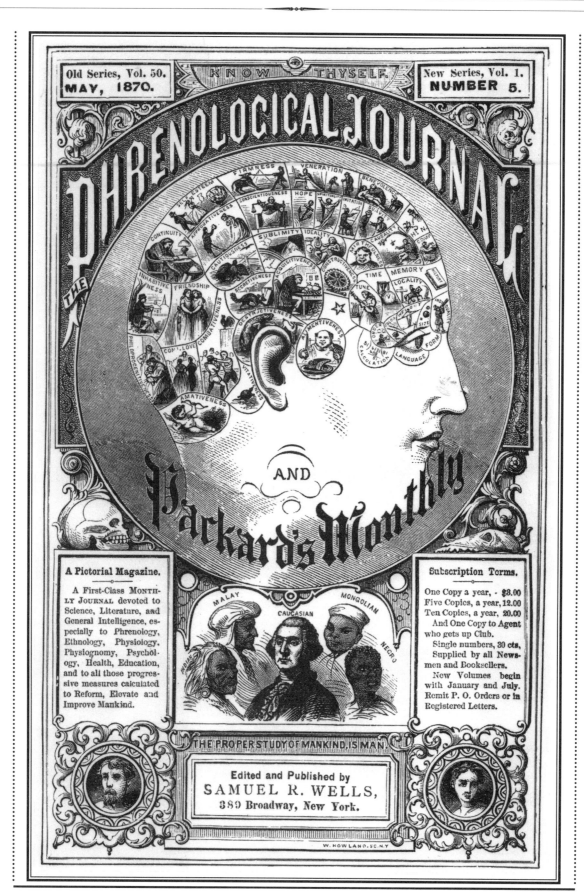

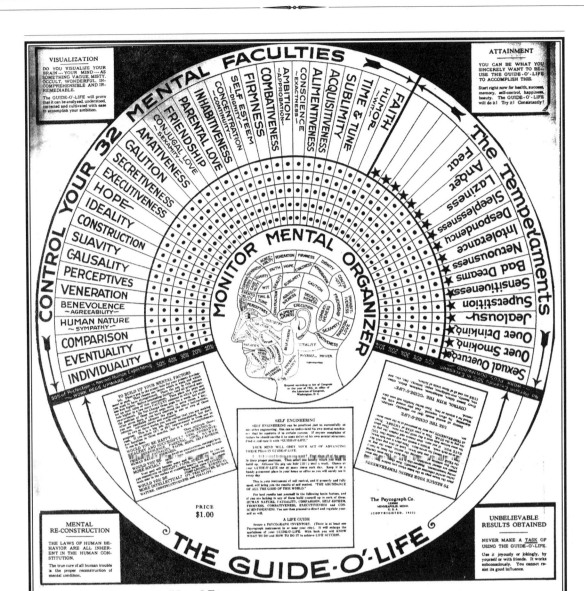

Definitions of the Mental Factors

INDIVIDUALITY, Observation—desire to see and examine for yourself.
EVENTUALITY, Memory of facts and circumstances.
COMPARISON, Inductive reasoning—analysis—illustration.
HUMAN NATURE, Perception of character and motives of others.
BENEVOLENCE, Kindness—goodness—sympathy—philanthropy.
VENERATION, Reverence for sacred things—devotion—respect.
PERCEPTIVES,
 SIZE, Cognizance of magnitude—measuring by the eye.
 WEIGHT, Balancing—climbing—perception of the law of gravity.
 COLOR, Perception and judgment of colors, and love of them.
 ORDER, Perception and love of method—system—arrangement.
 CALCULATION, Cognizance of numbers—mental arithmetic.
CAUSALITY, Applying causes to effect—originality.
SUAVITY, AGREEABLENESS, Pleasantness—persuasiveness.
CONSTRUCTIVENESS, Ability to formulate mentally or actually.
IDEALITY, Refinement—love of beauty—taste—purity.
HOPE, Expectation—enterprise—anticipation.
EXECUTIVENESS—force—energy—Leadership.
SECRETIVENESS—Discretion—reserve—policy—management.
CAUTION, Prudence—provision—watchfulness.
AMATIVENESS, Love between the sexes—desire to marry.
CONJUGAL LOVE, Matrimony—love of one—union for life.
FRIENDSHIP, Adhesiveness—sociability—love of society.
PARENTAL LOVE, Regard for offspring.
INHABITIVENESS, Love of home—being in your own town, state, country.
CONCENTRATIVENESS—Ability to think deeply and to analyze thoroughly.
SELF-ESTEEM, Self-respect—independence—dignity.
FIRMNESS, Decision—perseverance—stability—tenacity of will.
COMBATIVENESS, Resistance—defense—courage—opposition.
APPROBATIVENESS, Ambition—display—love of praise.
CONSCIENTIOUSNESS, Integrity—love of right—justice—equity.
ALIMENTIVENESS, Appetite—hunger—love of eating. Most Americans eat too much and are diseased and starving. Learn about wrong and right foods. Send for "Right Living" and save and prolong your life.

ACQUISITIVENESS, Accumulation—frugality—economy.
SUBLIMITY, Love of grandeur—infinitude—the endless.
TIME and TUNE—Cognizance of duration and succession of time—punctuality. Sense of harmony and melody—love of music.
HUMOR, MIRTHFULNESS—Perception of the absurd—jocoseness—wit—fun.
FAITH, SPIRITUALITY, Intuition—faith—"light within"—credulity.

COPYRIGHTED 1932—BY FRANK P. WHITE, MINNEAPOLIS, MINN.

YOU

You can be self-guiding, self-directing and self-sustaining. You should proceed immediately to develop any faculty that hinders you from doing your best. You have an absolute right to do your best if you are sincere. It is not only your right but your duty. To do your best you may have to develop certain faculties that are now crippling you. The way to develop a faculty is to specially use it. To specially use it is to first clearly understand it. Second, to intelligently, systematically and continuously put it into use. You can do this if you will thoroughly use the "Guide-O'-Life." You can specially call into action a faculty as certainly as you can intentionally and individually use one arm and not the other.

You have control over your body to a great degree in directing your hands and feet. You can have the same individual control over your faculties. You can direct them intelligently, systematically and at your pleasure. Therefore, you can specially use one or more faculties and not specially use the others. **This causes a corresponding additional amount of blood to flow directly to the brain organs of the faculties used.** This is a basis of special brain growth. This particular part of the brain receives additional blood and this contains the elements out of which new cells, fibers, arteries and veins are built. This may all be added to the amount of brain than you have already in this particular part. This is brain growth.

THE GUIDE O' LIFE accompanied Psycograph readings to help clients understand and improve themselves.

including poet Walt Whitman, who met the Fowlers in 1849 and became a longtime believer in phrenology.

Following in the Footsteps of the Fowlers

Meanwhile, other phrenologists opened shops in other parts of the United States or traveled from town to town earning money by doing personality readings. Phrenologists tried to note differences in the head sizes and body types of people from different parts of the world, and they even wrote about the phrenology of animals, including dogs, apes, and horses. Many phrenologists also practiced "physiognomy," an older system that linked personality traits to facial features (including eye color, ear size, and nose length), as well as the shape of the body as a whole.

Phrenologists advised parents how to raise their children based on head size and shape. Over time, phrenology became increasingly popular as part of the larger self-improvement, health, and hygiene movements in the United States, including the anti-tobacco movement, dress reforms against tight-waisted women's clothing, water cures, and the humane treatment of prisoners.

Phrenology provided American physicians with a rational and practical framework to explain and treat mental illness. Instead of searching for religiously based explanations such as possession by evil spirits, the *American Journal of Insanity* began reporting that lack of exercise or too much tobacco might damage specific regions of the brain. Those physicians who believed in the principles of phrenology sometimes used

leeches to drain blood from portions of the head believed to correspond to overdeveloped characteristics, such as "Combativeness."

Into the 1850s, phrenology books and articles regularly discussed the healing powers of mesmerism and the existence of clairvoyance, which was associated with the phrenological region of "Spirituality" (or "Faith"). But this support of spiritualism didn't last. Phrenology publications later warned that such feelings were too speculative and were signs of injury to the brain. During this period of growing skepticism, phrenological publications moved away from discussion of miracle cures, although they still included large amounts of easy-to-use medical information, promoting the benefits of eating a healthy diet or getting enough exercise.

In the 1851 book *A Defense of Phrenology* (published by the Fowlers), A. Boardman wrote: "We look upon phrenology as among the first of human sciences in interest and importance–as a science which not only furnishes us with the true physiology of the brain, but of a science pregnant with more important influences than the revelations of Galileo."

As the nineteenth century progressed, phrenologists proposed more faculties than the initial faculties proposed by Gall and Spurtzheim. New people trained to become phrenologists, either as apprentices or by studying at the American Institute of Phrenology–which the Fowler company established in New York City in 1866, and which offered coursework in phrenology and anatomy. Ironically, although many prominent phrenologists warned against impostors and charlatans within the field, a

number of scientists had already grown frustrated with the science. By now, European and American physicians were condemning all phrenologists (or "bumpologists"), and complained about their inconclusive evidence. The phrenologists' certainty in the accuracy of their intricate map of the brain prevented them from doing further research on the subject.

Phrenology Receives a Blow to the Head

The "science" of phrenology suffered a critical blow to the head in 1861 when French anthropologist Paul Broca announced convincing evidence that the area of the brain that governed speech was not localized under the eyeballs, as Gall had thought. When responding to critics, the phrenologists often compared themselves to astronomers who, too, had been attacked by what one phrenologist called the "pseudo learned." In the years that followed, early neuroscientists found further evidence that regionalized activity within the brain was not configured as Gall had described. The phrenologists, for example, did not know about the distinctions between the right and left sides of the brain.

But longtime phrenologists continued to believe that their system was based solidly on fact. In the 1875 book *The Mysteries of the Head and Heart Explained,* J. Stanley Grimes wrote: "When you begin to examine strangers, do not guess at anything; confine your remarks to the organs and combinations that are so decidedly developed or deficient that if phrenology is true you cannot be mistaken."

In some respects, the phrenologists sent their customers mixed messages, encouraging them to be skeptical, to learn more about science and health, and yet to accept a set of conclusions about the body and mind that most physicians no longer believed to be true. So it is no surprise that more people came to the conclusion that the phrenologists had been mistaken, especially as the fields of psychology, psychiatry, and neuroscience expanded during the late nineteenth and early twentieth centuries. By this time, most phrenologists and phrenology publications had gone out of business.

Today, intelligence tests and vocational testing have replaced phrenology as a way to measure aptitude and reasoning skills. Meanwhile, practitioners of "reflexology" have filled the shoes of the phrenologists, so to speak, by studying personality traits not by looking at the shape of someone's head, but by analyzing their feet. Additionally, neuroscientists know substantially more about the ways that specific parts of the brain control specific skills. In 1999, for example, Canadian scientists reported that the physical structure of Albert Einstein's brain was well developed in the area now believed to control mathematical reasoning. Although people no longer study phrenology the way that Franz Gall did two hundred years ago, they remain fascinated in finding links between the body and the mind.

Psycograph—Phrenology's Foremost Device

Phrenology was in its dying days during the early twentieth century, as even the general public was beginning to doubt the notion that you could judge someone's intelligence and character by the size and shape of their head. But Henry C. Lavery of Superior, Wisconsin, was no skeptic. Not only did Lavery believe phrenology was true, but he was so dedicated to this field of study that he created new interest in phrenology by inventing a complicated device in 1905 called the Psycograph, which could measure the shape of a person's head and then give them a lengthy assessment of their personality based on those measurements.

In 1931, Lavery went into business with Frank P. White, who had taken his life savings of $38,000 out of the stock of a local sandpaper manufacturer (called 3M) to finance a new company operating the Psycograph. Whereas

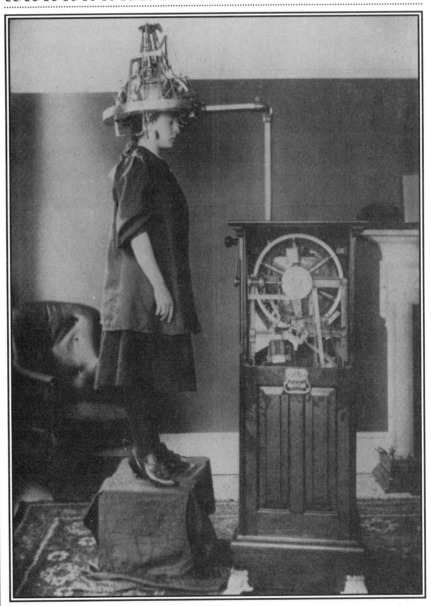

THE FIRST PSYCOGRAPH MADE BY LAVERY, PATENTED IN 1905. IT WEIGHED 1,000 POUNDS AND HE COULDN'T GET IT OUT OF HIS HOUSE.

an experienced phrenologist in the past might require an hour to feel the customer's head and write down the measurements of each area, the Psycograph could give someone a detailed personality printout in only five minutes! Accurate or not, the Psycograph was both a gimmick and a labor-saving device.

The Psycograph consists of 1,954 parts housed in a metal carrier with a motor-driven belt inside a wooden cabinet containing statements about 32 different mental faculties. For each category, the Psycograph prints out a measurement on a 1 to 5 scale, ranging from "Deficient" to "Very Superior." There are 160 statements in all, with up to 32 appearing on each printout.

The scores are determined by various probes, each with five contact points in the headpiece, making contact with the head. The customer sits in a chair connected to the machine and the headpiece is lowered and adjusted to fit snugly. The operator then pulls back a lever that activates the belt-driven motor, which then receives low-voltage signals from the headpiece and stamps out the appropriate statement for each faculty, beginning with "Individuality" and ending with "Faith." The customer sitting in the chair does not feel any type of shock or sensation during the measurement, other than the round ends of the probes and the weight of the headpiece. When wearing the Psycograph headpiece today, people report a wide range of sensations, saying the prongs feel ticklish, massaging, or strange.

Because the Psycograph printouts are based on actual head measurements, people with large

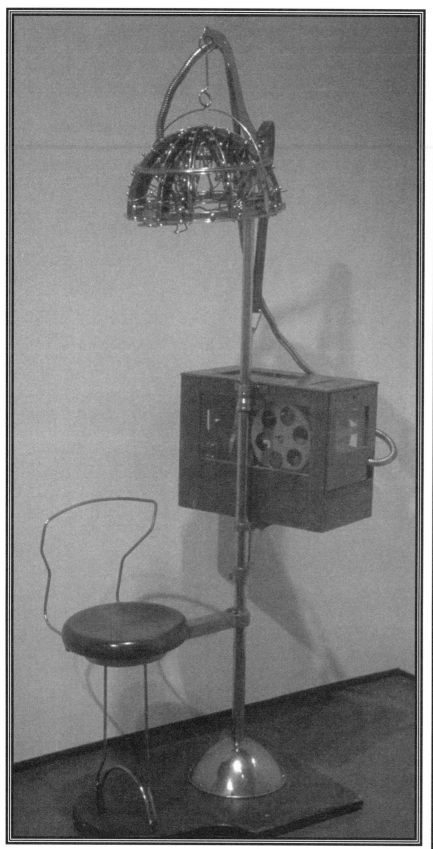

THE PSYCOGRAPH.

heads tend to get high scores. With the number ranking of each area comes a piece of advice. Because the Psycograph measures head sizes, not brainwaves, it cannot tell that a human is sitting in the chair, or just how far the prongs are pushed out. So a large watermelon will appear to be very superior in many areas, while an orange will be deficient in those same categories.

Some sample statements appear below:

5 EVENTUALITY—Very Superior—Be tolerant of other people who lack the keen sense of eventuality which you possess. Do not burden memory with use-less detail.

2 VENERATION—Low Average —Respect for authority might well be developed. See that material interests do not entirely supplant the moral and ethical.

3 PERCEPTIVES—Average— In general your judgment of size, weight, color, number and order is satisfactory. Specific interests may neces-sitate more development.

3 SUAVITY—Average—You can be pleasant, polite, and tactful with others, but with many people you achieve more by exercising more diplomacy and courtesy.

2 CONSTRUCTIVENESS— Low Average—The studied use of tools, instruments, and mechanical construction will aid to develop this. Learn to adjust and adapt.

2 IDEALITY—Low Average— Don't be too "matter of fact" about cultural things of life. Turn attention more to an appreciation of the fine and beautiful.

3 EXECUTION—Average— Your energy tends toward average achievement. Situations may demand severe measures. Cultivate thorough-going action.

3 SECRETIVENESS— Average—Guard against imprudent speech and action. Frankness may sometimes be a handicap.

Sincerity may not need to be advertised.

4 CAUTION—Superior—Self solicitude is admirable if not carried to extremes. A habit of apprehension should not prevent normal and beneficial activity.

continued on page 146

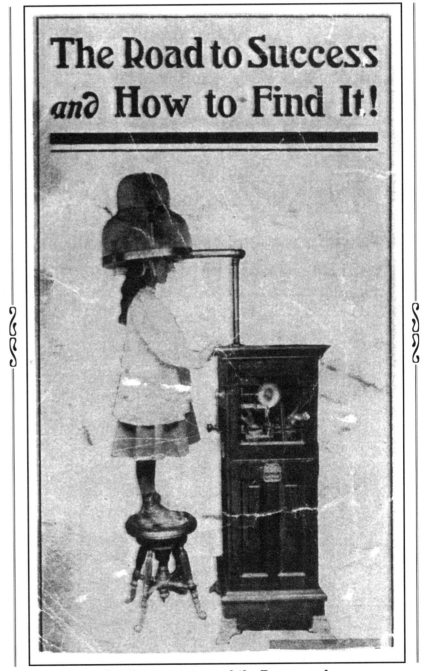

The Road to Success and How to Find It!

Another prototype of the Psycograph.

PSYCOGRAPH
KNOW THYSELF!

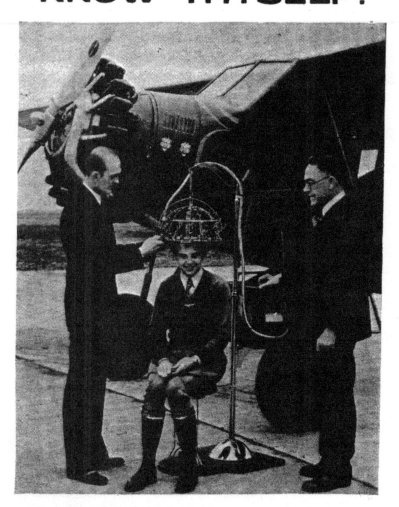

Measures thirty-two mental faculties and prints record, rating each faculty from 1 to 5, with an explanation of each development. It will bring out your strong and weak characteristics. It will help parents understand their children. Vocational chart given with each measurement. No one sees your reading but you.

SEE YOURSELF AS OTHERS SEE YOU!

Henry C. Lavery (right), self-proclaimed "profound thinker" and inventor of the Psycograph, watching a pilot being assessed. To find out about his mechanical skills, perhaps?

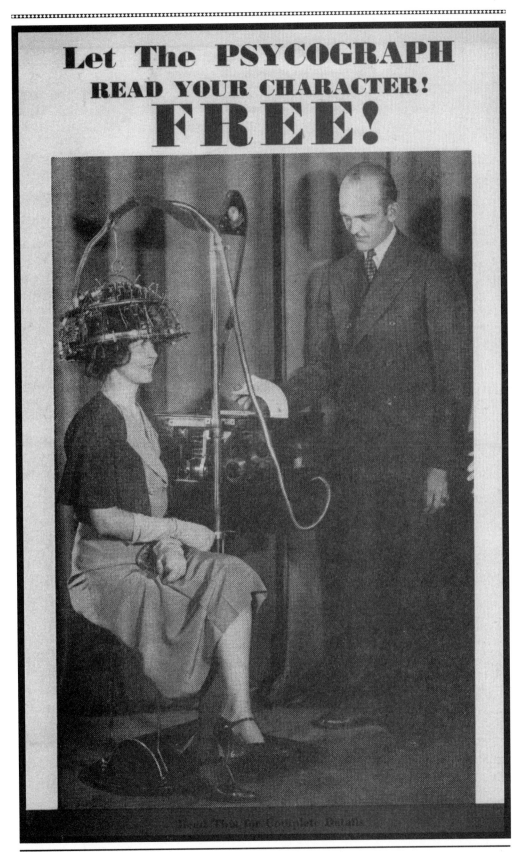

Brochure used to promote Psycograph readings in theaters.

3 AMATIVENESS—Average—You have capacity for a healthy affection of a mate. Exercise appreciation of love and strive for congenial companionship.

2 SEXAMITY—Low Average—A normal love life is essential to health and happiness.

Cultivate your erotic nature. Don't allow your mate to be love-starved.

3 INHABITIVENESS—Average—Appreciation of home may not prevent you from traveling to distant fields if more inviting.

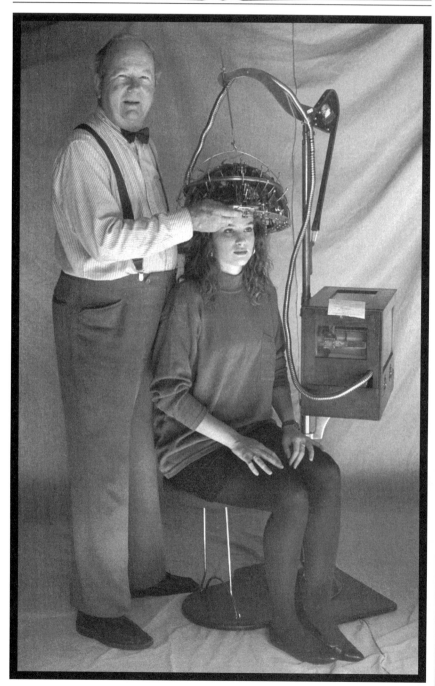

 Bob McCoy interviews a potential museum staff member.

Domestic tendency may be cultivated.

1 FRIENDSHIP—Deficient—You need to be more gregarious and sociable. Superficial interest in people not enough. Concrete friendship is superior.

5 CONTINUITY—Very superior—Great capacity for consistent application. Power of association of ideas should be balanced by ability to disconnect.

1 DIGNITY—Deficient—Sublimate your feeling of inadequacy and inferiority by expressing your value to society in many small services to many people.

4 FIRMNESS—Superior—Learn to yield when flexibility is of mutual benefit. Stability of character is invaluable when used constructively and unselfishly.

4 COMBATIVENESS—Superior—Don't go around with a chip on your shoulder, but maintain your defenses. Continue to overcome obstacles. Be aggressive but just.

4 APPROBATION—Superior—Love of display and respect for public opinion may be maintained if not offensive. Continue to win admiration.

4 EXACTNESS—Superior—Your tendency to be accurate and pain-staking will serve you well if you do not demand the same degree from all others. Be tolerant.

1 ACQUISITIVENESS—Deficient—You should cultivate a desire for possessions and a sense of material value. Visualize wealth and personal property values.

4 SUBLIMITY—Superior—A high degree of appreciation

of the magnificent and stupendous gives you exaltation and nobility. Exercise this quality consistently.

3 WIT—Average—Try to get fun and mirth out of life. Smile and joke with others and improve your wit. You need to appreciate more of the ludicrous in life.

In addition to getting a personality printout, customers also received a chart they could use to calculate their success rate for numerous careers, from "Aviator" to "Zeppelin Attendant," as different occupations needed different personality traits. For example, "Radio Announcer" needed a good amount of "Wit," but a "Detective" did not. A "Stenographer" needed

to do well in "Exactness," whereas a "Sailor" needed good "Perceptives."

About 40 Psycographs were built, and the local business in Minneapolis flourished. The machines were leased to entrepreneurs throughout the area for $2,000 down plus $35 a month. They were popular attractions for

continued on page 151

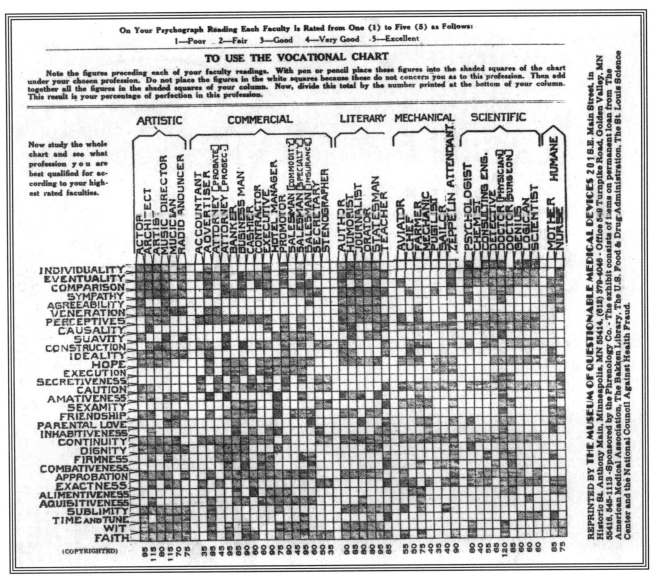

The Vocational Chart.

BASED ON THE PSYCOGRAPH READING, A CLIENT COULD FILL IN THE SHADOWED AREAS TO FIND A SUITABLE VOCATION.

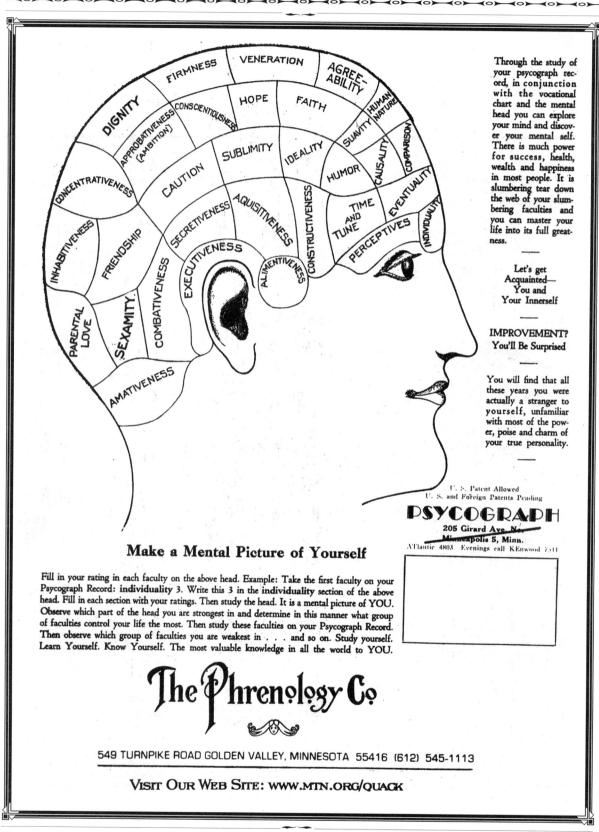

Through the study of your psycograph record, in conjunction with the vocational chart and the mental head you can explore your mind and discover your mental self. There is much power for success, health, wealth and happiness in most people. It is slumbering tear down the web of your slumbering faculties and you can master your life into its full greatness.

Let's get
Acquainted—
You and
Your Innerself

IMPROVEMENT?
You'll Be Surprised

You will find that all these years you were actually a stranger to yourself, unfamiliar with most of the power, poise and charm of your true personality.

U. S. Patent Allowed
U. S. and Foreign Patents Pending

PSYCOGRAPH
205 Girard Ave. N.
Minneapolis 5, Minn.
ATlantic 4803　Evenings call KEnwood 7311

Make a Mental Picture of Yourself

Fill in your rating in each faculty on the above head. Example: Take the first faculty on your Psycograph Record: individuality 3. Write this 3 in the individuality section of the above head. Fill in each section with your ratings. Then study the head. It is a mental picture of YOU. Observe which part of the head you are strongest in and determine in this manner what group of faculties control your life the most. Then study these faculties on your Psycograph Record. Then observe which group of faculties you are weakest in . . . and so on. Study yourself. Learn Yourself. Know Yourself. The most valuable knowledge in all the world to YOU.

The Phrenology Co

549 TURNPIKE ROAD GOLDEN VALLEY, MINNESOTA 55416 (612) 545-1113

VISIT OUR WEB SITE: WWW.MTN.ORG/QUACK

The reverse side of the vocational chart shows the character trait associated with each part of the head according to Dr. Gall.

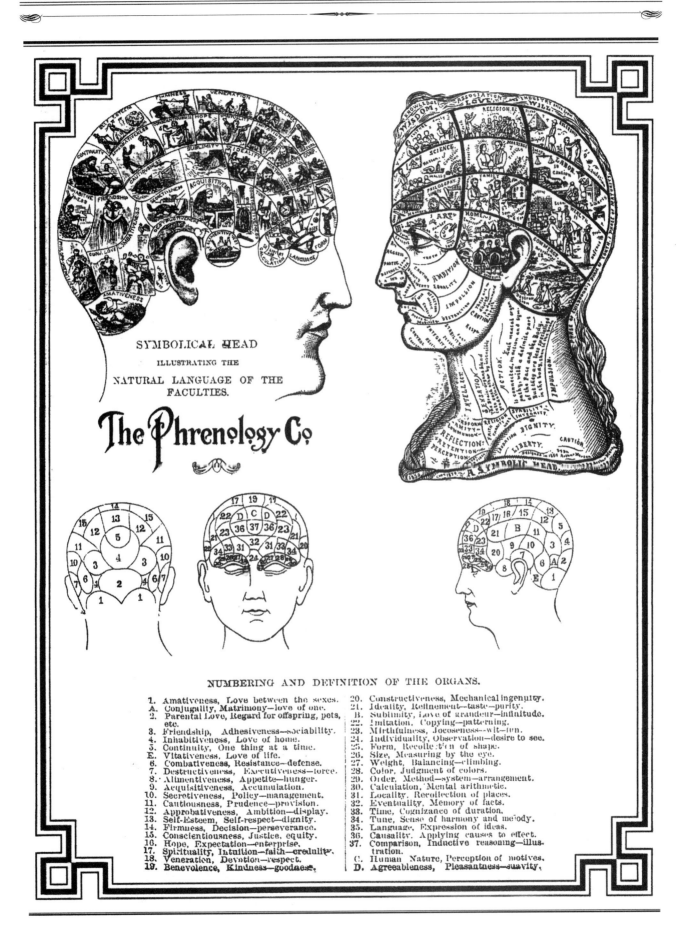

SYMBOLICAL HEAD

ILLUSTRATING THE

NATURAL LANGUAGE OF THE
FACULTIES.

The Phrenology Co.

NUMBERING AND DEFINITION OF THE ORGANS.

1. Amativeness, Love between the sexes.
A. Conjugality, Matrimony—love of one.
2. Parental Love, Regard for offspring, pets, etc.
3. Friendship, Adhesiveness—sociability.
4. Inhabitiveness, Love of home.
5. Continuity, One thing at a time.
E. Vitativeness, Love of life.
6. Combativeness, Resistance—defense.
7. Destructiveness, Executiveness—force.
8. Alimentiveness, Appetite—hunger.
9. Acquisitiveness, Accumulation.
10. Secretiveness, Policy—management.
11. Cautiousness, Prudence—provision.
12. Approbativeness, Ambition—display.
13. Self-Esteem, Self-respect—dignity.
14. Firmness, Decision—perseverance.
15. Conscientiousness, Justice, equity.
16. Hope, Expectation—enterprise.
17. Spirituality, Intuition—faith—credulity.
18. Veneration, Devotion—respect.
19. Benevolence, Kindness—goodness.

20. Constructiveness, Mechanical ingenuity.
21. Ideality, Refinement—taste—purity.
B. Sublimity, Love of grandeur—infinitude.
22. Imitation, Copying—patterning.
23. Mirthfulness, Jocoseness—wit—fun.
24. Individuality, Observation—desire to see.
25. Form, Recollection of shape.
26. Size, Measuring by the eye.
27. Weight, Balancing—climbing.
28. Color, Judgment of colors.
29. Order, Method—system—arrangement.
30. Calculation, Mental arithmetic.
31. Locality, Recollection of places.
32. Eventuality, Memory of facts.
33. Time, Cognizance of duration.
34. Tune, Sense of harmony and melody.
35. Language, Expression of ideas.
36. Causality, Applying causes to effect.
37. Comparison, Inductive reasoning—illustration.
C. Human Nature, Perception of motives.
D. Agreeableness, Pleasantness—suavity.

The Evansville Press

SATURDAY, AUG. 5, 1933

Chief Wiltshire Uses 'Head Reading' Machine To Check Up on Policemen

A. P. Eberlin Finds He Is Qualified for His Job After Test

"Look up, not down; forward and not backward," was the sage advice which the Victory Theater "Psycograph" machine passed on to A. P. Eberlin, Chamber of Commerce secretary-manager.

For Mr. Eberlin had his "head read" Thursday on this mechanical "head-feeler" which runs its delicate fingers over your cranium and then sets down on a typewritten sheet what your bumps denote.

For instance, Mr. Eberlin has little or no hope, just about average faith and average wit, the machine says.

However he rated high in dignity. Eberlin is firm, too, almost to the point of stubbornness at times, the psycograph warned him. He has a great capacity for constant application to work, it showed.

Eberlin qualified for his present job as an executive by drawing a mark above 70. And the machine operator reveals that plenty of "big shots" fall far below that mark.

Police Chief Wiltshire is another who was "psyched."

High Individuality

The chief too rated low in hope and faith but he batted out a fine average, the highest that can be recorded, in individuality.

The Psycograph pointed out that he kept most of his ideas to himself and that he is fond of good food.

But after these good characteristics, the gadget showed that Wiltshire's "respect for law and order may suffice in general but that cultivation along specific lines may be of value."

Soon after Chief Wiltshire returned to his office, streams of patrolmen invaded the theater and also demanded tests.

It seems that the chief wanted to find out whether or not his officers are fitted for their jobs.

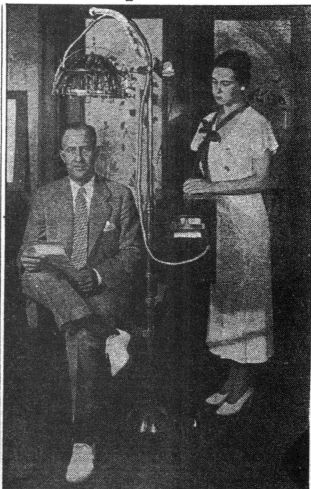

Here is Arthur P. Eberlin, Chamber of Commerce secretary, who rated a 73 on the "Psycograph," a mechanical device being exhibited at Loew's Victory Theater, which is designed to reveal all your characteristics. Miss Mildred Kriger is operating the machine.

(Whether there will be any changes in the department as the result of these tests, the chief hasn't revealed.)

The psycograph machine will be demonstrated to theater patrons from 2 to 5 p. m. and 7 p. m. to 11 p. m. daily for the next six days.

EVANSVILLE PRESS (Indiana) article describing how the Evansville Police Department and other city officials were evaluated by the Psycograph.

theater lobbies and department stores, which found them to be good attractions during the Great Depression. In 1934, two enterprising promoters earned $200,000 after setting up shop in the Black Forest Village at the Century of Progress Exposition at the World's Fair in Chicago.

But the success didn't last. Scientists had debunked phrenology more than 50 years beforehand, and the public interest in the Psycograph faded. Only a handful of Psycographs currently exist, two of which are usually in working order, as they are being used for entertainment at the Museum of Questionable Medical Devices in Minneapolis, Minnesota.

Wilhelm Reich—The Power of Orgone Energy

Wilhelm Reich, the self-described discoverer of "Orgone" energy, died in prison in 1957, but his two-sided reputation has lived on. On one hand, many people remember Reich for the first half of his career, as a groundbreaking European psychiatrist and political activist who followed his convictions in spite of great opposition. On the other hand, many people remember Reich for the second half of his career, when he was living in the United States, utilizing unproven "life energies" to cure disease, and warding off alleged government conspiracies and UFOs. Needless to say, Wilhelm Reich spent much of his life feeling misunderstood.

Reich was born in Dobrzynia, Galicia, Austria, in 1897. After earning a medical degree from the University of Vienna in 1922, he began working with renowned psychoanalyst Sigmund Freud, famous for his work on the unconscious. Reich's early research built on some of Freud's ideas, but Reich emphasized further connections

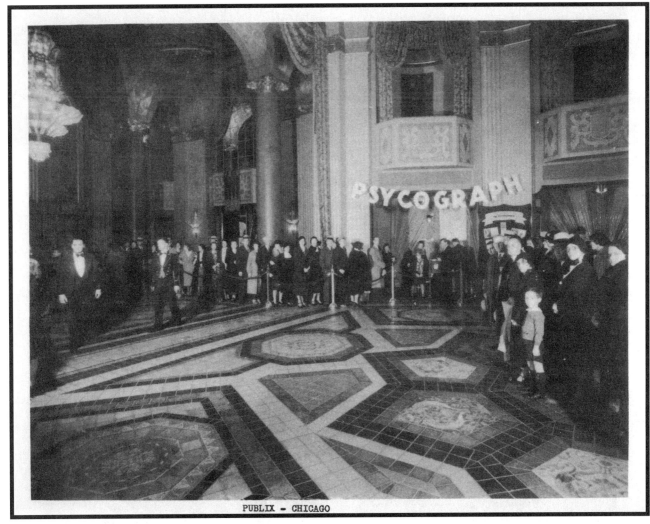

OPERATORS WERE SO SUCCESSFUL IN THE WELSH VILLAGE AT THE WORLD'S FAIR THAT THEY MOVED TO A HOTEL IN CHICAGO.

between the mind and the body more than most psychiatrists of his day. For example, Reich described a type of defense mechanism called "character armor," which linked physical tension to psychological tension. In addition to studying the psychology of individuals, Reich grew interested in the psychology of societies. He felt that morality and political progress could not take place until a society was sexually healthy. Today, many scholars say that at this point in his career, Reich was a genius ahead of his time. But that didn't last.

In spite of his promising early work, Reich's Marxist politics and views about sexuality gradually alienated him from the other psychiatrists in Vienna. In 1930, Reich left for Berlin, Germany, but he was not happy there either. He was an opponent of German fascism, arguing that it was mentally unhealthy and stemmed from sexually repressed neuroses. These strong opinions put him in jeopardy when the Nazis came into power, so Reich fled to Scandinavia, and then moved to the United States in 1939.

For two years Reich worked in Manhattan as an associate professor at the New School for Social Research. But life did not get easier for him. Had he died at this point, instead of in 1957, he might have been remembered only in positive terms. But this was not to be. Not long after moving to the United States, Reich announced that he

⇒ THINKING "INSIDE" THE BOX—ORGONE ENERGY ACCUMULATOR ⇐

Building an Orgone Energy Accumulator, like the one Wilhelm Reich began using in 1940, is not an overwhelming task. Accumulators were large enough to hold a medium-sized adult seated on a chair. (Dimensions of the box were approximately 4½ feet high, 2 feet wide, 2½ feet deep). Sheet iron lined the inside of the Accumulator, and the outside was made out of wood or celotex. The door on the front of the box could close shut, and a window on the door let in light and air. Why the Orgone wouldn't seep out through the window or the crack in the door remains a mystery.

According to Reich, the organic components of the box help to store up Orgone energy, and can cure numerous medical problems, including anemia, arthritis, colds, hay fever, ulcer, skin abrasions, and most forms of cancer in its early stages.

Supposedly, patients begin to feel warm sensations while sitting inside the box, as their bodies begin to soak up Orgone energy. Then their faces redden and their body temperatures rise. When they start to feel a slight dizziness or nausea, that means they have absorbed all of the Orgone energy they can handle. But these negative symptoms should disappear after leaving the box and getting some fresh air. The entire process should take only 10 to 30 minutes.

Patients were warned not to overdo their Orgone treatments! Under no circumstances should they spend hours in the Accumulator or fall asleep inside. Absorbing too much Orgone energy supposedly could cause vomiting and do severe physical damage. The Orgone Energy Accumulator was one of the few quack devices that apparently could give you too much of a good thing.

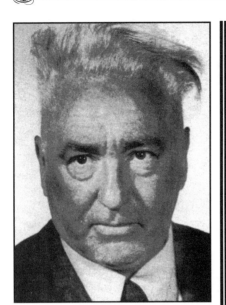

WILLIAM REICH

had discovered a special form of energy called "Orgone," which linked humans to the physical universe. This so-called discovery irrevocably damaged Reich's career and professional reputation.

According to his theory, Orgone falls to earth from outer space but is only partially detectable through conventional laws of physics–which perhaps explains why no physicist had ever heard of it. Reich said that Orgone is the energy released during sexual orgasm and that it has natural healing powers. Therefore, absorbing large quantities of Orgone could make a person healthier. Additionally, Reich said that Orgone influences the weather and makes the sky and ocean look blue. (Scientists already had explanations for weather patterns and the color of the sky and ocean, and no one working outside of Reich's influence ever confirmed the existence of Orgone.)

In 1940, Reich began telling patients that they could be treated for life-threatening diseases as well as psychological problems by sitting in an easy-to-build box called an Orgone Energy Accumulator, which stored up the vital healing energy. Patients could use the box in a therapist's office, or rent one, or purchase a box for home use (see sidebar on page 152). From a mechanical standpoint, the Orgone Energy Accumulators were harmless: they were simple boxes that did nothing at all. However, by the mid-1950s, officials in the Food and Drug Administration worried that the boxes indirectly caused harm, as people would sit in the boxes instead of seeking out the medical attention they needed, especially for cancer and other serious diseases.

By this time, Reich had left his job, established the Orgone Institute in Forest Hills, Long Island, and set up a publishing outlet in Greenwich Village. As time went on, Reich spoke increasingly about international

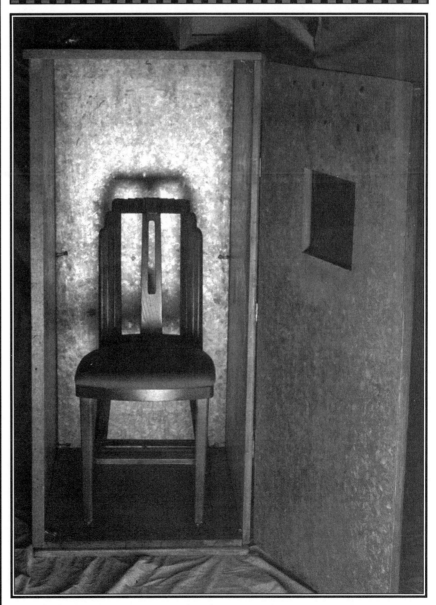

THE ORGONE ENERGY ACCUMULATOR.

conspiracies to suppress knowledge about Orgone. He also spoke about hostile extraterrestrials that threatened the earth. Other psychiatrists grew sincerely concerned about Reich's mental health.

In 1954, the FDA ordered Reich to stop shipping the Accumulators across state lines. He defied the order, went on trial, and was found guilty of contempt of court. He was fined $10,000 and sentenced to two years in prison. In 1957, a few weeks before his release, Reich died of a heart attack in the Lewisburg Federal Penitentiary in Pennsylvania. He was 60 years old.

But that did not put an end to Orgone. A group of followers who remained dedicated to Reich's ideas started a journal about Orgone energy in 1967, and founded the American College of Orgonomy in Manhattan the following year. In 1987, the college relocated to Princeton, New Jersey. In addition to using the Orgone Energy Accumulator, they also use another device that Reich designed, called a Cloudbuster, which is just as powerful and about as easy to assemble as an Orgone box. Cloudbusters have large hollow metal pipes that can pull down Orgone energy and affect weather patterns when pointed at the sky without using any chemicals or physical force. Supposedly, they also are useful weapons against hostile flying saucers.

Confident Quackery— The Road to Success

Physical ailments aren't the only reasons people have turned to quack remedies. Many people have sought out unconventional treatments to gain new confidence and psychological strength. The Bureau Scientifique Francais in Montreal, Canada, reminded the public that success in business and in romance depends on self-confidence, as shy people often go needlessly overlooked by others. But there was hope!

The Bureau's 1913 "Road to Success" program was designed to help the timid overcome their bashfulness, increase their personal power, and lead more fulfilling lives. For $3, customers could order 12 simple "Auto-Suggestion" lessons to complete at home and 53 "Anti-Bash" tablets from the Bureau's offices in Montreal. The

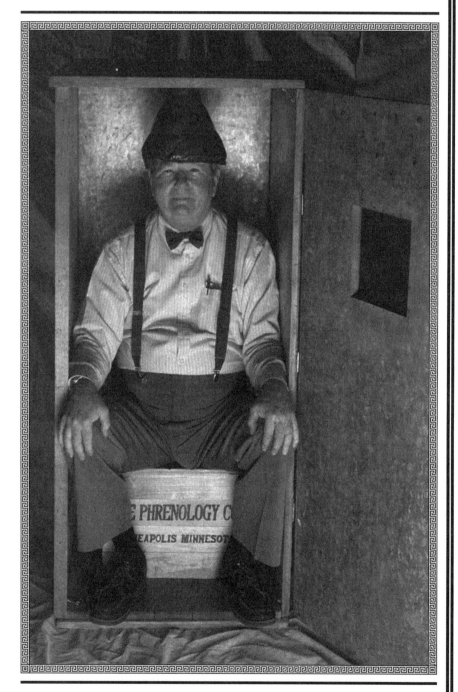

Bob McCoy sitting inside the original Orgone Energy Accumulator, which was used in Reich's 1954 trial.

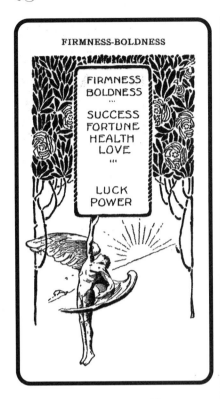

FIRMNESS-BOLDNESS

tablets supposedly would act upon the nerves and keep them at a normal state.

According to the company's promotional material, the pills were developed by eminent doctors and specialists in the nervous system following 30 years of research, and would help keep your "mind clear" and your "imagination fruitful." The company's advertisements also included the following bold statements to help convince potential customers that they, too, should be more bold:

"Free yourself from bashfulness, this plague of humanity, which tortures its victims by pin pricks, and prevents them from making use of their good qualities of heart and mind, and destines them to die without those around them having ever realized their inestimable qualities.

"It is useless for you to be young, to have fruitful aspiration in your soul, and to possess

excellent financial, moral, and intellectual qualities, which seem to reserve a brilliant future for you, if you are always powerless before the ghost of bashfulness, which binds you like a slave in its invisible chains and prevents you from obtaining the success to which you have a right, either in business, or in love."

Still not sure if the "Road to Success" tablets are for you? Well, the Bureau Scientific Francais developed a detailed list of 30 signs that might indicate bashfulness, which the company defined as a disease that affects the nervous system and, in turn, all of the senses. If you suffer from bashfulness, you might "feel a

certain uneasiness" in the following situations:

When at the table with strangers.
When you are introduced to someone.
When you play the piano.
When you sing.
When speaking in private company or in public.
When asking to use the lavatory.
When you have a favor to ask.
When you have an exam to pass.
When you are at a dance.
When in the presence of the priest or the minister.
When in the presence of the doctor.
When in the presence of the lawyer.
When entertaining your guests.
When you pass on a street where you are known.
When asked to remain over night when visiting.

It seems safe to assume that most people would answer "yes"

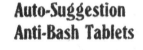
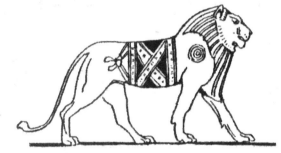

to at least a few of these statements. After all, isn't everyone a victim of bashfulness at one time or another? However, after treatment, according to the Bureau, "a dominating influence emanating from firmness, gracefulness and distinction, will radiate from your whole person, which is the natural lot of all persons well-balanced, both mentally and physically." Amen to that, so say we all!

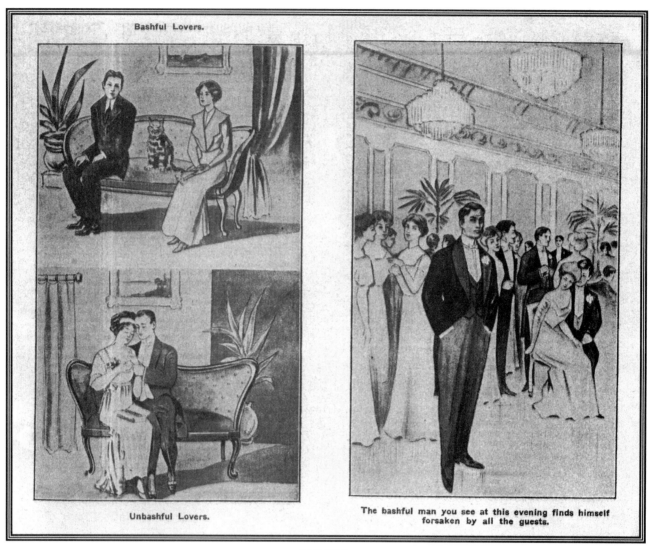

Bashful Lovers.

Unbashful Lovers.

The bashful man you see at this evening finds himself forsaken by all the guests.

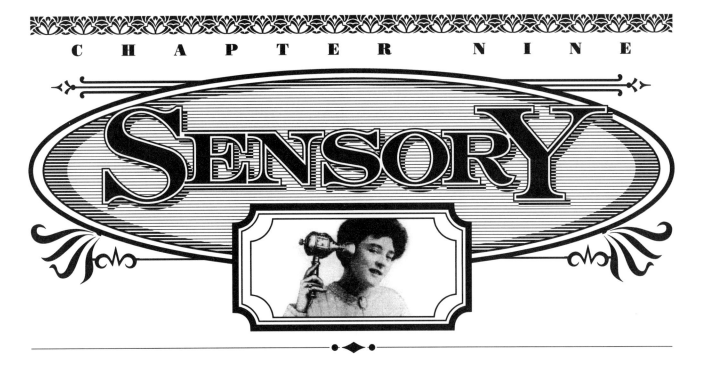

Sensory

DEVICES TO CLEAR YOUR HEAD.

Actina

I n the mid-1880s, "Professor" William C. Wilson was in New York City peddling the Actina Pocket Battery, the premier example of a quack vision and deafness device at the turn of the twentieth century. One hundred ten thousand Actina Batteries were sold for ten dollars from approximately 1885 until 1915 by Professor Wilson's N.Y. & London Electrical Association.

The Actina was a chrome finished metal cylinder about three inches long with a copper ribbon spiraling around the exterior of the device. At both ends was a screw cap. The center of the cylinder contained a piece of muslin soaked in sassafras, mustard oil, belladonna extract, ether, and amyl nitrate. To "recharge" the battery, consumers mailed the Actina to the company along with one dollar, and the muslin was again soaked in this pungent preparation. Samuel Hopkins Adams, writing critically of the Actina in "The Great American Fraud" published in Colliers, said, "The Actina, upon being unpacked from the box in which it is mailed, comports itself like a decayed onion. It is worth the $10 to get away from the odor."

The 1886 patent application describes the Actina as "a portable device to be carried in

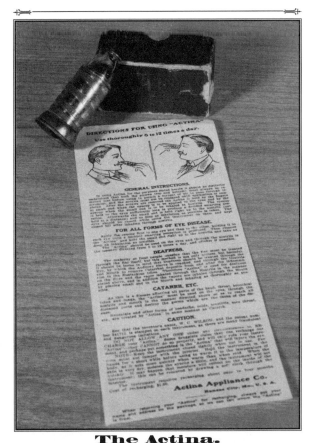

The Actina.

A 1915 FRAUD ORDER DECLARED THAT THE ONLY
EFFECT OF THE FUMES FROM THIS APPLIANCE WAS
TO MAKE THE EYES WATER AND THE NOSE RUN.

the pocket, which consists of a vaporizing device to be applied to the body for the purpose of stimulating the blood vessels or nerves to remove congestion, and to increase and render more active the circulation at the point where the device is applied."

Company advertisements were not so conservative. The Actina was called "a perfect galvanic and ozone battery" with alleged electricity produced by skin contact with the zinc and copper. Sweat was required to activate the battery: "The salts and acids of the perspiration through the skin producing, with the metals and chemicals with which the instrument is charged, a perfect galvanic and ozone current." In actuality, the device had no electrical properties.

Advertisements claimed the Actina would effectively cure all known diseases of the eye, including glaucoma, cataracts, and even color blindness, thus restoring normal vision. The treatment consisted of removing both screw caps and placing the large cup end of the Actina on the closed eyelid every half hour for cataracts, or every hour for glaucoma, for "as long as the patient can bear the pain."

Deafness and ringing in the ears were treated by introducing the small end of the Actina into the nostril and breathing in. This would supposedly cure the catarrh (congestion)–which the inventor claimed was the universal cause of these conditions and in fact of *all* diseases. Angina, cancer, diabetes, gonorrhea, tuberculosis, and other diseases were treated with the Actina in combination with special electromagnetic clothing, such as Electro Conservative Garments– also sold by Professor Wilson.

Professor Wilson relocated his company from New York to Kansas City in 1890 and sold his interest around 1900. After the attack in *Colliers* and the passage of the 1906 Pure Food and Drug Act, the company was reorganized as the Actina Appliance Company. It dropped its allegations that the Actina was an electrical device; nonetheless, the AMA Investigative Bureau continued to receive complaints about the Actina. In 1915, the Postmaster General issued a fraud order which prevented the device from being sold through the mail. This effectively stopped the sale of the Actina.

Quack Hearing Aids

The Actina is just one of dozens of quack hearing aids which were abundant in the early decades of the twentieth century. "Considering its strictly specialized nature," wrote Dr. Arthur Cramp of the AMA Investigative Bureau, "the number of faddists and fakers in the deafness cure field in proportion to the total number of medical empirics is large." As for why there was an excess of deafness quackery, Dr. Cramp offered no opinion. Hearing aid technology had progressed very little in over a century: ear trumpets, listening tubes, auricles, and cornets were still common. These devices worked only slightly better than cupping a hand behind the ear. Amplification appeared in hearing aids around 1900, but these devices were quite expensive, especially in contrast to the quack cures. Appearance was also a factor: legitimate device makers strove to

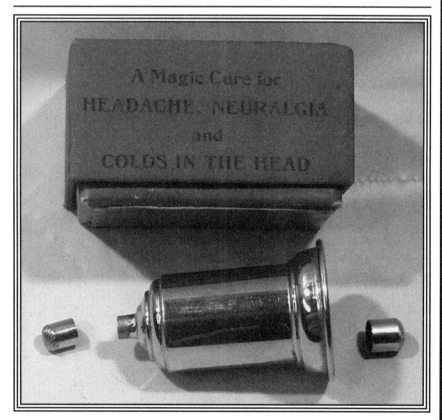

An Actina knock-off called "The Magnetic Vaporizer Magic Cure" (1900). It supposedly restored eyesight and cured deafness.

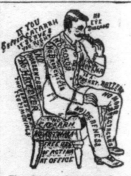

The above cut represents our method of curing all diseases of the Eye, Ear, Head or Throat with the Actina Battery.

THE GREAT EYE RESTORER
—AND—
CATARRH CURE
"ACTINA"
PRICE, $10.00.

THE BLIND SEE!
THE DEAF HEAR!

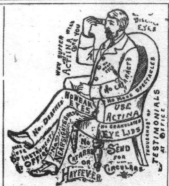

The above cut represents our method of curing all diseases of the Eye, Ear, Head or Throat with the Actina Battery

"ACTINA" is not a simple inhaler, but a perfect Galvanic and Ozone battery, the effects being produced by perfect contact with the skin of the fingers with the zinc element and the skin of the nose with the copper element and its chemical action. The salts and acids of the perspiration through the skin producing, with the metals and the chemicals with which the instrument is charged, a perfect galvanic and ozone current. When used on the eye, the elements are reversed, the zinc on the eye and the copper on the fingers. The price of the instrument complete is $10.00, and the one instrument will cure fifty or more persons in a family of any eye, ear, head or throat disease and will last for years.

This wonderful Electro-Chemico Invention is a new departure in the Oculist's Art. Physicians, Surgeons and Oculists, from Galen down to the present time, have sought a remedy outside the Optician's skill, but have perfected none.

Prof. Wilson, the Electrician, and inventor of the Magnetic or Magneto-Conservative Clothing system of the world, has discovered in "Actina" the Odic-force and vitalizing influence, ever present in all forms of life, animal and vegetable, and after experiments upon himself and intimate friends is now in a position to meet any physician and explain the character of this great discovery.

Fashion and the optician's interests have hitherto been the talisman which led the unsuspecting victim of temporarily weakened vision to the temple of experimentalizing oculists. Eye-glasses of various forms have been adopted, but adoption and adaptation are two different things; hence it is that thousands of ladies and gentlemen of middle age are now doomed to life long artificial aids to eye sight under the present system, and nature, thus violated, recoils upon her unhappy detractors by compelling a continuous change of power in the several lenses from year to year, until the natural laws of vision are distractingly outraged, and total blindness is often times the result. Therefore, avoid all artificial aids to sight, and use Nature's own remedy "Actina."

"ACTINA"—A MARVELOUS INVENTION WHICH IS MYSTIFYING THE OCULISTS, OPTICIANS, AND PHYSICIANS OF AMERICA AND EUROPE.

The Electric Light and Telephone are mere toys in value compared with the wonderful "Actina." "Oh, bosh!" say some of our thoughtless readers. But is it not a more useful and wonderful machine that will make the **deaf hear** and the **blind see** than all the steam engines and telephones? Yes, doubting reader, all is true we write and *hundreds of thousands so testify to the facts.*

Just as the people a few short years ago were mystified by the advent of the steam engine, steamship, the telegraph, telephone and electric light, so are the people almost awe-stricken at the remarkable effects of "Actina." By its use *the blind see, the deaf hear, and catarrh is rendered a thing of the past.* Of what value is the practice of medicine when after hundreds of years of experiment a case of catarrh has never been cured by medicine? This is also true of hay fever and neuralgic headaches. Then, again, the Oculists will tell you that myopia or nearsightedness can never be cured. They thus admit their own failures, while they are obliged to be silent when they see the thousands cured by "Actina." "Actina" never fails to cure all forms of diseased eyes, catarrh, headache, loss of voice, ringing in the ears, deafness, asthma, sore throat, colds, bronchitis, lung affections, without medicine or operations of any kind. Read the following remarkable testimony. We could print thousands of such if space would permit.

CATARACT REMOVED.

PLEASANT HILL, AUGUSTA, MAINE, March 11, 1902.

Gentlemen—My eyes had troubled me for some time and I had to change my glasses quite often. In the spring of 1895 I began to have serious trouble with them; they were badly inflamed and very painful. Our physician examined my eyes and said I had a cataract on my left eye; and said not to have anything done to it as long as you can see out of the other eye; when that fails go to the hospital and have the cataract taken off. For three months I was confined to a dark room with my eyes bandaged, and my food had to be brought to me. And had it not been for Actina being advertised in Word and Works, I should have been blind to-day. I sent for it and commenced to use it the first day of July, 1895, then I could only discern light from darkness, could not see the form or features of anyone. I had not used it a week before the pain was all gone, and they have never pained me since; and to-day I can see nearly as well with my left eye as I can with my right eye. I can read quite fine print, knit, and do my work without the aid of glasses. I would not part with my Actina for any sum of money if I could not get another.   Respectfully yours,
MRS. DEBORAH B. BURGESS.

Send for Prof. Wilson's Treatise on the Eye and on Diseases in General—Free on Application.

NEW YORK AND LONDON ELECTRIC ASSOCIATION, Manufacturers,
929 Walnut Street, Kansas City, Mo.

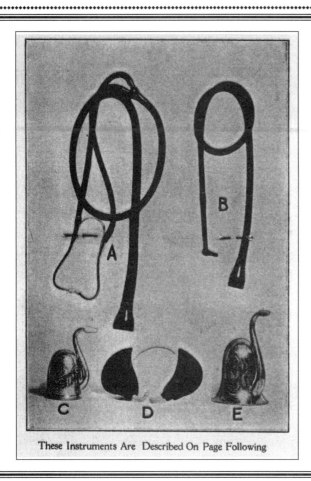

These Instruments Are Described On Page Following

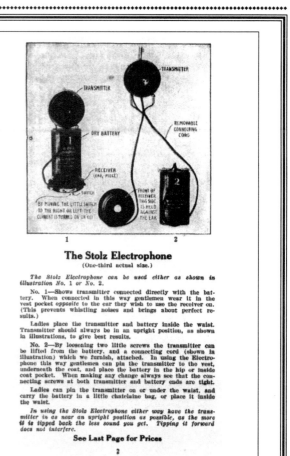

The Stolz Electrophone
(One-third actual size.)

The Stolz Electrophone can be used either as shown in illustration No. 1 or No. 2.

No. 1—Shows transmitter connected directly with the battery. When connected in this way gentlemen wear it in the vest pocket *opposite* to the ear they wish to use the receiver on. (This prevents whistling noises and brings about perfect results.)

Ladies place the transmitter and battery inside the waist. Transmitter should always be in an upright position, as shown in illustrations, to give best results.

No. 2—By loosening two little screws the transmitter can be lifted from the battery, and a connecting cord (shown in illustration) which we furnish, attached. In using the Electrophone this way gentlemen can pin the transmitter to the vest, underneath the coat, and place the battery in the hip or inside coat pocket. When making any change always see that the connecting screws at both transmitter and battery ends are tight.

Ladies can pin the transmitter on or under the waist, and carry the battery in a little chatelaine bag, or place it inside the waist.

In using the Stolz Electrophone either way have the transmitter in as near an upright position as possible, as the more it is tipped back the less sound you get. Tipping it forward does not interfere.

See Last Page for Prices

2

Auricles, trumpets, and hearing tubes were still being used in the early 20th century. Devices like the Stoltz electrophone sought to amplify using telephone technology.

design hearing aids which were relatively inconspicuous; quacks sold inconspicuous hearing aids which didn't work.

Patent medicines remained popular as deafness cures. Most were ear oils targeted to cure catarrhal deafness, or hearing problems caused by congestion. Leonard's Ear Oil sold, by A. O. Leonard, was an emulsion of mineral oil, soft soap, camphor, and eucalyptol. After being prosecuted in New York, and Ohio, and at the federal level, Mr. Leonard switched to selling ear "drums." Aurine Ear Balsam, a preparation of glycerin, boric acid, aromatic oils, and a local anesthetic, sold for two dollars

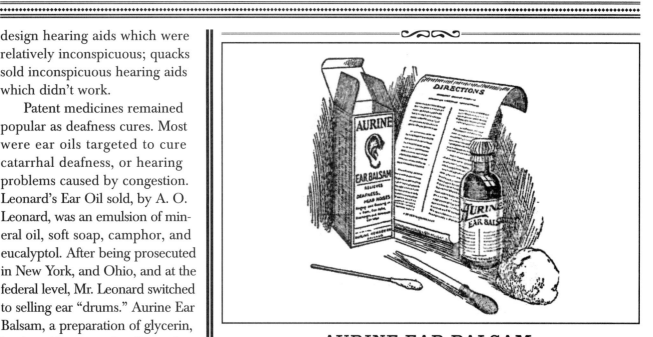

AURINE EAR BALSAM.

an ounce. Deafness nostrums included a "snake oil cure"; Virex, marketed by Dale Laboratories in Kansas City, was originally sold as "Rattlesnake Oil." Virex contained no snake oil–its major ingredient was oil of turpentine! Dale Laboratories was one of 27 patent medicine concerns owned by its operating group. Virex was declared a fraud and banned from using the mails in February 1926.

Quack devices for hearing loss also focused on curing catarrhal deafness. George P. Way of Detroit directly attacked the problem with his "Blowena." About two inches high, the Blowena was a rubber pipe with an elongated bowl which held a few drops of a pungent preparation. The top of the pipe

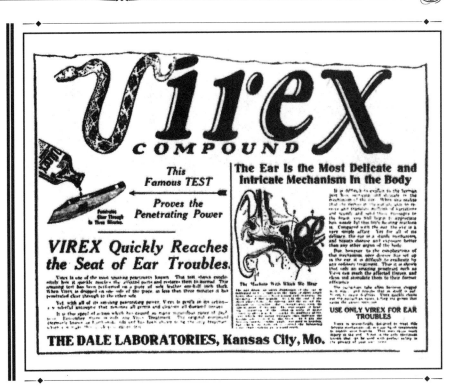

"BLOWENA"

For Catarrhal Deafness

As a very large per cent of DEAFNESS is caused by CATARRH, DR. WAY has invented a very unique instrument for this particular trouble. We call this instrument "BLOWENA," because we blow in the instrument by placing the curved end in the mouth, and the other end in one of the nostrils, and blow. The inside of this instrument has a silk sponge that is saturated with a medicine, and in blowing, this warm medicated air is forced up into the ear and nose cavities, and through the eustachian tube.

Our Medicated Ear Drum
Pat. July 15, 1908

It is unequaled as a sure relief for catarrh, hay fever, cold in the head and influenza, or any irritation of the nose and throat, but particularly for CATARRHAL DEAFNESS.

In using this instrument, the patient blows gently until he feels the vapor passing through the tubes to the eye. The vapor then passes through the posterior nares down into the throat. There is instant relief upon the first use, and, with continued use, the above diseases can be cured. There is a soothing, healing effect upon the throat where the membranes are inflamed through dropping of mucus or from dryness.

You will find great comfort in the use of this MAGIC BLOWER. It can be used several times a day by different members of the family, and can be carried in the vest pocket. One or two drops of the remedy from the bottle we send with every instrument, dropped on the sponge inside of the blower, is sufficient to last a week or two.

To cure soreness of the throat, you place the curved end in the mouth as before, but remove the open top by unscrewing it, draw a long breath, then swallow. You will notice that the vapor will give you instant relief upon the diseased parts of the throat.

This instrument is made of polished hard rubber and will last a life time. The little bottle of medicine we send with every "BLOWENA" will last for six months, and can be refilled at any time for 50 cents.

Wonderful results have been accomplished by parties using this Catarrh cure while wearing our Ear Drums, because it reduces the tissue and clears the cavities leading to the nose, throat and eustachian tube.

The price of this instrument is $3.00 sent post paid. Address,

GEO. P. WAY, 18 Adelaide St., DETROIT, MICH.

We earnestly recommend this Instrument to be used in connection with the Ear Drums

The Blowena was a device to cure catarrh. It was sold for $3 as an adjunct to George Way's artificial ear "drum."

bowl fit into the nostril, while the stem of the pipe was inserted into the mouth so the customer could blow her congestion and deafness away! In 1930, the Blowena sold for three dollars; refills on the aromatic drops were fifty cents. Mr. Way also sold medicated ear "drums." It wasn't clear from his advertising that his 1908 Way Ear Drum was designed to fit deeply into the ear canal; thus, a forceful insertion might rupture the ear drum.

The Morley Phone, "A Miniature and Invisible Device for the Relief of Deafness and Head Noises (non electrical)," could be worn with elegant formal ware without detracting from one's appearance. Unfortunately, it didn't work as a hearing aid. The Morley Phone was oiled silk, ¼ inch in diameter, with a silk thread running through the middle. The device was patented by Mrs. L. H. Vickers, who gave her rights to George Vickers, one of the three principles of The Morley Company. This company began

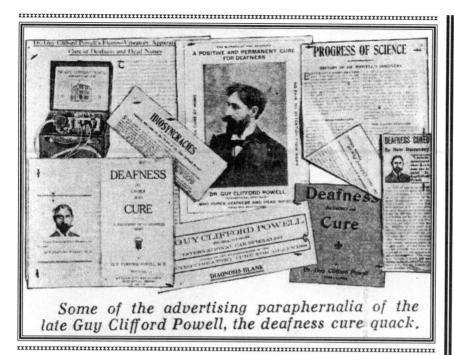

Some of the advertising paraphernalia of the late Guy Clifford Powell, the deafness cure quack.

operating some time in the late nineteenth century and, in 1900, became a Delaware corporation. The worthless Morley Phone was sold until 1936.

In 1926, Dr. Arthur Cramp of the AMA wrote in Hygeia, "The scope of deafness quackery and pseudomedicine is so broad, and the number of fads, faddists, fakes and fakers in the field is so great that a book might be written on the subject."

National Watch and Jewelry Co.

In 1909, Juda Ritholz of Chicago formed the National Watch and Jewelry Company. The firm incorporated in 1911 and experienced tremendous growth after World War I. Between 1921 and 1923, the company's net worth almost doubled from $205,500 to $392,448, while 1923 sales were reported to be $2 million! By this time Mr. Ritholz's sons had joined the business: Matthew Ritholz, who had worked for his father for a number of years; Samuel J. Ritholz,

an engraver by trade; and Benjamin D. Ritholz, a young attorney. The company was known for neither watches nor jewelry; its fortune

was made by selling eyeglasses through the mails.

Since most Ritholz spectacles sold for $2.95 to $4.95 a pair, this company had to sell 12,000–48,000 pairs a month to realize annual revenues of $1 to $2 million. It did so with aggressive marketing. The Ritholz family recruited an independent sales force with promises of earnings of $100 a week. New agents received a free pair of glasses and became eligible for cash bonuses and a chance to win a new Ford sedan. Distributors' kits started at $1.98 and commissions were $1 on every pair of eyeglasses sold. They flooded the marketplace with postcards, advertising various spectacle styles and recruiting agents as well. Consumer incentives included $1 off coupons, free purses, and "surprise gifts." Finally, they provided their own competition.

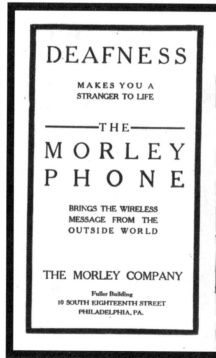

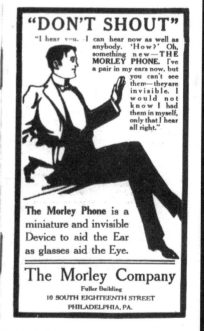

The *AMA Journal* stated in 1913, "The indiscriminate sale of a device of this sort, especially under exorbitant prices and under false and misleading claims, is not simply an injury to the purse, but a distinct menace to the health of the deaf."

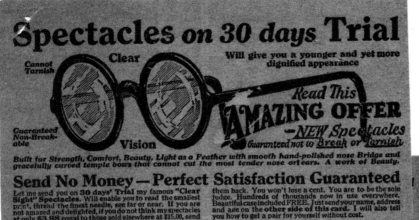

The Ritholz Spectacle Company, the Capitol Spectacle Company, and True-Fit Optical Company, all claimed to be "The World's Largest Mail Order Agency Spectacle House." This was true since they were all operated by the Ritholz family along with U.S.

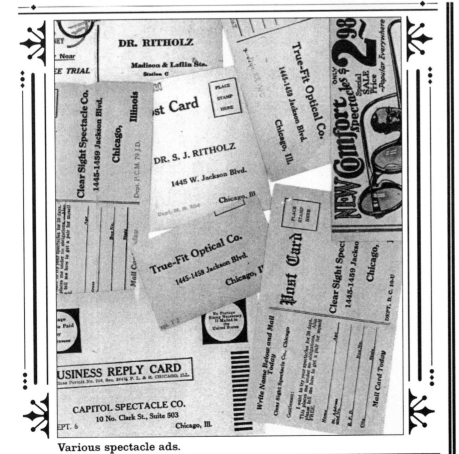

Various spectacle ads.

Spectacle Company, Nu-Way Optical Co., B. D. R. Spectacle Co., Dr. S. J. Ritholz, S. P. Spectacle Co., and a dozen others. If a consumer didn't want the $4.95 pair, he could get the $3.98 pair from another company. Likewise, if the consumer had a bad experience with one company, he could order from another—and unknowingly still be doing business with the Ritholz family. This proliferation of company names later came in handy when the AMA and government sought to shut the Ritholz companies down.

A company of this size couldn't fail to attract the attention of quackbuster Dr. Arthur Cramp of the AMA Investigative Bureau, also headquartered in Chicago. Dr. Cramp was outraged by the Ritholz companies' allegations that they could prescribe eyeglasses by mail order. The Ritholz companies

continued on page 167

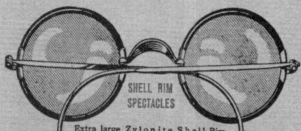
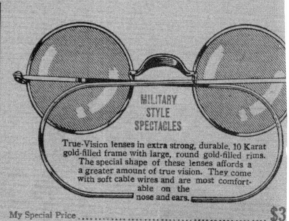
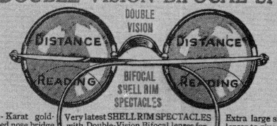
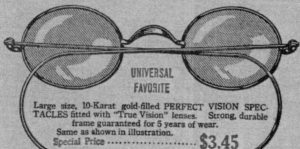

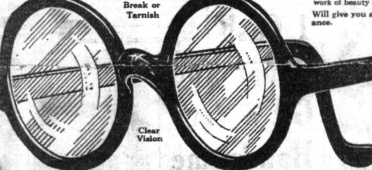
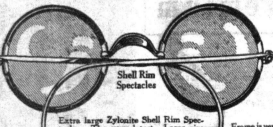

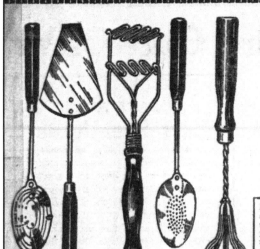
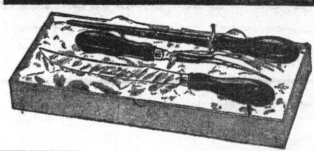
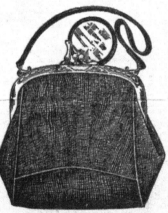
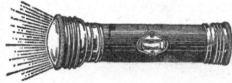
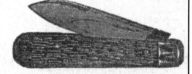

used a prescription formula which combined the consumer's age and the number of years glasses had been worn. For the most part, the Ritholz eyeglasses were the same as the reading glasses of different strengths currently sold in drugstores. Customers were offered a 10-day free trial, and those dissatisfied with their "prescription" were encouraged to take a "vision test," fill out a questionnaire, and return this information along with the unsatisfactory pair of glasses.

RITHOLZ
EYE VISION TEST

TEST TYPE FOR TESTING EYES.

1. If you cannot read this small print distinctly your eyesight is failing.
2. When the eyes are fatigued by reading they should receive attention.
3. If your spectacles fit the eyes they are resting.
4. If your spectacles magnify you cannot see as well after using.
5. Spectacles should improve your eyesight.
6. Vapor treatment clears away all dimness.
7. Floating specks indicate weakness.
8. Beware of strong glasses.
9. Strong glasses ruin eyes.
10. Avoid the knife.
11. Everybody
12. Should treat
13. Causes&
14. Restore
15. SIGHT

The "Exchange Instructions" were quite specific:

In either case it is not my fault, but you may return them, and answer all questions on the Exchange Blank and place the $4.98 all into the same package with the glasses and stick 8 cents worth of postage stamps on the outside of the package and it will be sure to reach me safely. You positively must stick 8 cents worth of postage stamps on the package no matter what your postmaster or Rural Carrier may tell you, as I know positively that if you don't the package will positively not be delivered to me in Chicago.

Therefore be sure and stick not less than 8 cents worth of postage stamps on the package if you return it for any reason, and it will be sure to meet me safely. You will, of course, notice that I used only 4 cents of stamps because I sent the package without any handwriting in (the flap was just fastened down by the prongs) and I therefore could sent it at the Parcel Post rate. You must, however, place 8 cents worth of postage stamps on the package if you return the spectacles for any reason, as the package must be sealed and sent as first-class mail (at letter rates) otherwise it will be lost and you will be responsible.

A 1924 credit report noted, "Many return the glasses accompanied by a dollar and are sent another pair. Others who remit complain of tardiness in obtaining return of their money in consequence of not having been satisfied with the goods. Not withstanding existing conditions, however, profits realized from those who accept and remit [payment] yield substantial incomes to the owners of the business."

The United States Post Office began its campaign against the Ritholz companies in October 1921 and reached an agreement that the selling of spectacles by mail would be abandoned. It wasn't. The Post Office tried again in 1922 and 1925. Dr. Cramp added his voice to the protest, publishing articles in *JAMA* and *Hygeia* during the summer of 1925. In 1928, the Post Office again received a pledge that the mail order spectacle sales would be abandoned, and again they were not. In 1932, the Post Office produced thousands of consumer complaints charging the Ritholz concern with fraud. In 1933, another agreement was reached which provided for refunds to 1,200 Ritholz customers, an agreement the Post Office later judged "not faithfully executed in accordance with its terms."

In April 1934, the Federal Trade Commission issued a cease and desist order prohibiting the sale of the "Marvel Eye Tester," a device invented by a Ritholz employee which was judged to be "injurious to the wearer of . . . spectacles." Evidently, the "eye tester" was made from ground window glass. Charged in this order were International Optical Co., Tru Sight Optical Co., Optical Spectacle Co., Nu Way Optical, U.S. Spectacle Co., Dr. Ritholz & Sons, Inc., and "Benjamin D., Morris I., Samuel H., F. and Ante Ritholz as individuals and co-partners."

In November 1934 and February 1935, the Post Office again charged the Ritholz companies, this time with fraud. At the 1935 hearing, the Post Office argued that it was not possible

to fit spectacles via mail order. Further, the United States Post Office charged that: 1) Ritholz lenses were inaccurate and poorly ground, 2) lenses were incorrectly placed in the frames, 3) that some lenses were chipped, cracked, splintered and off-center, and 4) some Ritholz bi-focals were manufactured by gluing an additional piece of glass to the bottom portion of the lens.

The Post Office obtained a fraud order banning Ritholz Optical, Dr. Ritholz Optical Company, and Dr. Ritholz Optical Company, Inc. from the mails, a resolution not entirely satisfactory to Dr. Cramp, who wrote in *Quackery and Nostrums*:

"The story was a sorry one. How many millions of dollars the Ritholz concerns took out of the pockets of ignorant but hopeful people is not of record. From the public's point of view, the tragic situation is that closing the mails to the various company

names and to the manager and the sales manager was a rather feeble punishment to the Ritholz fakers who, individually, can still use the United States mails. It would seem that if ever there was a case which called for criminal prosecution, this was it."

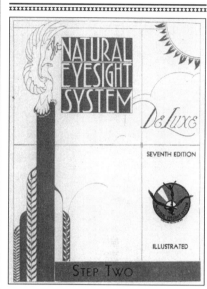

THE NATURAL EYE NORMALIZER CAME WITH FIVE BOOKLETS DESCRIBING TREATMENTS.

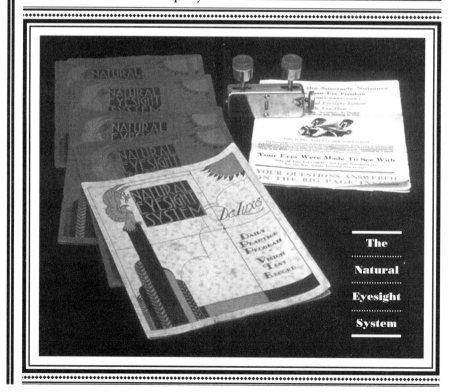

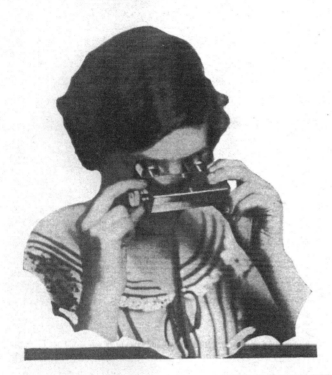

EYE NORMALIZER TREATMENTS

TREATMENT WITH THE NATURAL EYE NORMALIZER

The Natural Eye Normalizer runs with ease and gives your eyes that delightful treatment which relaxes, relieves and restores. It is operated by a simple "Twist of the Wrist."

STEP TWO　　　　　　　PAGE 17

Using The Natural Eye Normalizer.

The Natural Eye Normalizer

The Natural Eye Normalizer— a metal device finished in chrome with rubber gaskets fitting the eyes—was manufactured by the Natural Eyesight Institute during the 1930s. The device came with five booklets describing treatments and containing logs to record eye exercises. Users were also advised to sleep outside in moonlight, sunbathe nude between 11 a.m. and 2 p.m., and walk like a bear on hands and feet twice a week!

The "patient" put the device over the eyes, shutting out all light. The handle on the side of the device allowed the gaskets to rotate slightly to massage the eyelids. In theory, the device was supposed to relax the eyes, thereby eliminating all vision problems. The device had no effect on vision problems. Urbane Barrett, owner of the Natural Eyesight Institute, was convicted of mail fraud in 1937, a year before the U.S. Food and Drug Administration was authorized to regulate medical devices.

The Bates Method

In 1920, William Horatio Bates, M.D., published *The Cure of Imperfect Eyesight by Treatment Without Glasses*. Dr. Bates, an EENT specialist, believed that "all persons wearing glasses are curable without them." Dr. Bates claimed that nearsightedness, farsightedness, and astigmatism could be eliminated if the patient learned "central fixation," or seeing the center of vision without staring (focusing). To achieve this, he encouraged covering both eyes with hands or a blindfold and concentrating on the center of the blackness. He also believed in exercising the eyes, moving them back and forth rapidly so that figures seemed to swing. His theory received a boost in 1917 when he published "A New

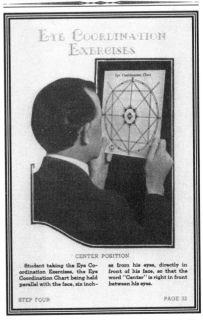

EYE COORDINATION EXERCISES

CENTER POSITION

Student taking the Eye Coordination Exercises, the Eye Coordination Chart being held parallel with the face, six inches from his eyes, directly in front of his face, so that the word "Center" is right in front between his eyes.

STEP FOUR　　　　　　　PAGE 23

Eye coordination exercises with The Natural Eye Normalizer.

Exercises from the The Natural Eyesight System booklet.

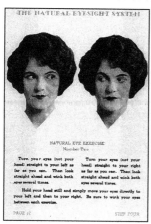 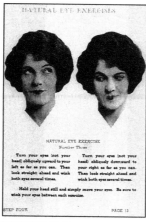 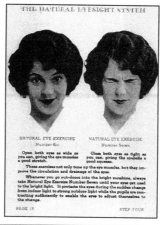 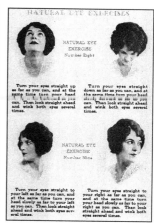

Course in Eye Training" in collaboration with Bernarr MacFadden, a major proponent of exercise at the turn of the century. In July 1919, Dr. Bates began publishing "Better Eyesight," a periodical judged to be advertising for himself so it was not granted magazine rates by the Postal Service. The Bates theory was exposed in "Science and Sensationalism," published by the *Journal of Ophthalmology*. Dr. Bates died in 1931.

The Bates theory lived on and its number of proponents grew. In 1956, Dr. Philip Pollack, a Manhattan optometrist, wrote *The Truth About Eye Exercises* which again exposed the flaws in the Bates System. This book was forgotten while the Bates theory was not. Today, the Bates theory is used to promote pinhole eyeglasses and other vision quackery.

Pinhole Eyeglasses

During the 1980s, the Bates theory was revived, ironically, in combination with aerobic exercise. Aerobic exercise was a healthy fad during the 1980s, a time when average Americans outfitted in aerobic body suits and wearing aerobic athletic shoes joined health clubs and gathered at juice bars after attending classes in low-impact or high-impact aerobics. "Aerobic" seemed to be everywhere. Why not in vision quackery?

The Aerobic Exercise Kit was produced and distributed by Natural Vision International Ltd. of Manitowoc, Wisconsin, from 1988 to 1993. Their headline read, "There's never been a better time to ELIMINATE Glasses and Contacts!!" For $99.95, consumers could purchase the Deluxe Vision Kit containing an Instruction Manual, "Aerobic Glasses," a reprint of the William Bates book, a palming mask (blindfold), an "Aerobic" eye patch, and an Eye Progress chart. The glasses were a pair of plastic dime store sunglasses with dozens of small holes in the lenses. Forego the blindfold, patch, and Bates book and the cost was reduced to only $69.95. The product claimed to help nearsightedness, farsightedness, astigmatism, presbyopia, and hypersensitivity to light.

In the early 1990s, the Food and Drug Administration com-menced action against Natural Vinson National Syndications, Inc. of New York, and Professional Product Research Co., Inc., of Brooklyn—all distributors of pinhole eyeglasses—for making false claims. The FTC charged that "the use of pinhole eyeglasses does not result in long-term vision improvement in these vision problems; pinhole eyeglasses do not cure, correct or ameliorate specific vision problems; they are not an adequate substitute for prescription lenses or contact lenses; and the defendants' eye-exercise programs do not strengthen muscles or improve vision; nor do they reduce or eliminate the need for prescription lenses."

The FTC further charged that pinhole eyeglasses were not an adequate substitute for sunglasses. The FTC prevailed and in October 1993, these three companies and four individuals related to these firms agreed to cease making false claims for the glasses and accept future sanctions. Professional Product Research and National Syndication agreed to provide consumer refunds with National Syndications establishing a $313,000 escrow fund for this

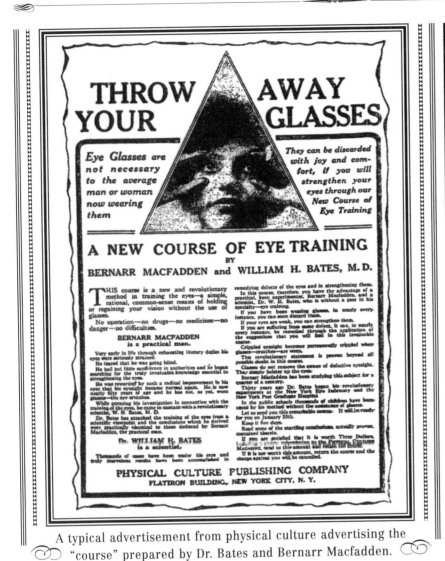

A typical advertisement from physical culture advertising the "course" prepared by Dr. Bates and Bernarr Macfadden.

glasses "when walking, driving, playing sports or engaging in ANY activity when your side vision is necessary."

Memory Band

The Memory Band was promoted as "Dependable Brain Hygiene, Great Boon to Students, Technicians, Inventors, Office-Keepers & Other Brain Workers." If your brain didn't need cleansing, the device also claimed to cure toothache, nasal bleeding, nasal inflammation, heavy head, poor vision, congestion of the brain, ringing in the ear, and "other illnesses."

The memory band consisted of a honeycomb of 68 triangles arranged four to a row which comprised the "radiator" at the front of the band. The purported operation of this device was that the radiator captured and emitted surplus heat, causing a vibration which stimulated the brain system, thereby increasing circulation to the brain in the process. "Brain fatigue," the accompanying literature explained, "is thus instantly

purpose. In May 1994, catalog marketer Life-style Fascination, Inc. reached an agreement with the FTC to cease making false claims for "Aerobic Eye Exercise Glasses."

RGX Vision-Improving Glasses were a similar product sold in the 1990s. RGX's claims were:

1) See clearer instantly
2) See better without eyeglasses
3) Magnification without use of magnifying lenses, and
4) Decreased glare from computer monitors

RGX warned that their glasses would not protect eyes from the sun and cautioned not to wear the

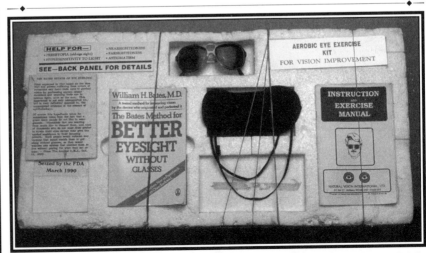

The manufacturers of the Aerobic Eye Exercise Kit claimed that multiple pinholes in lenses were an adequate substitute for prescription glasses or contacts, and that using their product would improve one's vision.

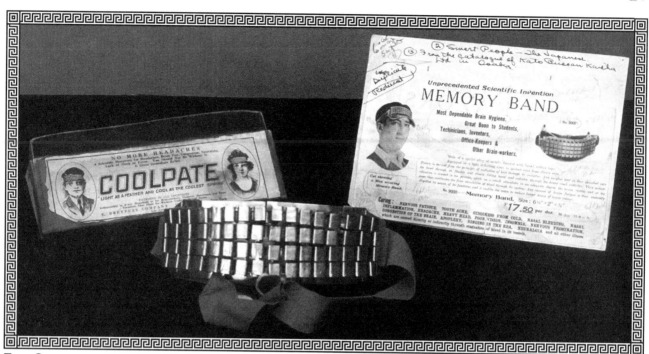

THE COOLPATE, MADE IN 1902, WAS COPIED IN 1912 BY A JAPANESE MANUFACTURING COMPANY AND RENAMED THE MEMORY BAND.

dispelled by means of its functions and it enables the users to endure longer hours of brain labour." The Memory Band sold for $17.50 a dozen.

Never Ear Candle Alone!

This advice from Quality Health Products, an ear candle supplier, should have read "Never Ear Candle . . . Period!" for ear candling can be downright dangerous! Imagine hot liquid paraffin dripping into your ear! A 1996 survey of 122 otolarynologists turned up 21 reports of ear injury caused by ear candles, with burns the most common injury, followed by temporary hearing loss and perforated ear drum. In March 1999, the Video Otoscopy Forum posted on the web "Untoward otological and audiological consequences of ear candling" as a warning to consumers and health care professionals. This article presents a case study (including graphic pictures) of a woman who suffered a burn and temporary hearing loss after using ear candles. She healed after a plate of candle wax was lifted off her tympanic membrane.

Even T.C. Naturals Ear Candles has posted a consumer alert on the internet. The company feels "it is our responsibility to warn the public of a type of ear candle that is not only fraudulent, but also the use of which could lead to permanent injury." Of course, this purveyor of ear candles argues that the warning applies to competitors' products, not to the T.C. Naturals brand–but at least it is an admission within the industry that ear candling is dangerous.

Ear candles, also called aural candles or ear cones, are not really candles at all. They are cone-shaped cylinders, about 10" long, made of muslin dipped in paraffin or beeswax. A paper plate is cut so that it will fit around the candle, and the candle is inserted in the ear and lighted. The burning of the muslin-paraffin cylinder is supposed to cause a vacuum to "remove ear wax build-up." There are about two dozen other health claims for the device, most related to ear or sinus problems, including eliminating ear infection and the need for ventilating tubes in children's ears. As the candle burns, the wax melts. For some reason, the sellers of ear candles would have us believe that melting paraffin only flows down the outside of the cylinder. Ashes, partially burned lint, and paraffin may accumulate in the ear. Dr. Daniel Seely of Spokane, Washington, conducted a clinical trial using ear candles on eight subjects: he found no negative pressure (vacuum) from burning the cylinder and no evidence of cerumen (ear wax) in the burned residue.

The Center for Devices and Radiological Health (CDRH), in addition to finding no scientific evidence to support ear candling, has determined "the label of the product contains inadequate directions for use since adequate directions cannot be written for the product's purported use. CDRH considers the product to be dangerous when used according to its labeling, since the use of a lit candle in the proximity of a person's face would carry a high risk of causing potentially severe skin/hair burns and middle ear damage."

The Food and Drug Administration has been trying to stop the sale of ear candles since at least 1993, when about $6,000 worth of ear candles and related items were seized from Quality Health Products of Fayette, Ohio. Since then, U.S. companies have received warning letters, and imports of ear candles from Canada and Italy have been blocked. Regrettably, hundreds, perhaps thousands, of distributors and retail outlets continue to carry these dangerous items.

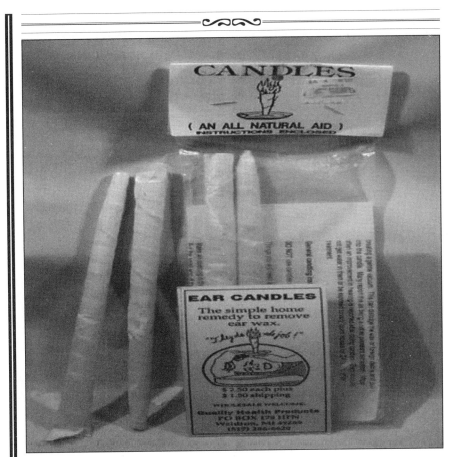

Ear candles.

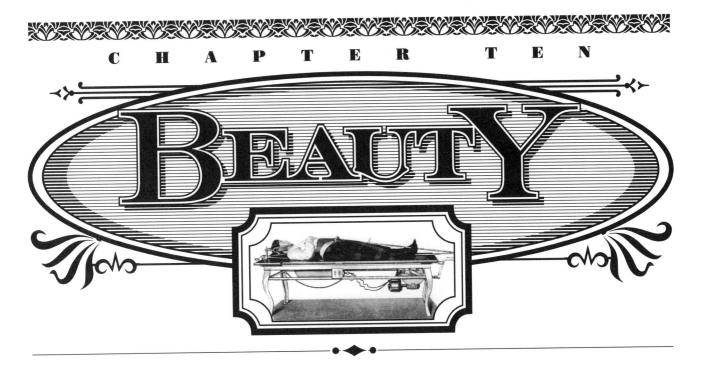

BEAUTY

FROM QUACK STRAPS TO NIP & TUCK.

Plastic surgery has displaced the quack straps and other devices that folks used to use in an attempt to alter their bodies. The Health Appliance Company produced a chin reducer consisting of nothing but straps. Height increasers were also made of straps, as were ear straighteners (though one ear straightener was simply gum to hold the ears flat to the head!).

The 1930s' Sculptron, the "New Science of Rhinoplasticology," was a metal nose straightener billed as the "perfect Grecian instrument." The Sculptron sold for six dollars, though the price fell to five dollars, three dollars, and finally two dollars. The company sold eight hundred thousand devices before being shut down by the U.S. Postal Inspectors.

The Trados New Nose Shaper was similar to the Sculptron. This brass device contained five small metal plates which could be adjusted with screws. A tiny wrench came with the device. Users were cautioned:

"Too strenuous pressure at the beginning of the treatment would interfere with the regular course of the blood circulation which would temporarily redden the nose at the points of pressure. This pressure should be VERY SLIGHT at the start of the treatment and increased a trifle each week."

How many weeks of treatment were required, the Trados company didn't say.

continued on page 178

Scientific Height Increasing

L. GLOVER
(Specialist)

459 San Carlos Avenue

SAUSALITO, CALIFORNIA

Dear Friend:

Don't let people tell you that height is entirely a matter of heredity. If you could go back, say, twenty generations, you would find that you had just as many tall ancestors as your six feet tall companion.

It is obvious, then, that something concerning you individually, or maybe your parents, has kept you from growing.

The reasons are many, but they are not completely hereditary, as I have explained. The mere fact that height can be increased is a proof that the individual will respond to his particular treatment. Most people carry themselves badly. They allow their bodies to sag. They are always sitting around. Even when standing they allow the body to collapse upon itself. Even those who hold themselves erect frequently allow the spinal column to collapse upon itself. Often, in spite of any amount of ordinary exercise the bones are not permitted the loosening or given the stimulation to growth and elongation. Now, as we all know, the spinal column is composed of thirty-three bones. Between each bone and the next is a layer of cartilage, which separates the vertebrae. In the faulty method of standing, lack of exercise, or, rather, lack of scientific height increasing exercise, or any of the many habits which prevent development of height, these vertebrae are pressed upon each other. Thus the cartilage is prevented from assuming its normal condition, and the bones being pressed together, are prevented from elongating, as it is their natural function to do.

Obviously, if this condition develops, and the vertebral column itself is prevented from growing and developing normally, we have a condition where the whole spine and central nervous system are affected. Can we, therefore, expect the bones of the arms and legs to develop fully? There is in Nature a law of correlative development. If you retard the development of important parts, there is a correlative effect upon other parts. This is particularly so with regard to the nervous system, and the body is kept in a uniform condition in this way. When you contract the spinal column you affect the central nervous system; and the body, to protect itself, promotes a correlative lessening of development in other parts. This, of course, applies specially to the bone tissue, for we are dealing with the bony structure of the spinal column and its effect upon other bony structures.

So it is, that in any system of scientific height increasing we must use this knowledge of the spinal column; we must counteract these habits which have prevented the development of the spinal column and its cartilagenous places, but at the same time we must give such treatment as will stimulate the growth of the bones of the body efficiently.

With regard to the development of the bones, I would like to refer to a recognized authority on Physical Education as to the importance of the development of the bones and its effect on the increase in height. The authority is Edwin Checkley, who probably the most careful teacher of physical culture. He says (see page 62 of "Checkley's Natural Method of Physical Culture"):

"The bones are not insensible material but contain a blood system, a life and sensitiveness equal to that of the other parts of the body. They are, in fact, as much dependent upon exercise for health as the muscles. Moreover, a bone may be increased in dimensions by exercise, so that the chances of increasing the height and building out the frame by carrying the body in the best manner will be aided by the actual growth or properly exercised bones."

The object, therefore, of this Special Course will be to give you such treatment as will promote more bone development and elongation, first of all by directing nourishment to the bones, and especially the spinal structures and also to give the bones the maximum opportunity for growth by special stimulation.

Don't be a "runt" any longer. Avail yourself of this opportunity now, and let science make you the fine figure Nature intended you to be.

You cannot estimate the value of extra inches in cash. Can you tell exactly how much it will mean to you to meet everybody, on all occasions, being able to look them STRAIGHT in the eye, instead of having, as at present, to slide up unnoticed? You know how much you are losing by being short, don't you?

Do away with your handicap of being short. Come right along now, and let us get started. The fee—why it is absolutely negligible considering the value that increased height means to you.

Fill in your form now.

Sincerely yours for increased height.

L. GLOV

THIS DEVICE CONSISTED OF TWO CANVAS BANDS SEWN TOGETHER AT EACH END. IT WAS PLACED LIKE A HALTER ABOUT THE HEAD OF THE USER, WHO WAS THEN SUSPENDED FROM AN OVERHEAD BEAM!

IMPROVE ⟨On⟩ NATURE

With These Dynamic Figure Enhancing Devices.

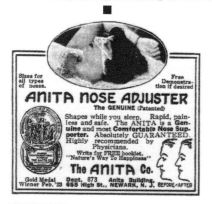
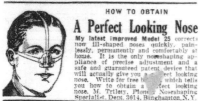
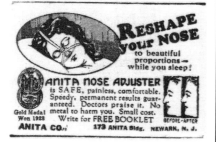
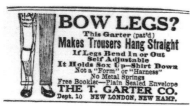
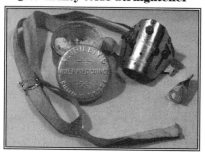
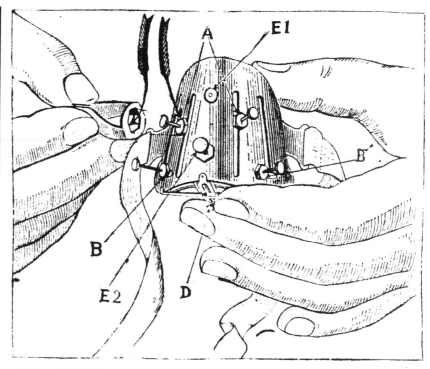

BEFORE placing my New Nose Shaper "Trados" Model 25 in position, same should be adjusted by means of the attached key as follows: For noses resembling illustrations No. 1 and No. 2, as shown on next page, the hexagonal screws A (see double arrow on copy) should be loosened, moved toward the middle of the slit and re-tightened. Then the screws B should be adjusted to wherever the pressure is needed. Screw D should be moved as far as possible toward the inside of Shaper. Then the appliance is placed on the nose as shown in picture herewith and fastened at the back of head by means of straps and buckle. Now tighten the screws A, E2 and D enough to obtain only a SLIGHT PRESSURE.

Too strenuous a pressure at the beginning of the treatment would interfere with the regular course of the blood circulation which would temporarily redden the nose at the points of pressure. This pressure should be VERY SLIGHT at the start of the treatment and increased a trifle each week.

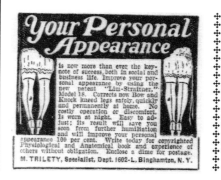
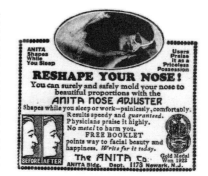

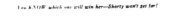

SHORT FELLOWS DON'T GET FAR

But You Can Make Other Folks Look UP To You

IN business . . . in love . . . big men generally win! No two ways about it—the tall, well built, healthy looking fellow gets a long lead on the little fellow—and the lead usually counts big at the finish.

It requires a **dominating** personality to make a good first impression—and first impressions count.

When two men are competing for business—who gets the first interview? The big man—every time.

When two men are after the same job—who gets the first chance to tell the boss about himself? The big man—every time.

One of the biggest concerns in Chicago has a rule that no man shorter than five feet eleven inches can get a job on

its selling force! Why? Because big men can sell faster and make more money—and this concern wants money-makers.

You can get into the class of big money-makers by being tall, healthy and well built!

The old theory that you stop growing when you are nineteen years old has been blasted! Science has found the way to add inches and pounds to every man.

You, too, can be a big man making others look up to you—and getting the advantages that come to big men.

My methods are sure! They are scientifically correct! They have worked on hundreds and hundreds of men and women! They are perfectly natural, based on laws of Nature!

You owe it to yourself to start on this now—today. You owe it to your future, to your health, to your welfare, to fill in the Coupon on the next page and TO MAIL IT TODAY!

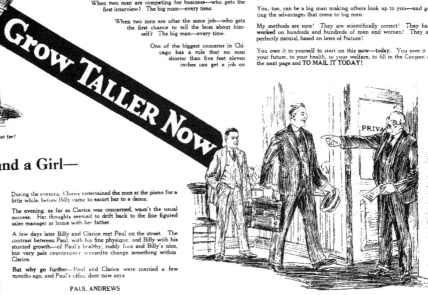

You KNOW which one will win her—Shorty won't get far!

Grow Taller Now

The Story of Two Men and a Girl—

Gossip around town had it that pretty Clarice Young would soon become the wife of Billy Gaston. They were constantly together—playing golf, riding in Billy's new roadster—dining at the Country Club.

Clarice was the belle of the town, pretty, talented, popular.

Billy was fortunate in that his father had thoughtfully made a fortune before being taken by an attack of pneumonia.

Nothing, it seemed, could break this match.

Just when the town was preparing for what promised to be the season's biggest social event, Clarice's father brought his new sales manager out to dinner one night.

Paul Andrews, the new man, was a fine, tall, healthy, clean-cut chap, who in his college days had made something of a reputation as a football star. He was not rich by a long way—a mighty long way at that.

During the evening, Clarice entertained the men at the piano for a little while, before Billy came to escort her to a dance.

The evening, as far as Clarice was concerned, wasn't the usual success. Her thoughts seemed to drift back to the fine figured sales manager at home with her father.

A few days later Billy and Clarice met Paul on the street. The contrast between Paul, with his fine physique, and Billy with his stunted growth—of Paul's healthy, ruddy face and Billy's nice, but very pale countenance, seemed to change something within Clarice.

But why go further—Paul and Clarice were married a few months ago, and Paul's office door now says

PAUL ANDREWS
Vice-President

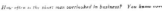

How often is the short man overlooked in business? You know very well.

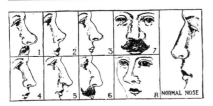

1   2   3   4   5   6   7   8 NORMAL NOSE

FOR NOSES RESEMBLING ILLUSTRATIONS No. 3, No. 4, No. 5, loosen the four hexagonal screws A and B and move toward the lower end; slide screw D toward the middle then tighten all six screws slightly. For noses with an exaggerated droop which need more than ordinary pressure to raise them, I will supply a special device* which can be attached to screw E1 then slipped through a strap which goes straight over the head and fastens at the back with the other straps.

When correcting broad noses screws B are the main ones in operation.

If a sloping nose (bend to one side) is to be corrected (see illustration 8) move the hexagonal screw A of the right side (looking upon the apparatus) toward the middle and screw A of the left side downward.

From the above explanation, it will be easily perceived that my appliance can be adjusted to fit the user's particular case by means of these screws and straps.

IF you use TRADOS MODEL only once a day, it is preferable that you use it at night just before retiring for at least 30 minutes and even longer if you wish results quickly. It may also be worn at different intervals during the day; for instance, if you sit down to read for 20 or 30 minutes you can wear the appliance without the least inconvenience, and in a short time you will be simply delighted with the results you will have obtained from its use.

Others Grew Taller—So Can You

IF you really knew, and realized, the good work that my COURSE IN SCIENTIFIC HEIGHT INCREASING is doing from day to day, you would be only too anxious to avail yourself of the opportunity of getting it right now.

I am anxious to convince you that height can be increased, and I feel that the best way to do this is to show you that it is being increased, every day, by those scientific measures I have adopted in my COURSE FOR SCIENTIFIC HEIGHT INCREASING. I am quoting a few recent reports made to me by some of my pupils who have benefited by the instructions I gave them during their Course.

The second report on this sheet has just reached me, and shows what can be done, after only two months' training and faithful following of the instructions I give. Suffering from underweight, in addition to the annoying lack of stature, you can imagine the genuine delight of this pupil at the results he has been able to obtain by faithfully following, for two months only, my instructions. He has a lesson yet to come, and this speeds up results on the height increasing.

Of course, you may not be underweight. The opposite may be your trouble. MY

INSTRUCTIONS WILL HELP YOU TO NORMALIZE YOUR WEIGHT.

I can absolutely and positively assure you that all my instructions are calculated, in addition to increasing the height, to have a beneficial effect on the general health. In fact, the first remark made by my pupils is that they FEEL BETTER and full of pep. The health improves, and that in no uncertain manner. My instructions give you an enthusiasm to live, and to achieve your ambitions. They "make you feel better"; they "make you feel different," as one pupil puts it. The more you do them, the better you enjoy them. They inspire your interest and your best efforts.

I would like you to come in right now, and let us get started. The earlier you start the better results you may expect to get. I will mail you the first lesson and the apparatus you will need immediately upon receipt of your order, together with remittance of only $8.75. This fee, low as it is, is inclusive, and covers the whole of your Course. For this amount, you will receive three installments, at intervals of a month apart, the second and third being sent to you in response to your reports.

Won't you let me hear from you now—NOW?

In conjunction with the Course I use a highly scientific apparatus, which enables me to secure a loosening of ALL the bones and segments. While I am doing this I give the bones and the body generally a scientific growth stimulus. Thus I use every means that Nature has available for increasing height, and consequently achieve the most remarkable results.

GAINS FOUR INCHES IN TWO MONTHS (Pupil, age 20)
Mr. L. Glover,
Dear Sir:
I have followed your instructions for the second lesson in your course. I have increased my height very much. I now measure 5 feet 5 inches tall. My height before starting your course was 5 feet 1 inch. I am expecting your final instructions.
Yours truly, J——S——, New York.

GAINS FIVE INCHES IN TWO MONTHS (Pupil, age 23)
Mr. L. Glover,
Dear Sir:
I am very delighted with your course. It is one month since I began your course and from the time that I began until now I gained eight pounds and one inch in height. I am very sure that at the end of your course I shall be of normal height.
Yours sincerely, M——P——, South Orleans, Mass.

Mr. L. Glover,
Dear Sir:
I have continued to follow your course carefully and I am thrilled with the wonderful results. I have gained 4 more inches and 18 more pounds and I can hardly wait for the last lesson.
Sincerely yours, from your faithful pupil,
M——P——, South Orleans, Mass.

GAINS S...INCHES IN TWO MONTHS (Pupil, age 22)
Mr. L. Glover,
Dear Sir:
Am now ready for the final treatment of your course, which I must say is wonderful. I have gained 5½ inches since taking your course. I am a real man now and can't recommend your course too highly. It is just wonderful. My age is 22 years. I am today one of the greatest ball players in the country but the lack of size held me down in past years, but your course has helped me greatly. I can hardly give you enough praise. Here's hoping that others will benefit from your course as I have.
Respectfully yours, L——D——G——, St. Louis, Mo.

GAINS SEVERAL INCHES (Pupil, age 35)
Mr. L. Glover,
Dear Sir:
Since I started taking your course in HEIGHT INCREASING I have gained several inches. I feel much better than I did at first, and I know the course is doing me good. I feel much better all over, and think I am ready for my next lesson.
Yours truly, E——F——T——, Kentucky.

(ORIGINALS ON FILE)

$1,000.00 CHALLENGE I will pay $1,000.00 to anybody who can prove that the above and any other testimonials used by me are not absolutely genuine.

My Course Does the Work—Hundreds of Letters in My Files Prove It. Reference—Bank of Sausalito.

GET BUSY WITH YOUR COURSE NOW

Slimming Soap & Salt

Losing weight in the bathtub was a fashionable idea in the 1930s. Slimming soaps and bath salts abounded. As Charles D. Solomon wrote in *The Traffic in Health*, "People will believe anything. Nostrum makers know that. Consequently, they concoct powders

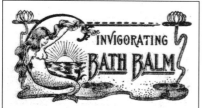

Its use is indispensable after the bath.

This new preparation has so many very decided advantages that one thorough trial will make everyone its friend and voluntary advertiser. It affords rational skin culture, the quality of which so decidedly influences health and vigor.

It is composed of pure, fine penetrating oils, combined with ingredients that are cleansing, healing and nourishing to the tissues, and is very highly recommended for use on the Face, Neck and Bust, for the prompt and healthful filling out of these parts, and the removal of wrinkles and facial blemishes, and for use over the body when the skin is rough and dry, and should be used for healing and softening the skin after exposure to the sun or wind. Invaluable for sunburn, chafing, chapping or any roughness of skin. Its use on the feet at night will relieve all aching and prevent corns.

After a bath it stimulates the return of the blood to the surface and prevents any possibility of taking cold. It also removes scaly deposits, pimples and eruptions, leaving the skin pure and velvety by replacing the natural oil which has been lost by the renovating process of the bath, thus securing the necessary eliminations to insure a delicate texture and peach like loveliness. The protecting and invigorating influence of this magical balm cannot be imagined without a trial. By it the finishing touch of renovating is completed and circulation fully restored. All foreign secretions are liberated, excreted or disinfected, leaving the body exquisitely clean, pure and sweet. Nothing better to use on the face after shaving. Price $1.00.

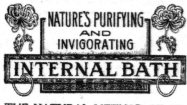

THE NATURAL METHOD OF OBTAINING HEALTH AND BEAUTY.

and soaps with which fat is to be worked or rubbed away."

These products had great names like Everywoman's Flesh Reducer, Fatoff, La Mar Reducing Soap, and Lesser Slim Figure Bath Tablets. Mont Kar Slimming Soap was simply a small hand bar of soap containing a lot of impurities which appear to be pumice and sand. The bar is so laden with impurities that it would dissolve almost instantly. Louisenbad Reduction Salts consisted of table salt, Glaubers salt, and potassium

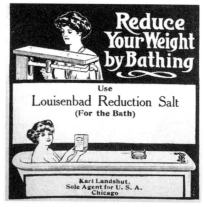

The Journal of the AMA advised that two baths per week would produce no appreciable reduction in weight in any individual who was not extremely dirty.

chloride. Either product would have been hard on the skin. The U.S. Postal Inspectors exposed these products in the 1930s. While these cosmetics seem laughable today, they don't appear any less

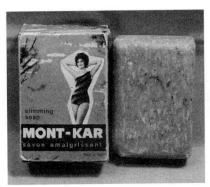

MONT-KAR SOAP.

credible than the thigh reducing cream popular in the early 1990s.

Massage That Fat Away!

The dream of a machine that will exercise for us has been around since at least 1857, when Swedish Dr. Gustav Zander invented mechanical exercise devices—in part because physical therapy was labor intensive. The belt-driven Zander machines sought to mimic actual exercise, including bicycling and rowing. U.S. hospitals added "Zander rooms," which were later closed when the machines produced no therapeutic effect. By the 1890s, Dr. John Harvey Kellogg at the Battle Creek Sanitarium was a proponent of mechano-therapy, improving Zander designs as well as inventing machines of his own. The popularity of these machines declined by World War I, but the dream of automated mechanical no-work exercise refused to die: these machines have reappeared once a generation with popular comebacks in the 1930s, the 1950s, and the 1980s.

The vibrating belt massager and the roller massager were typically found in spas and salons. "Without physical effort, your body is brought in shape by a selective massage," professes a distributor of these machines today. The 1999 therapeutic claims

have a familiar ring: the belt massager and roller are said to "degenerate cellulite, purify, stimulate metabolism and circulation, increase oxygen, activate the lymph and digestive systems, remove toxins, strengthen skin, relax tension and cramps, and reduce girth." Claims in the 1930s, when thousands of these machines were sold, were that they would reduce weight and prevent or cure arthritis, bursitis, stroke, multiple sclerosis, or heart trouble, and relieve

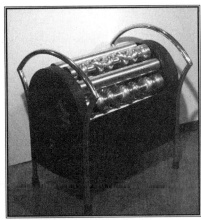

ABOVE:

The aluminum rollers on this beautifully made rolling machine rotate to supposedly roll fat off the buttocks, thighs, or belly of the user.

BELOW:

Dana has been using this for weeks. It feels good, but her measurements have not changed!

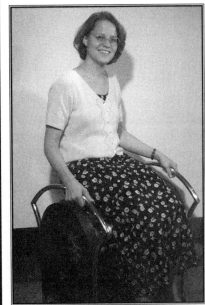

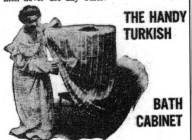

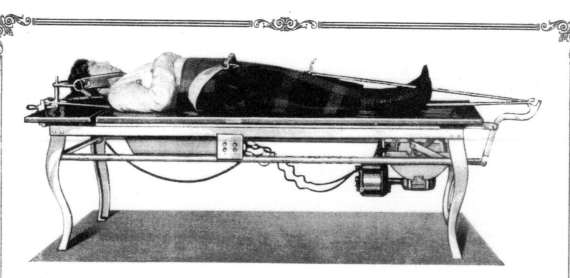

The couch is a handsome piece of apparatus, occupying a floor space of 7 ft. 6 in. by 30 inches, upholstered in brown Spanish, hand buffed leatherwove. The legs and frame work are finished in brown, with the upper metal parts nickle plated, and the underneath metal parts aluminized.

The patient does not slide on the machine, but the top on which the patient lies moves on ball bearings with the patient. **In this top is an opening six inches wide directly underneath the** spine, **under which is fastened the light container, giving to the spine the action of light and heat.**

The machine is attached to any light socket, and started by means of a toggle switch on the side of the couch. There is a separate switch for the lights so that you can have light without traction, or traction without light, if you desire.

There is a slot in the head piece so that by reversing the harness the patient can take traction face down, allowing the operator to give spinal manipulation or use high powered light, during traction.

Our Ten Year Guarantee:

"Any mechanical part or parts of a Riesland Therapeutic Traction Couch which break within ten years from date of purchase, ordinary wear and tear excepted, will be replaced free of charge."

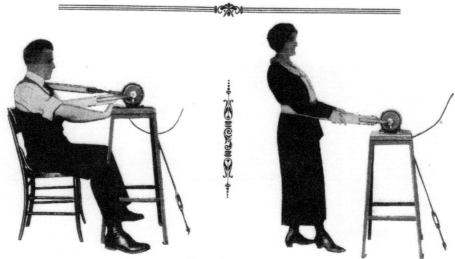

Patent Applied For

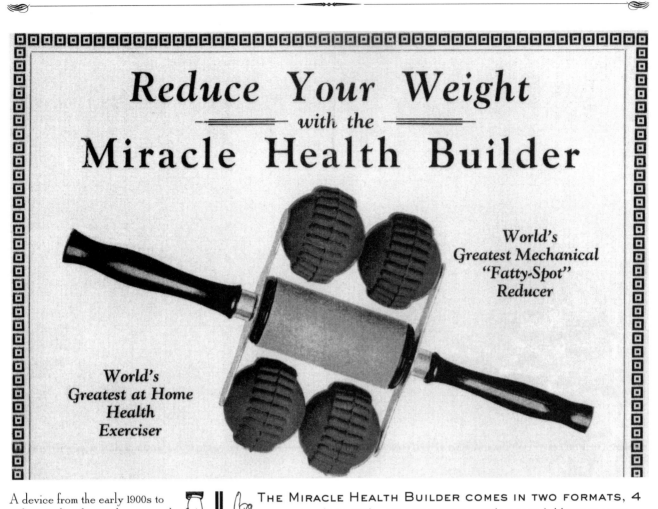

Reduce Your Weight
—— with the ——
Miracle Health Builder

World's Greatest Mechanical "Fatty-Spot" Reducer

World's Greatest at Home Health Exerciser

A device from the early 1900s to make muscles alternately tense and relax to lose weight via electrodes clamped on the body.

☞ THE MIRACLE HEALTH BUILDER COMES IN TWO FORMATS, 4 IN A ROW (BELOW), OR SIDE BY SIDE (ABOVE.) USERS LIKE THE FEEL, BUT THEIR FATTY-SPOTS HAVE PERSISTED.

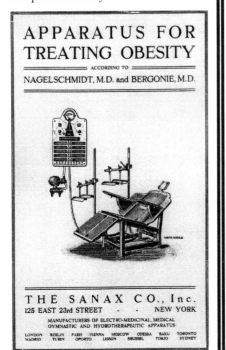

backache, headache, menstrual cramps, and nervous tension. The 1990s' devices are fun to use but, in terms of exercise, weight loss, and health benefits, they are as worthless as those of a century ago.

The hand-operated Miracle Health Builder, "World's Greatest Mechanical 'Fatty-Spot' Reducer" by Miracle Laboratories, was promoted as a cure for "that deadly malady constipation . . . a principal cause" of excess weight. "Reduce or Repent" was the Miracle motto. The device was actually a good quality hand held massager— it just wouldn't cause weight loss as claimed.

Body wraps are a related product which also fail to cause

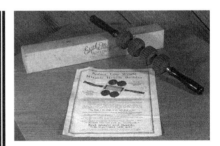

weight loss. Salons and spas charge $75 or more to spread lotion on the body and wrap customers in plastic or muslin for an hour-long treatment. Body wraps for home use are nothing more than a lotion or cream and plastic wrap, such as that used in the kitchen. This scam finds believers because body wraps can cause a slight and temporary reduction of body mass— before and after measurements

PUBLIC BEWARE!

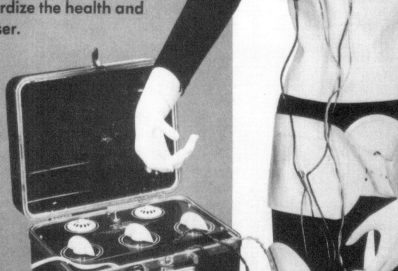

WARNING AGAINST RELAXACIZORS

All persons who use a Relaxacizor device for muscle exercise and other purposes are hereby advised and warned that the device has been found to be dangerous to health by a United States District Court. Relaxacizor devices have been distributed since 1949, and approximately 400,000 units have been sold.

The Court found that the Relaxacizor may:

1. Aggravate many medical conditions in susceptible persons;

2. Have a serious potential for damage to the heart and other vital body organs; and

3. Be capable of causing a miscarriage, and otherwise may jeopardize the health and even the life of the user.

For further information write to:
U.S. Department of Health, Education, and Welfare
Public Health Service
Food and Drug Administration
5600 Fishers Lane
Rockville, Maryland 20852

* GPO : 1970 O - 406-433

may differ by a fraction of an inch. Generally, the difference is caused by water loss from perspiration. The water in the skin will be naturally replaced within hours, thus eliminating the alleged weight loss.

Fitness Machines: Electronic Muscle Stimulators

Since the middle of the twentieth century, electronic muscle stimulators (EMS) have promised to do our exercising for us. These machines consist of an electric source—a battery or electric motor—with contacts applied to muscles. The machines send a current into the muscles, causing an involuntary muscle contraction. The involuntary contractions, it is promised, will tone the muscles! Often, the machines also claim to cause weight loss or reduce body mass.

In a current alert, the Food and Drug Administration lists six applications of EMS machines:

1 Body slimming and trimming
2 Body shaping and contouring
3 Weight loss
4 Bust development
5 Wrinkle removal
6 Cellulite removal

The alert states that the FDA "has seen no scientific data to support the use of EMS devices for these conditions and purposes." The FDA does recognize that EMS devices are useful for "muscle reeducation, relief of muscle spasm, increasing range of motion, disuse atrophy therapy, increased local blood circulation, and immediate postsurgical simulation of calf muscles to prevent venous thrombosis." Use of EMS machines for these conditions requires a

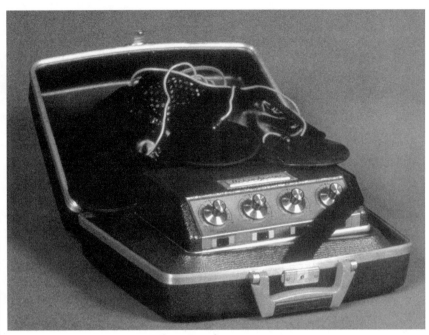

The Relaxacizor

prescription. EMS machines sold to laymen without prescription are considered misbranded.

The Relaxacizor (1949-1970) may be the most dangerous EMS machine ever sold in the U.S. because of its relatively powerful transformer. The Relaxacizor was invented by electrical engineer William J. Browner in 1938. He partnered with salon owner Burton Skiles, but production of the machines was held back because of materials shortages during World War II. The machine experienced tremendous post-war popularity; by 1956 more than 800 people were employed by the Relaxacizor organization.

The Relaxacizor was featured in better magazines throughout the 1950s. *Vogue* proclaimed "a wonderful new machine for passive exercising . . . whittle away excess inches while you relax." Bernice Peck, Health and Beauty Editor of *Mademoiselle,* was a fan. In 1951, she gave the Relaxacizor a two page spread, and in 1954, she wrote, "This since 1951,

is my lazy way to slim back again from size 14 to 12 . . . I simply lie there lazily, half hour a day, reading resting, watching TV . . . After a week of daily treatments that re-establish the measurements I want, I taper off . . . ." Ralph Boss, writing in the October 1956 edition of *Coronet* was equally complimentary: "It is an ingenious little gadget which, amazingly, allows you to take the exercise you need, at home, laying down and completely without effort. You can read a book, smoke a cigarette, doze—and exercise without moving a muscle yourself . . . . With the dials set high, an hour with the Relaxacizor gives muscles exercise equivalent to a round of golf, a five-mile walk or an afternoon on horseback."

A February 1959 article in *Esquire* magazine, "Keeping Fit at 40 Fathoms," reported that the U.S. Navy ordered thirteen specially built transistorized Relaxacizors for an experiment called "applied research" by Lt. Commander John H. Ebersole of the

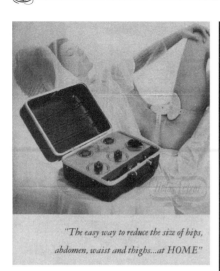

"The easy way to reduce the size of hips, abdomen, waist and thighs...at HOME"

Another version of the Relaxacizor. These devices have had enduring appeal— and profitability!

U.S. nuclear submarine, *Seawolf.* The *Seawolf* stayed underwater for 60 days in 1958, and during this time thirteen crew members used their quarter size Relaxacizors for one half hour a day, six days a week. The average loss of around the waist was one inch with a maximum loss of three inches reported. There was speculation that the experiment in the submarine might be applied to "human behavior in another area: namely forthcoming travel in space ships."

Over 400,000 Relaxacizor models of varying sizes were sold between 1949 and 1970. The device sold for $100 to $400. In 1970, a federal judge found this device capable of inducing heart failure and possibly contributing to "gastro-intestinal, orthopedic, muscular, neurological, vascular, dermatological, kidney, gynecological, and pelvic disorders." The court also found the device might aggravate epilepsy, hernia, multiple sclerosis, spinal fusion, tubo-ovarian abscess, ulcers, and varicose veins. The court prohibited

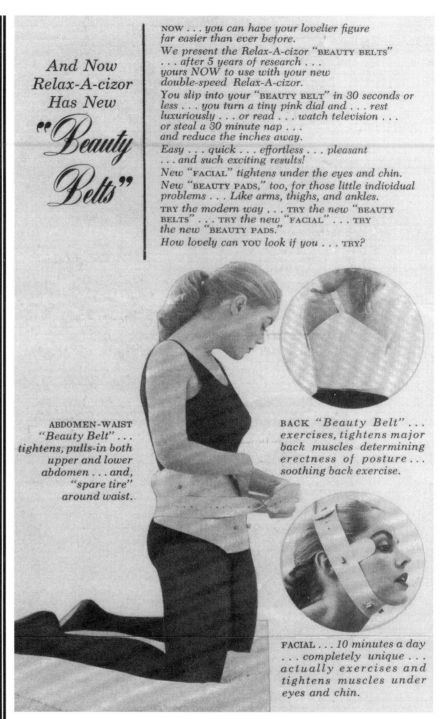

And Now Relax-A-cizor Has New "Beauty Belts"

NOW . . . you can have your lovelier figure far easier than ever before.

We present the Relax-A-cizor "BEAUTY BELTS" . . . after 5 years of research . . . yours NOW to use with your new double-speed Relax-A-cizor.

You slip into your "BEAUTY BELT" in 30 seconds or less . . . you turn a tiny pink dial and . . . rest luxuriously . . . or read . . . watch television . . . or steal a 30 minute nap . . . and reduce the inches away.

Easy . . . quick . . . effortless . . . pleasant . . . and such exciting results!

New "FACIAL" tightens under the eyes and chin.
New "BEAUTY PADS," too, for those little individual problems . . . Like arms, thighs, and ankles.

TRY the modern way . . . TRY the new "BEAUTY BELTS" . . . TRY the new "FACIAL" . . . TRY the new "BEAUTY PADS."

How lovely can YOU look if you . . . TRY?

ABDOMEN-WAIST "Beauty Belt" . . . tightens, pulls-in both upper and lower abdomen . . . and, "spare tire" around waist.

BACK "Beauty Belt" . . . exercises, tightens major back muscles determining erectness of posture . . . soothing back exercise.

FACIAL . . . 10 minutes a day . . . completely unique . . . actually exercises and tightens muscles under eyes and chin.

sales of the Relaxacizor except by prescription.

The Nemectron, for "precision slimming," is another EMS device from the 1950s. The Nemectron would have been a great weapon against the effects of aging . . . if only it had worked. Seized by the U.S. government

in 1959, the device allegedly could give you a younger-looking appearance by regenerating tissues and toning the body. By "duplicating the body's own natural pattern of electricity" it provided "a type of precision slimming unattainable by the usual methods of exercise, drugs, or

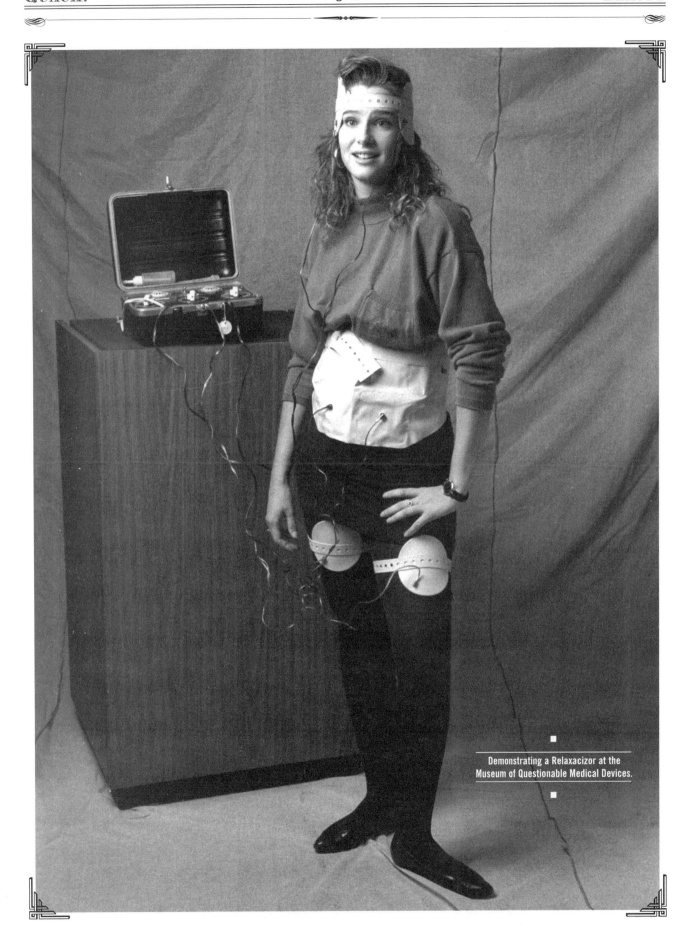

Demonstrating a Relaxacizor at the
Museum of Questionable Medical Devices.

diet." Using electric current through the rings, it allegedly dissolved fat which was "eliminated through natural body functions."

The Nemectron had other uses, too. It claimed to reduce or enlarge bust size (your choice?), a claim typical of EMS devices. As a rejuvenator, the machine strengthened feet, rejuvenated nerves and glands, removed double chins and dowager's hump, and could clear up your complexion—so there was no threat of struggling with acne as your skin got younger.

The Electro Body Toner by Slimnomics was not to be used

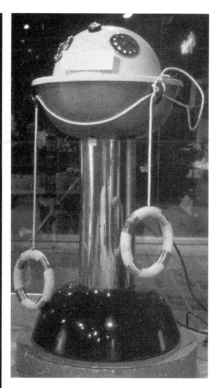

TWO Views of the Nemectron——————— RIGHT AND BELOW

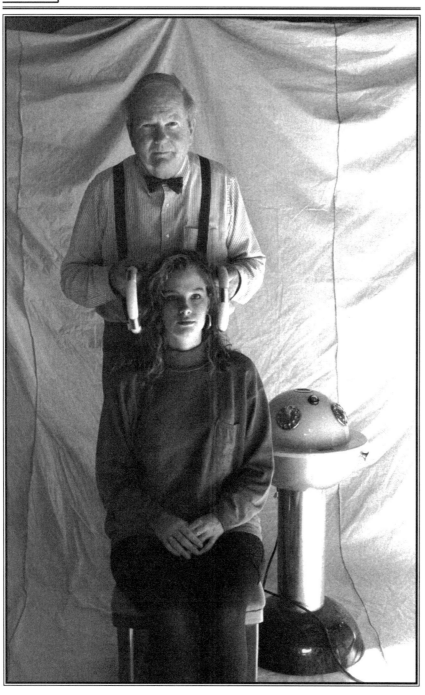

by people who were pregnant or had pacemakers, a heart condition or heart disease. Users with "intra-abdominal, gastrointestinal, orthopedic, muscular, neurological, vascular, dermatological, kidney, gynecological and pelvic complaints or disorders" were advised to check with doctors before using the device. Thirty years after the Relaxacizor's heyday, the ads for the Slimnomics device claimed: "The Electro Body Toner exercises your muscles while you relax. It is easy to use and small enough to carry with you, anywhere you go, so you can use it any time you are relaxing, reading a book or magazine, visiting with friends or watching TV." The 1980s' Electro-Body Toner resembled a 1960s' transistor radio. Running off a 9-volt battery, it didn't contain enough power to do much of anything.

The T.E.N.S. Sanidad of the 1990s also looked something like an old-fashioned transistor radio. This compact device, manufactured

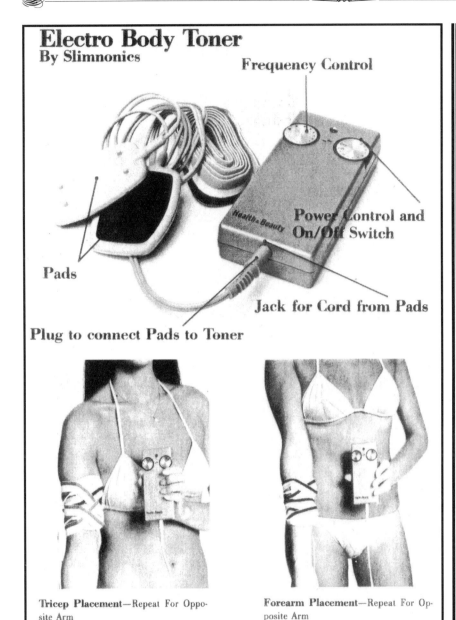

Electro Body Toner
By Slimnonics

Frequency Control

Power Control and On/Off Switch

Pads

Jack for Cord from Pads

Plug to connect Pads to Toner

Tricep Placement—Repeat For Opposite Arm

Forearm Placement—Repeat For Opposite Arm

ABOVE: THE ELECTRO BODY TONER.

BELOW: THE T.E.N.S. SANIDAD.

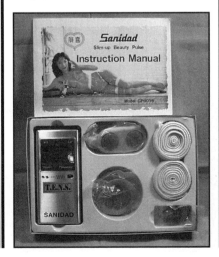

outside of the U.S., sought to cash in on the look and name of a device used to counteract chronic pain manufactured by a reputable U.S. company. The T.E.N.S. Sanidad came with two sets of pink and black rubber pads, two lead wires, two fixing bands (cloth belts) for attaching pads, a 9-volt battery, and a dual sponge pad for dipping in water. Treatment was advocated for 10 to 20 minutes, once or twice daily. The device was not to be used by those

"in which bleeding may occur, with a weak heart, concerned with their blood pressure, in their menstrual period or just before or after childbirth, with other illnesses, who have been instructed by their physicians not to use electrical instruments."

Conditions this device claimed to treat were:

- Fatigue
- Stiff neck
- Muscular aches and pains
- Stiff muscles
- Neuralgia in old people
- Lack of exercise
- Eye strain
- Farsightedness
- Headache
- Insomnia
- "Pseudo-nearsightedness"
- Eyelid wrinkles
- Breast enlargement
- Appetite stimulant
- Increase female charm
- Growth stimulant
- Night incontinence
- Hemorrhoids
- Constipation
- High blood pressure
- Indigestion
- Sore throat
- "For a loud voice"
- Hand paralysis
- Toothache

It's an impressive list for a small box powered by a 9-volt battery!

The 1990s also produced an EMS designed and marketed exclusively for men, the "Fitness Machine." The 1996 Model EE-400 was called the Executive Briefcase Model. According to its advertising, it was the most advanced exercise system available. The Food and Drug Administration disagreed. On April 14, 1999, FDA investigators accompanied the U.S. Marshall to the offices of Executive Fitness Products in

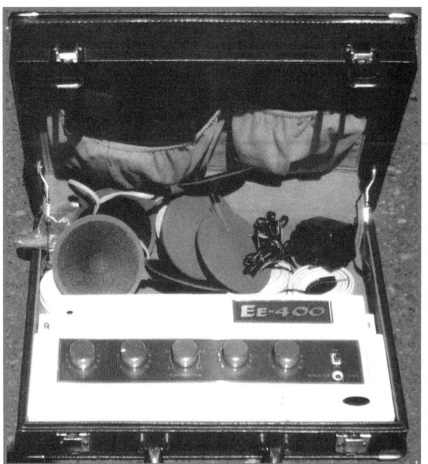

The Fitness Machine—Executive Briefcase Model—was advertised as the most advanced exercise system you could buy. In 1999, the FDA disagreed and ordered the devices to be destroyed.

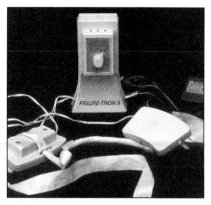

The Figure–Tron, with battery-operated vibrating pads. Seized by the FDA in 1966 and declared fraudulent.

Atlanta, Georgia, to assist in the seizure of hundreds of these devices with an estimated retail value of $200,000. The Ultratonic series manufactured by Executive Fitness, when used on the chest, were considered potent enough to have the potential to stimulate the heart and cause cardiac arrhythmias which could lead to injury or death. The devices were ordered destroyed.

Bust Developers

There is no exercise regimen, no diet, no herbal cure, no cream, and no machine which will increase breast size. Nonetheless, bust developers continue to occupy a niche in the marketplace of quack products. The "magic" is in the marketing, as this wonderful ad copy from the Venus-Carnis company illustrates:

How I Obtained a Beautiful Bust

By an Accidental Discovery

AFTER MASSAGE, CREAMS, WOODEN CUPS, ELECTRICITY, VACUUM APPLIANCES AND INTERNAL DRUGS HAD ALL FAILED TO PRODUCE ANY RESULTS.

AN ABSOLUTELY CERTAIN METHOD FOR DEVELOPING THE BUST TO ANY DESIRED SIZE.

By MARGARETTE MERLAIN

Had I not suffered from ill-health and a generally debilitated condition of the system, the precious secret which I now propose to reveal might have for ever remained hidden from me, and I might have gone through life without satisfying that craving for a beautiful, firm, well-rounded bust, which I now possess at over 37 years of age.

I obtained the superb bust development which I now have in less than one month by following the same simple treatment which I recommend to you. I accomplished this result

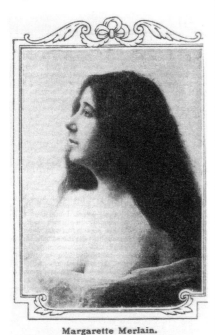

Margarette Merlain.

without any discomfort, trouble, or loss of time, after all other methods had failed to do me any good.

I Longed for a Beautiful Bust

Trouble, worry, and illness robbed me of whatever bust development I

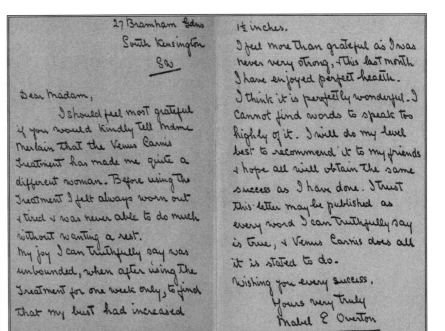

A testimonial for the Venus Carnis bust developer from a satisfied customer.

enjoyed during my girlhood, and I was so anxious to possess a beautiful, firm, well-rounded bust that I tried practically all kinds of remedies, including massage, cold creams, wooden cups, electricity, vacuum appliances, and internal drugs, but each and every one of them absolutely failed to do me any good. I then became thoroughly disheartened, and made up my mind that there was absolutely nothing that would develop the bust.

My health was generally bad. I felt tired and weak all the time, and I consulted several doctors and specialists for the purpose of obtaining something to build up my general health, but the medicines which they gave me were either too strong or were not suited to my condition. At last I heard of a certain rare herb which was said to posses marvellous medicinal properties for strengthening the entire system. It appeared to be so simple and harmless that I was at first skeptical of obtaining any

benefit from its use, but I took it faithfully, for I had become thoroughly discouraged, and, like a drowning person, was ready to grasp even at a straw.

Within a few days of commencing to take this simple remedy, I began to feel much stronger and more vigorous. After I had been taking the preparation for a week, I noticed a peculiar pricking sensation in my bust, and upon an examination I found to my utter astonishment that the flat, flabby bust which had hung so lifeless and of which I was so thoroughly ashamed, had now become much firmer and more solid, and had considerably increased in size. I could scarcely believe the evidence of my own eyes, and I had no idea that the remedy which I had been taking was in any sense responsible for the result, but I presumed it was due solely to some peculiar accident. I kept on taking the remedy, however, on account of its wonderful benefit to my health.

The Strange Effect of a Rare Herb.

After I had been taking the remedy mentioned above for a period of two weeks, I noticed that my bust had become firm and solid and had wonderfully increased in size. One day I happened to mention this fact to an eminent chemist, who was a friend of mine, and who had supplied to me the rare herb which I had been taking. He asked me about the effect produced on my bust, and after I finished he turned to me with the remark: "Madam, you have indeed made a most wonderful discovery, which is likely to prove a blessing to every woman lacking in bust development . . . ."

An Absolutely Certain Method for Developing the Bust.

My chemist friend explained that inasmuch as I had already obtained such a wonderful development of the bust from the use of the tonic remedy which I had been taking, he would like to have me employ two other methods in connection with the remedy, for a period of two weeks, and note the result. He thoroughly explained the methods to me, which he desired me to employ, and I followed his instructions faithfully for a period of two weeks. Day by day I watched my bust grow in size, until in less than 30 days' time I had obtained such a superb bust development that I could scarcely believe my own eyes when I looked upon the wonderful transformation that had been made. This was over one year ago, and although I am now a woman over 37 years of age, my breasts are firm and solid, and if anything, even larger than I could possibly wish them to be. They are so firm that they require

absolutely no support whatsoever. In fact, I have never seen any woman at my age who had such firm, solid breasts as I now possess, and when I contrast them with the flat, flabby ones which had hung so lifeless before I took this treatment, I cannot help thinking that a miracle has truly been wrought.

Friends Sought My Secret.

Madame C—whom I had known for many years, and who said that her bust had been flat and masculine looking all her life—saw the marvellous bust development which I had obtained, and begged me to give her my secret. I confess that I was rather anxious to see if the results of the treatment would be as marvellous in creating a bust where there

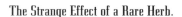

A FEW LATE TESTIMONIALS.

"VESTRO FULLY DEVELOPS AND RESTORES HEALTH."

The Aurum Medicine Co., Chicago, Ills.   PURLE, MO., Jan. 5, 1903.
Dear Sirs:—I have used Vestro and cannot find words enough to recommend it to poor, weak, wasted and ill formed women who are plodding wearily along with no other thought than that hopeless despair.
Vestro not only fully developed my bust, but it improved my health and appearance in every possible way.
I was a great sufferer from painful menstruation—it was so bad that I was compelled to take morphine for about five days every month. I was not able to do housework for over three years, and now I am able to do all my own work without the slightest pain and bearing down sensation, and all from the use of Vestro.
If you think that this letter will be of any service to you in relieving other women, you may publish it in full with my picture if you wish.   MRS. AUGUST DRANER.

"VESTRO VERY SATISFACTORY IN EVERY RESPECT."

Aurum Medicine Co., Chicago, Ills.   74 W. High St., SPRINGFIELD, O., Jan. 18, 1903.
Dear Sirs:—I have used your Vestro for about four weeks and find it *very satisfactory in every respect.*
It has no equal for *rounding out the neck and bust.*   Very truly,   MISS F. WATKINS.

"PERFECTLY DELIGHTED WITH VESTRO. HEALTH BENEFITTED."

The Aurum Medicine Co., Chicago, Ills.   BEAVER DAM, WIS., March 19, 1903.
Gentlemen:—I am perfectly delighted with Vestro; I cannot say enough in its praise. After using only one month's treatment my bust is developed more than two inches; Vestro has not only developed my bust but has been of great benefit to my health in general.
Very sincerely,   EDNA M. BEECHER.

"AN INCREASE NEVER DREAMED OF IN ONE MONTH."

Aurum Medicine Co., Chicago, Ills.   RIGGS, CARTER CO., KY., Feb. 13, 1903.
Dear Sirs:—It is with the greatest pleasure I write you these lines in praise of your wonderful Vestro which after using one month with such improvement *and an increase never dreamed of.* I wasted much money on swindlers buying different developers and the *vacuum process* which did me no good whatever.
Yours truly,   MISS E. J. W.

never had been one, as in renewing the former fullness and beauty of my own bust. I gave her my treatment and thoroughly instructed her how to use it, and in less than one week after commencing its use, she came to me with a joyful countenance. Her bust, which had before appeared like two small flattened eggs, had now begun to grow, and was taking on new vibrant life and firmness. As she continued the treatment her bust steadily grew in size, and gave the treatment to several of my other friends, who were lacking in bust development, and without a single exception they were astonished and delighted, for it not only enlarged their busts, but gave them rested nerves and buoyant health.

What Miracle is this that has been Wrought?

After using my secret for developing the bust, several of my friends came to me with astonishment and wonderment in their eyes, crying: "What miracle is this that has been wrought? Surely you have made the most marvellous scientific discovery of the age, and you owe it as a duty to the world to give it to all women." While I could not help but feel the force of their argument, still I know of no way by which I could let others know of my discovery, without placing myself in the ranks of ordinary advertisers, who dwelt at length upon the merits of goods which I knew by actual experience to be absolutely worthless and without value. I thought of many plans, but none seemed to be sufficiently broad in its scope to give all women in every land the benefit of my discovery. At last I decided that I could bind no better plan than to frankly and truthfully tell the story of how I developed my own bust, and put it in the form of this little booklet, which I trust every reader will regard as confidential.

I Positively Refuse to Accept Money. This is My Free Gift to all Women.

Several of my friends advised me to sell my secret for developing the bust, stating that I could make thousands of dollars by so doing, but I am fortunately so situated that I have what money I require for my own maintenance, and after mature reflection, I decided to give my secret to the world, so that all women might benefit thereby. Therefore I have arranged with a thoroughly responsible company to manufacture the products required for this treatment, and furnish them to all ladies who

wish them at a stipulated price, and I have made them sign a contract agreeing not to charge over a certain stipulated amount in any instance, so that I might be absolutely assured that no one would be overcharged for the products required. I further made the Company agree to furnish 2,000 treatments at half price, in consideration of my giving them my secret, so that 2,000 women will benefit by this half price offer. The Company has also agreed with me to give away 1,000 treatments to women who are actually too poor to pay for them, upon proof being furnished to this effect. These are the conditions which I imposed before imparting my secret. I did not receive from the Company a single penny of money for my secret, but I preferred to impose the conditions above mentioned. I wanted to be sure in the first place that no one would be overcharged, or charged an amount in excess of a certain stimulated sum which I have named.

It is not one cent to me whether you purchase the treatment or not, as I do not receive any commission either directly or indirectly from the sales, and I do not receive any money from the Company, except a very small fee to pay for stenographic services in answering such letters of their patrons as they cannot very well answer themselves, and which I may be required to answer. These are letters to women who wish special advice. I feel that I shall be sufficiently rewarded by the gratitude which I know that women must feel from the wonderful benefits which they are bound to derive from this marvellous method for developing the bust.

Do not Take this Treatment Unless You Want Your Bust to grow.

On account of the wondrous beauty produced by my system of treatment, I have decided to call it the Venus-Carnis treatment, or "flesh

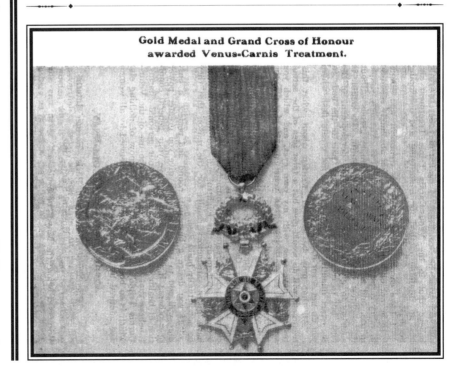

Gold Medal and Grand Cross of Honour awarded Venus-Carnis Treatment.

beautiful." It is not only a wonderful treatment for enlarging the bust, but it will grow new flesh and tissue on any part of the body which may be desired . . . .

Venus-Carnis Treatment Investigated by Committee of Paris Savants.

I submitted my treatment to a scientific society know as the Comitè des Savants de Paris, who appointed a commission of savants to investigate my discovery, and after investigation, they awarded it with the Gold Medal and the Grand Cross of Honour, together with diplomas certifying to its merit and efficacy. Surely such a tribute from judges of so high an order seems a positive indication that the Venus-Carnis treatment is entirely different from anything else that has ever been known to the world.

How to Gain Admiration Wherever You Go. A Beautiful Bust is Nature's Richest Charm.

If you want the admiration and adoration of others, you must possess a beautiful bust, for this is the emblem of true womanhood. With a bust full and well rounded, you are bound to create universal admiration. If your chest is flat and your bust is soft and flabby, only glances of pity will be turned in your direction. Pads and artificial appliances are extremely injurious to your system, and their presence is easily detected by others; no matter how ingeniously they may be contrived, pads never have the fascinating appearance of a living, throbbing bust.

The Mysterious Fascination of a Well Developed Bust.

It is a well-known fact that there is something mysteriously fascinating in a full, well-developed bust which creates a strange, feverish excitement among those who are thrown into contact with the woman possessing this delicate charm. Conceal such a bust from the view of others as carefully as you wish, by a gown, and still there is that quiver of beautiful flesh which lends an indescribable hypnotic effect to your every movement. With such a charm, you cannot fail to arouse to life the worship and adoration of men and the admiration and envy of women.

A Magic Effect upon Others.

Strange as this inexplicable power may seem, it is nevertheless true, as you have but to look upon the woman who is lacking in bust development to realize that she can never hope to possess the same influence over others as is within the power of her more fortunate sister, who rejoices in a full and voluptuous bust. A magic and instantaneous effect is created upon others by such a woman, for her presence inspires in them a keen appreciation for her perfect development . . . .

A Beautiful Bust Means More Than a Pretty Face.

A full throbbing bust is the charm which gives to woman her power to sway the hearts of men and turn the destinies of empires. It lends stateliness to the carriage that endures even after the marks of time have implanted their imprints upon the face. The woman who is entirely without the influence over others which is exerted by the woman with a well-developed bust and shapely form . . . .

Price of the Venus-Carnis Treatment.

The price of the complete Venus-Carnis treatment for a quantity which is designed to last for 30 days is $15. This price has been absolutely fixed by our contract with Madame Margarette Merlain, the discoverer. Under our contract with her this is the price which we have agreed shall be charged, and Madame Merlain gave us her secret without charge under our guarantee that we would in no case charge more than $15, and that we would publish this fact in all circular matter which we sent out, so that patrons may be absolutely protected.

The products required for the treatment are very expensive to manufacture, and Madame Merlain felt that without a contract of this kind the manufacturer might easily exact a charge of $25 or $50 for the complete treatment. Great credit is due to Madame Merlain for her generosity in giving up her secret absolutely without charge for the benefit of women who wish to develop their bust.

The Institut Venus-Carnis is permanently located at Pembroke House, Oxford Street, London, W; 17 Boulevard de la Madeleine, Paris; with money deposited at large banks in each city. As to honesty and reliability, the highest references can be furnished in all parts of the world.

Allure Bust Developer

Advertisements for the Allure Bust Developer claimed to "exercise the breasts by contraction and relaxation," thereby improving the circulation to "underfed" breast tissues so that the breasts would grow normally and naturally. The result would be a beautiful bust line and the restoration of

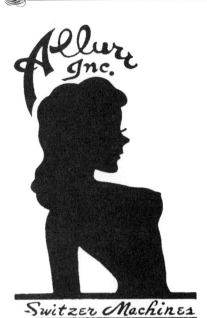

Logo for the Allure bust developer.
Look familiar?

youth, beauty, and glamour, without the use of surgery, hormones,
or creams. Most frightening was
the promise that regular use would
prevent breast cancer. The Allure
consisted of a pink metal cabinet
housing a motor which produced
a vacuum. Breast-shaped cups
were attached to tubing which
connected on the right-hand side
of the machine. The FDA Notices
of Judgment between 1958 and
1960, which effectively stopped
the sale and manufacture of the
device, cited inadequate directions for use plus potential health
dangers as the reasons for confis-
cation and destruction of the
Allure machines.

The foot operated breast
enlarger pump used calf power
to operate the device and cause
a vacuum. In 1976, ten million
women each spent $9.95 on this
device which caused only bruis-
ing. The earlier Abunda Beauty
bust developer was hydro-powered.
In her book, *The Technology of
Orgasm*, Rachel Maines explains

that when municipalities first began
supplying water to homes, meters
were not installed. With unlimited
use of water at no cost, hydropower
from the powder room faucet was
a cost-effective way to power early
vibrators and bust developers.

The Abunda, a pink plastic
breast-shaped cone, with a hose
that attached to the kitchen

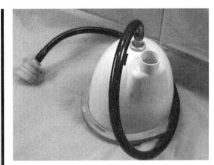

The Abunda.

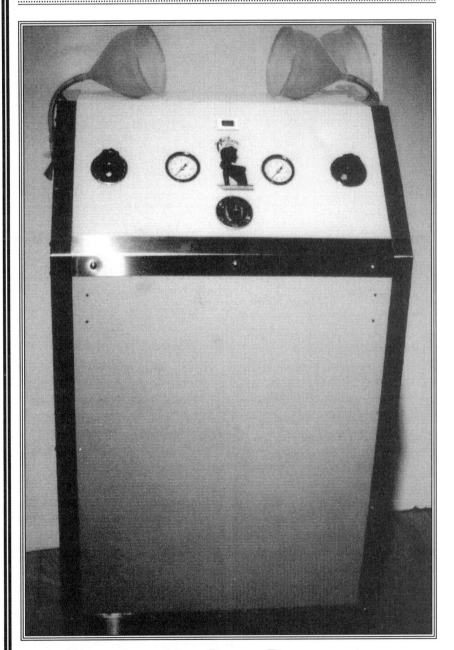

THE ALLURE BUST DEVELOPER

faucet and an outlet for the water to run into the sink, was advertised as the means to achieve a perfect bust by hydro-massage in the late 1950s.

On October 17, 1960 the U.S. Food & Drug Administration issued Notice of Judgment #5027 and seized 380 of the devices plus 89 display units at Albuquerque, New Mexico. The results of their investigation showed that it did not fulfill any of the promises made in its advertisements.

The promotional literature for the Abunda consisted of the following instructions and poetic description of its promise to the user:

INSTRUCTIONS

1.
Attach connection to kitchen water faucet.

2.
Surround right breast with cup, press firmly against rib cage.

3.
Turn warm water slowly, gradually increasing water pressure. Increase temperature to maximum point of comfort.

4.
Without removing unit from body, slowly reduce water temperature.

5.
Allow cold water to massage bust for two minutes.

6.
Transfer unit to left breast and repeat above procedure.

NOTHING compares to HYDRO-MASSAGE

Since the days of Athens and Rome, hydro-massage has been used successfully by millions. The restorative, healing, beautifying

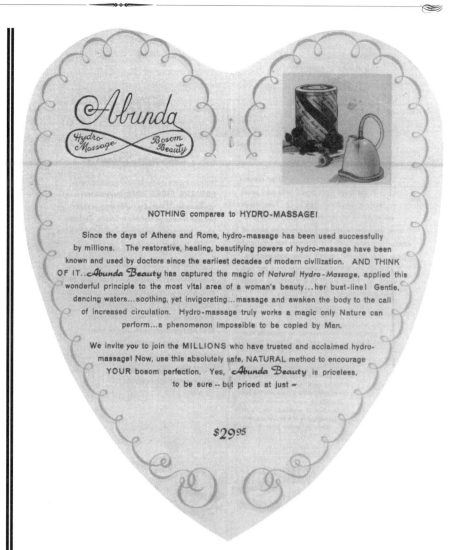

NOTHING compares to HYDRO-MASSAGE!

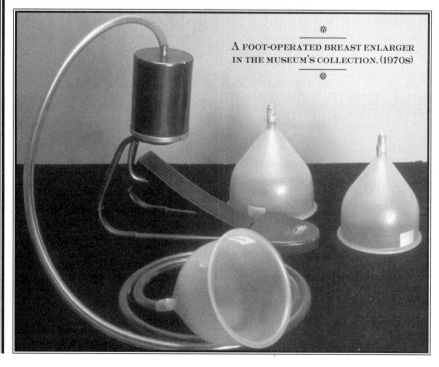

A FOOT-OPERATED BREAST ENLARGER IN THE MUSEUM'S COLLECTION. (1970S)

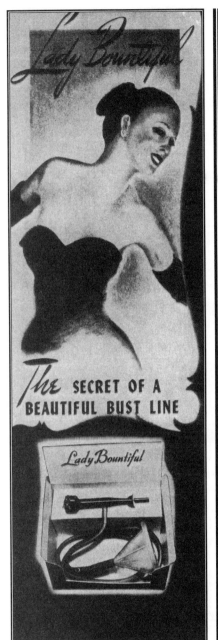

The SECRET OF A BEAUTIFUL BUST LINE

Lady Bountiful

Patent Applied For

Over a period of time we have noticed that the women who boast of the splendid satisfaction they have derived from their new bustlines, are those who have received instructions in its proper use; for that reason we either prefer to have a representative call at your home at your convenience or to have you drop in for a free demonstration.

Telephone or write for free demonstration at your convenience, at absolutely no obligation to purchase.

$25.00 complete
Plus State Sales Tax

LADY BOUNTIFUL
6404 Hollywood Blvd.
Hollywood 28, California
Telephone: GLadstone 4056

powers of hydro-massage have been known and used by doctors since the earliest decades of modern civilization. **AND THINK OF IT**. Abunda Beauty has captured the magic Natural Hydro-Massage, applied this wonderful principle to the most vital area of a woman's body . . . her bust-line. Gentle, dancing waters . . . soothing, yet invigorating . . . massage and awaken the body to the call of increased circulation. Hydro-massage truly works a magic only Nature can perform . . . a phenomenon impossible to be copied by Man.

We invite you to join the **MILLIONS** who have trusted and acclaimed hydro-massage! Now, use this absolutely safe, **NATURAL** method to encourage YOUR bosom perfection,

Abunda Beauty is priceless, to be sure—but priced at just **$29.95**

Roll-a-Ray Heat Massage With Infra Red

"Apply Heat Alone—The handy handle hooks anywhere and the rays can be pointed in any direction. Or massage alone—Just use Roll-a-Ray without connecting the electricity. Or Heat and Massage Both! Use massage and penetrating rays for loosening muscle and assisting in driving fatty tissues away."

So claimed the Roll-a-Ray, a molded brown plastic case with a handle, about 8 inches long, 7½ inches high and 4½ inches wide. On the bottom at both ends was a corrugated plastic roller; at one time these were made of rubber. Also on the bottom was a molded plastic mesh which protected a small 60 watt light bulb.

The advertisements claimed

The Lady Bountiful was another bust developer which attached to the kitchen faucet. The suction was produced when water ran past a tube connected to the breast hose, producing a modest vacuum. No water was used on the breast itself. The device was outlawed by the FDA in 1957.

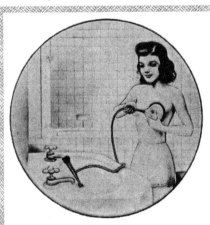

Easy To Use

(a) Attach vacuum unit to the COLD water faucet.

(b) Turn on the water — full force.

(c) Place plastic cup snugly over breast.

(d) Place thumb over the small opening on the tube near the cup, and hold the thumb there until the vacuum (created by the flowing water) pulls the breast out fully into the cup.

(e) After breast has been pulled into the cup, release thumb suddenly and allow the breast to return to original position.

(f) Continue this process — thumb alternately on and off.

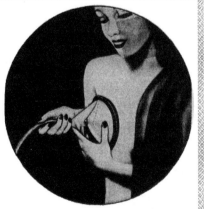

How To Fit the Lady Bountiful

The above illustration shows the proper position of the plastic cup on the breast. Note that when the right thumb is pressed firmly over the small opening in tube, the vacuum created pulls the breast out to the proper position. When the thumb is removed from the opening (note dotted line) the vacuum is released and the breast reverts to its former position.

The LADY BOUNTIFUL operates on the natural principle of a vacuum and uses the perfectly natural processes of exercise to develop tissue which has remained dormant and inactive.

The women who are most highly satisfied with the results they have received are those who have exercised with the LADY BOUNTIFUL faithfully over sufficient lengths of time. To these satisfied users there is no question but that LADY BOUNTIFUL has helped them attain a more symmetrical development.

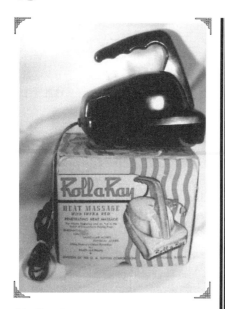

"Roll-a-Ray uses two of the most effective reducing methods employed by masseurs and Turkish baths—heat and massage. Now you can enjoy the benefits of both simultaneously in your own home. Just connect the Roll-a-Ray to your light socket and follow the directions for helping to remove fatty tissues. Many varied ailments respond to application of heat and massage. With their aid nature frequently steps in and relieves distress." The "varied ailments" were rheumatism, lumbago, and muscular aches. In short, the Roll-a-Ray pledged that a 60 watt light bulb would remove aches and pains while rolling the fat away!

The Food and Drug Administration didn't agree and the Roll-a-Ray was judged to be mis branded. The manufacturer, O.A. Sutton Corp. of Wichita, Kansas, was allowed to claim the seized devices. The court ordered that a 30 watt bulb replace the 60 watt bulb, that foil be placed in the cavity behind the bulb, that erroneous claims were to be removed from the directions and devices, and that substitute labeling approved by the FDA be used.

Vision Dieter Glasses

Will glasses with different colored lenses cause weight loss? Optometrist John D. Miller of Little Rock, Arkansas thought so and in the early 1980s manufactured Vision Dieter Glasses. Dr. Miller theorized that if advertisers used color to attract, color might also be used to repel or repulse.

He believed that his dual-tinted glasses caused a "very low-level confusion in the subconscious," resulting in rejection by the conscious.

Dr. Miller claimed that appetite control and weight loss would result if Vision Dieter glasses were worn for two hours a day (during the morning or afternoon but never at meals). The glasses were purported to also be effective for

Two examples of the Roll-a-Ray.

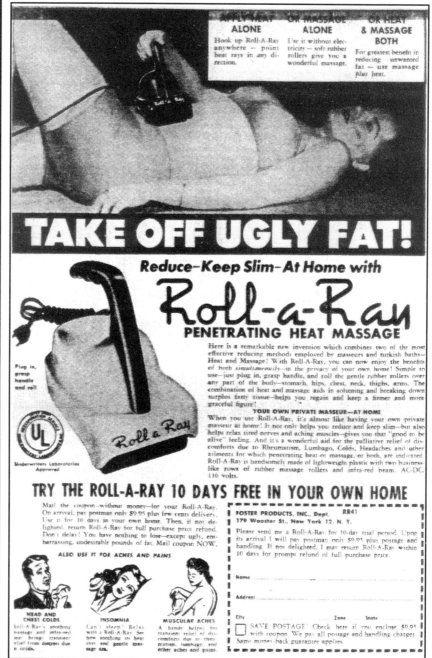

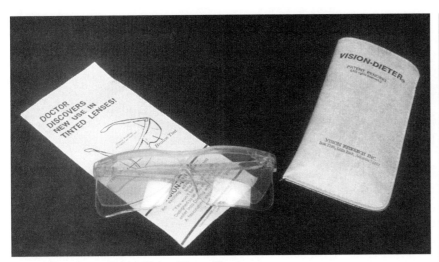

Lose fat on sight with the **Vision Dieter Glasses.**

nicotine and caffeine cessation. Promotional literature advertised that "independent laboratory tests" confirmed results! In part, this was true: 21 people wore the glasses for 20 days and the glasses were judged to be safe. The health claims were never tested. Little Rock FDA investigators began work on this case in September 1982, and in January 1984, the U.S. District Court, Eastern Division, ordered the destruction of the Vision Dieter glasses inventory, reserving 75 pairs for use in consumer education.

Acu-Stop 2000

"Congratulations! You've taken the first step to becoming a slimmer, trimmer and healthier person. This product you have just received, Acu-Stop 2000,

The Acu-Stop 2000.

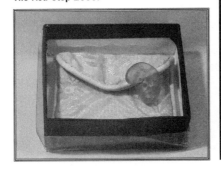

will enable you to make amazing changes in your life. You will eat less, you will eat healthier and you won't feel deprived!

"Acu-Stop 2000 is based on the Oriental principle of acupuncture, but without any pain or discomfort. The ear piece, which is almost invisible, will pinpoint pressure to those areas in your ear which regulate hunger. You will eat less and you will lose weight, fast! It's that simple."

So wrote Mike Powers, President of Acu-Stop 2000, in the early 1990s. Mr. Powers went on to explain that the Acu-Stop, a bit of rubber 1 inch by 1½ inches, with small nubs on top, was to be inserted in the right ear whenever the user felt hungry, and massaged for 2 to 3 minutes. This was the Acu-Stop 2000 weight loss system. Results were guaranteed within 30 days.

The economics of Acu-Stop 2000 were also quite simple: the small rubber device which cost about 17¢ to manufacture sold for $39.95 plus shipping and handling. In 1995, the U.S. Food and Drug Administration seized 19,000 Acu-Stops and destroyed them in a hospital incinerator. Original Marketing, Inc., which

did business as Acu-Stop 2000, its advertising agency, and two of its corporate officers entered into a consent agreement with the Federal Trade Commission in May 1995. By doing so, the companies and officers admitted no guilt. They did agree to provide refunds to consumers, escrowing a $50,000 reserve fund for this purpose, and as individuals, each posted a $300,000 performance bond agreeing not to market any weight loss or weight control product.

Baldness Remedies

The Crosley Radio Corporation manufactured at least two models of Xervacs, a baldness remedy invented by Andrè A. Cueto, beginning in 1936. Operators of barber shops, beauty parlors, and salons were told they might earn $75 a week giving half hour treatments with the device. The suggested treatment cost was $1 to $2; the machine sold for $150. In a 1936 sales letter, Powell Crosley, Jr., founder and owner of Crosley Radio, told prospective buyers

The Xervac.

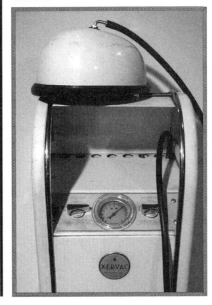

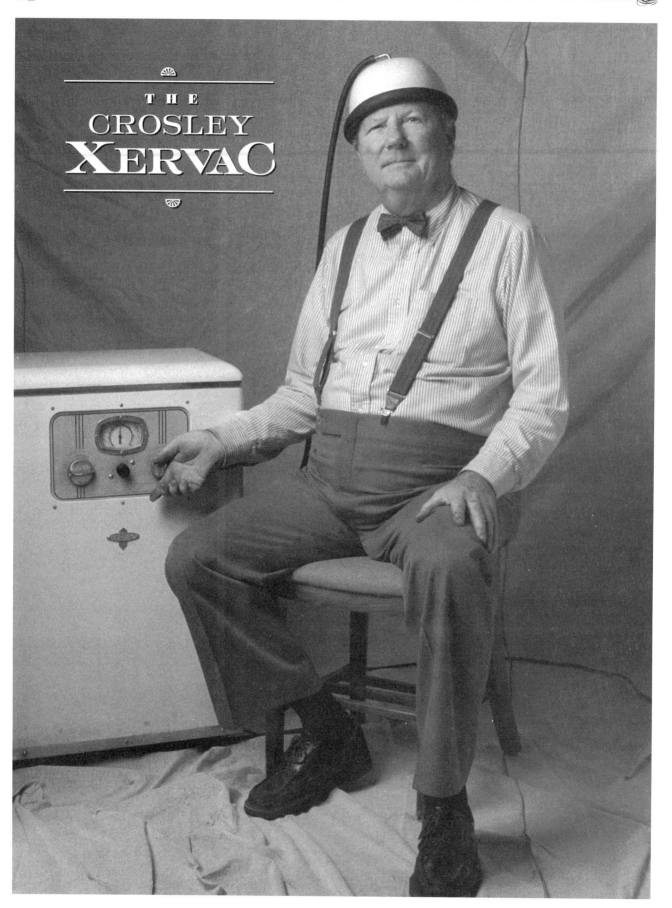

THE
CROSLEY
XERVAC

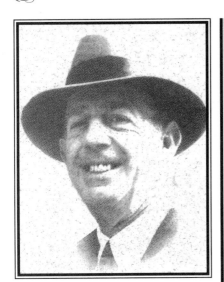

Powel Crosley, Jr.

Below: The Barclay Co. originally manufactured this product, called Tricopherous, in 1814. They claimed it cured baldness, sprains, dandruff, grey hair, etc.

"Until we started the development of the Xervac, we had no idea about the vanity of the human race."

Powel Crosley, Jr., born in September 1886, began his career with American Automobile Accessories, where he sold car gadgets by mail order. Mr. Crosley generated the first automobile radio and the first push-button radio. When he purchased the Cincinnati Reds in 1934, he developed electric lights to illuminate the ball field so working people could attend night games. Crosley also invented "compact cars, the Shelvador refrigerator, disc brakes, the 35mm camera, 4 different airplanes, and one product that he took off the market because

it was before its time, the fax machine!" The Crosley Xervac seems to be the least touted of his innovations.

The Xervac used a small vacuum force to massage the scalp and allegedly make hair grow. (The smaller unit alternated vacuum suction with blowing air.) The motor was housed in the cabinet, which was connected via a length of rubber hose to the helmet. A rubber helmet seal fit inside the helmet, and for thick hair an additional rubber head cap was supplied. Implicit claims for the device were arresting the "abnormal falling of hair" after five hours of treatment, hair growth in "previous fuzz" after 10 hours of treatment, and finally, "full

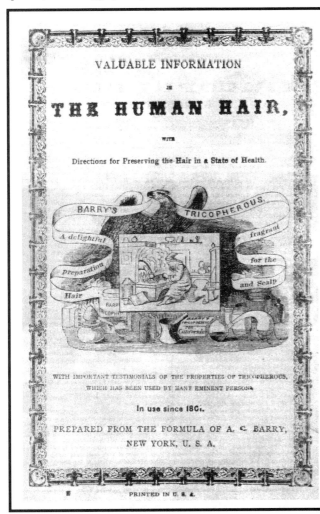

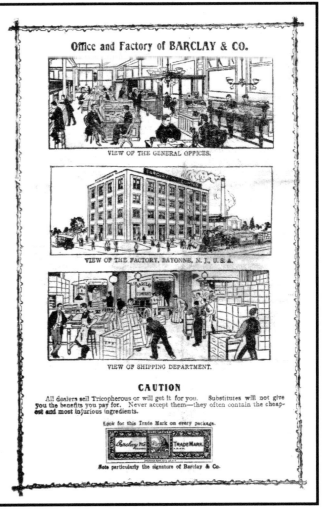

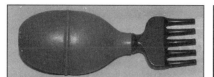

ABOVE: This comb had a built-in hair tonic dispenser for hair restoration.

OPPOSITE, RIGHT: Ointrasan—"A New Source of Profit for Your Shop." Instructions: "1st apply hot towel, then massage scalp, then spray on Ointrasan." It was expected to work so well that shops should plan on opening in the evenings for male customers! A professional bottle for 60 treatments cost $2.35, a 74% profit (1936).

growth of hair" beginning in the temporal regions, bald pate, and surrounding a widow's peak. Time required for full growth of hair was said to vary and it was noted that hair already present "grows at a faster rate." Treatments every other day were recommended. Even the CEO took treatments: Lew Crosley, grandson of Powel Crosley, Jr., recalls his grandfather "sitting in his bathroom each morning back in the '30s with that crazy helmet perched on his head and, no, it didn't do one bit of good."

Competing with Crosley in the vacuum baldness-remedy market was The Modern Vacuum Cap Co. of Denver Colorado. This company produced a vacuum cap with a manually powered pump. Treatments of 15 minutes twice a day were suggested. This company's claims were more tentative than Crosley's, for the instructions patiently explained: "Of course, some cases take longer than others, and especially where the scalp has been deprived of hair for years no person need expect a new growth immediately. It took months and possibly years to bring on this bald condition and to expect a luxuriant growth at once would be the greatest folly. If you are patient results are bound to come."

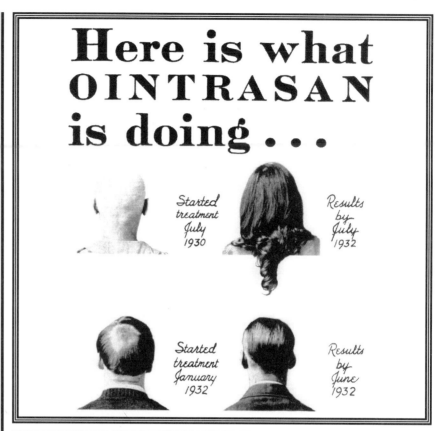

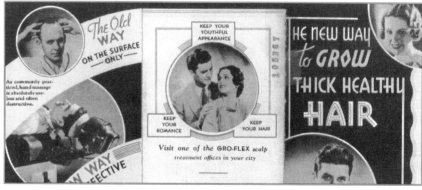

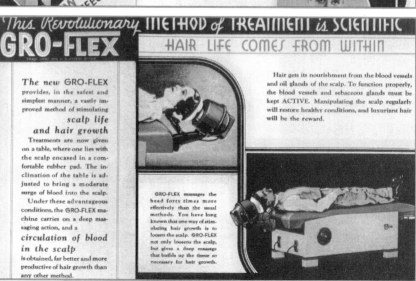

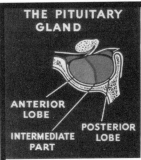 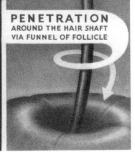

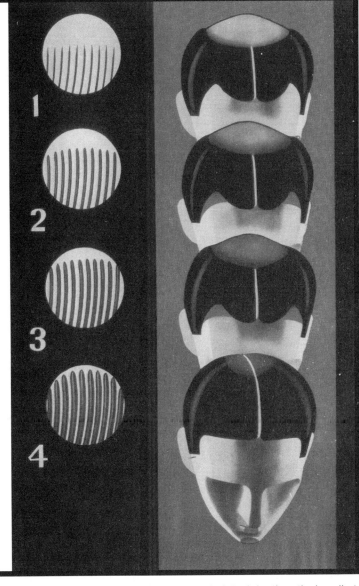

As Ultrasol treatment removes the Neo-keratin obstruction to the development of fuzz or thin short hair, to the fullest size inherent in the root, less and less of the scalp shows through. The relative "covering" value of a given number of hair over a given spot, as hair improvement may take place, is shown diagramatically,* in the circles on the opposite page: 1—Thin short hair. 2—Same hair improved. 3—Same hair further improved. 4—Same hair still further improved.

Men who have used Ultrasol report:

✓ How abnormal hair loss has stopped

✓ How fuzz has grown to mature hair

✓ How the scalp feels fresh, free from dandruff

✓ How dull, dry, faded hair becomes brilliant

✓ How new hair on gray heads is frequently of the original shade. This would indicate that the treatment may help to prevent premature graying

Although thousands of men and women have used the treatment and an impressive record of results has accumulated testifying to its effectiveness, the Institute cannot ethically presume to foretell the exact results of the treatment in any specific case. No two scalp conditions are alike. Therefore, the effective result of the treatment on the individual's scalp can be determined only by personal experience.

* Based on observation by Post Institute, of progressive hair improvement on a number of men and women over a three-year period.

[6]

Ultrasol was a cosmetic for hair that supposedly contained oil, lemon juice, eggs, sulfur, and pituitary gland extract—the latter being the active ingredient. However, there is not the slightest evidence to show that rubbing pituitary gland extract on a bald head will grow hair! (1936)

Many companies advertised by circulating post cards in public places, hoping people interested in the product would pick them up and send them in. Who could fail to be impressed by the luxuriant head of hair shown? Who would not want to try the Calvacura Method, given such results?

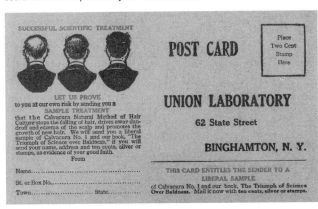

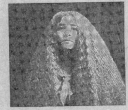

The Blud Rub from the 1940s is perhaps the most famous quack baldness cure in the Museum collection for it was featured in an oft-repeated episode of the *I Love Lucy* television show. Typically, the Blud Rub was found in a barber shop. The barber held the device in contact with the customers' head, moving it forward and backward and side-to-side. The disks (once covered with pads) rotated up-and-down, alternating sides. The theory was that scalp massage would make the hair grow.

X-ray Depilatory: The Tricho System

The most tragic, the most heartbreaking, of all quack devices manufactured in the U.S. may be the Tricho Machine and similar devices advertised as the Dermic Institute, the EpilaX-ray, Hair-X Laboratories, Hamomar Method, and Marton Method. These brand names represented the misapplication of X-rays as salon depilatories. And the Tricho System, with over 55 locations nationally,

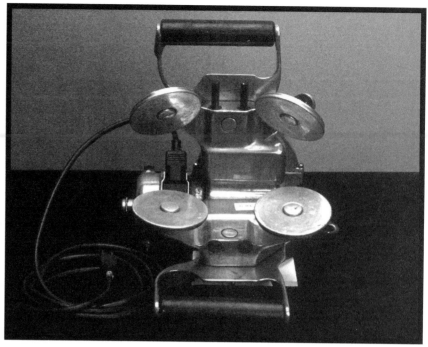

⟩ THE BLUD RUB ⟨

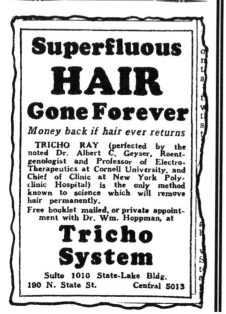

was by and far the largest source of these dangerous rays. The victims were overwhelmingly women in their late teens and early twenties. These young women, perhaps believing Tricho propaganda, propaganda which stated forthrightly that men are repulsed by superfluous hair and that marriage might be out of reach because of a hint of a mustache or dark hair on the legs, unknowingly put their beauty, their health, and their lives on the line. From the late 1920s through the 1940s and perhaps later, these women turned up in doctors' offices displaying the hideous results of X-ray depilation: hardened and wrinkled skin, receded gums, never-healing ulcerated sores over the face or legs, tumors, and, of course, cancer.

Certainly the radium cures of the same period were equally dangerous. But even the great radium quack, W. J. A. Bailey, is on record as believing in his product and as having used it himself. Mr. Bailey, a self-styled

expert and futurist, was not a doctor nor a scientist. That he made money off his radium products is known, though he did not become wealthy. Mr. Bailey was a believer.

Dr. Albert C. Geyser, designer of the Tricho machine, may have started out as a believer. His X-ray

□

DR. ALBERT C. GEYSER

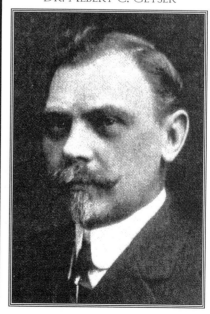

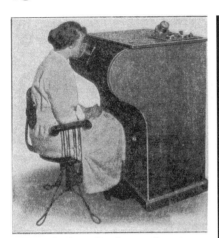

Patient placed in position for upper lip treatment.

depilatory contained a filter; he may have thought it would work. But the evidence suggests that if Dr. Geyser didn't know the dangers of his X-ray debilitation at the outset, the damaging results soon became apparent and he had the practice, the background, and the training to recognize the danger. He chose not to and continued to risk the health of vulnerable young women.

Dr. Geyser announced his new X-ray technique for removing unwanted body hair to the medical community via an article, "Hypertrichosis and its Treatment" in the medical journal, the *Urologic and Cutaneous Review,* Vol. XXVII, No. 8, 1923. At this time, he was Medical Director of the Tricho Institute, a business of his creation. His past credentials included Professor of Physiological Therapy and Chief of Clinic at Fordham University and Chief of the Electro and Roentgenray Clinic at Cornell College. Dr. Geyser was not only an M.D., he was an academician, and a scientist. In his article, he described his then-new device:

"It is now possible to produce, by the construction of special apparatus and the use of filters, rays that are almost homogenous in composition. With this end in view I had constructed for me a Roetngen-ray apparatus to do one thing only and that is the atrophying of hair bulbs and their follicles. . . . The *advantages* of the Roentgen-ray are that it is painless. Instead of destroying a few hairs at a time, all of them are treated at once. Instead of waiting years for a complete result only a few months are required. The time of treatment requires only a few minutes and is repeated once in two weeks. . . . In cases of severe hypertrichosis, where other methods of relief have failed or proven inadequate and the removal of hairs is paramount, the use of the Roentgen-ray from a modern apparatus giving not less than 60 K. V. is the method of choice."

Dr. Geyser was not as forthcoming with the general public. Advertisements for the Tricho System copiously avoided the word X-ray, for by the late 1920s some of the dangers of X-rays were known. Instead, the public was told "Today in TRICHO SYSTEM one wave length only is created and it is so short that it measures only one-third of an Angstom unit or one thirty-millionth (1/30,000,000) of the thickness of a ten-cent piece. These inconceivably short vibratory waves bombarding the hair papillae interfere with the function of the lymphoid cells of which the papillae are composed but without affecting the simple epidermic cells of the skin. . . . TRICHO SYSTEM, national in extent,

Above Left: A woman demonstrates the (thankfully) one-of-a-kind Tricho System for removing unwanted hair.

Right: A bogus medal "awarded" to the manufacturers of the Tricho System.

The Final Seal of Approval

PARIS! What visions that word conjures up in the feminine mind! Paris, that dictates fashions to the world—Paris, that makes the beautifying of women a fine art. Where is the woman or girl who would not like to get all her frocks and hats from Paris? Where is the woman or girl who will be satisfied with less if she can have French cosmetics and perfumes?

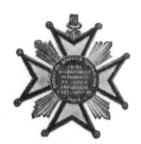

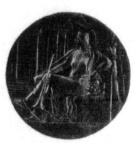

The Grand Prix, Medaille d'Or and Cross of Honor were awarded to Tricho System at the Exposition Generale Commerciale, Paris, 1925. No photographic reproduction can do justice to the beauty of these medals, tho the general appearance is clearly shown. Tricho System is justly proud of this award.

Paris has placed the seal of approval on TRICHO SYSTEM. At the Exposition Generale Commerciale in 1925, the Grand Prize and gold medal were awarded to TRICHO SYSTEM as the best and most efficient method known for the permanent removal of superfluous hair. TRICHO SYSTEM competed with hair removers of every kind and description from all over the world and the report of the Committee of Awards was unanimous.

The Grand Prix diploma and the form on which the Committee's report was made are too large to reproduce in this booklet, but both, together with the medals may be seen at the New York office. The award report with facsimile signatures of the Committee appear on the opposite page.

offers the one scientific, infallible method for the permanent removal of superfluous hair."

The Tricho System did not remain reserved for "severe hypertrichosis." Dr. Geyser leased his X-ray machines to salons, and provided beauty operators with a two week training course. Instead of two applications of X-rays, the Tricho System required a minimum of six treatments, with 15 to 20 generally recommended. Clients paid three dollars a treatment

Warnings about the relationship between X-rays and pre-cancerous skin conditions began appearing in the medical journals in 1925. In a 1925 address before the American Medico-Physical Research Association, Dr. Geyser discussed the dangers of X-ray depilatories (though claimed his device was safe.) At the 1929 annual meeting of the American Medical Association, doctors were asked to report injuries caused by the Tricho. A sampling of cases was published in *JAMA*:

"MISS S. R,, NEW YORK– Twenty Tricho treatments three years previously. Telangiectasia and atrophy both present and growing steadily worse. Painful ulcer as large as a silver dollar over left jaw.

"MISS H. K. (AGED 30), MILWAUKEE–Fifteen Tricho treatments between July, 1926, and April, 1927. Treatments resumed and four exposures given between July 1 and Septemeber 11, 1927. In October, 1927, patient first observed redness and pruritus, which increased in severity, resulting in painful ulcerations and disability. In December, 1928, hands and both legs showed extensive injury from the knees to the feet, with telangiectasia, atrophy and pigmentation. A deep X-ray ulcer below the right knee; smaller ulcers below the left knee and a number of atrophic adherent scars of previously healed ulcers. Patient wholly disabled for work, bed-ridden, and suffering severely.

"MISS D. M. (AGED 26), WASHINGTON D.C.–Took Tricho treatment for superfluous hair on hands, forearms, axilla, chin and outer portion of right lip. Developed numerous telangiectases of the hands and arms, atrophy and telangiectasis in both axillae, wrinkling of the skin of the chin, with atrophy and telangiectasis of the upper lip: also marked atrophy of the gum beneath the lower lip."

As late as 1947, women were still seeking medical treatment for problems resulting from Tricho treatments. Doctors Anthony C. Ciollaro and Marcus B. Einhorn in "The Use of X-rays for the Treatment of Hypertrichosis is Dangerous," (*JAMA* 135: 1947) reported: "Judging from conversations with dermatologists in different sections of the country and judging from the many cases of radiodermatitis seen in practice and in clinics, the number of cases of X-ray burns, cancer and death resulting from the treatments administered by the Tricho Institute must have run into the thousands. It is impossible to obtain or

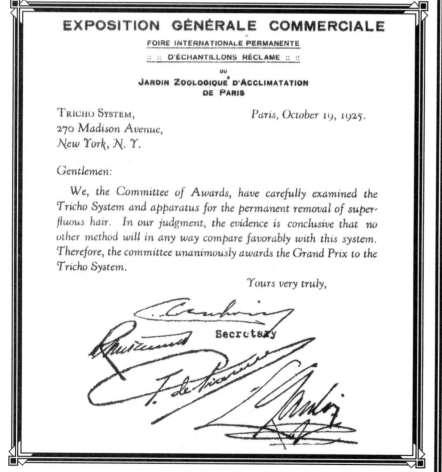

EXPOSITION GÉNÉRALE COMMERCIALE

FOIRE INTERNATIONALE PERMANENTE
:: :: D'ÉCHANTILLONS RÉCLAME :: ::
DU
JARDIN ZOOLOGIQUE D'ACCLIMATATION
DE PARIS

TRICHO SYSTEM,   Paris, October 19, 1925.
270 Madison Avenue,
New York, N. Y.

Gentlemen:

We, the Committee of Awards, have carefully examined the Tricho System and apparatus for the permanent removal of superfluous hair. In our judgment, the evidence is conclusive that no other method will in any way compare favorably with this system. Therefore, the committee unanimously awards the Grand Prix to the Tricho System.

Yours very truly,

Secretary

This letter notified the recipient of the award shown on the previous page. However, this award is completely phony. In London in 1914, Max Kaiser sold these awards to anyone willing to pay $400. He guaranteed that the buyer would receive either a "grand prize" or a "gold medal" at one of the numerous "International Exhibitions" of the day.

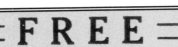
estimate the actual number because the cases were not reportable and therefore were not recorded."

Auto-Hemic Serum— A Cure for Laziness, Ugliness, Frigidity, and Many Other Conditions

In the early 1920s, a new therapy burst upon the scene. According to its literature it was "The Missing Link in Medicine"–possibly referring to the ease with which one may make monkeys of certain physicians. More specifically, although vague, the literature states that the patient was injected with a solution made by "attenuating, hemolizing, incubating, and potentizing a few drops of his or her own blood and then making further dilution according to needs of the case, as can be determined only by a physician skilled in its use."

Dr. L.D. Rogers, the inventor of this system, claimed that "without any great exaggeration, this new modified serum treatment is good for anything that is the matter with you, provided the cause is not organic, mechanical or bacterial." The AMA commented at that time, "One infers that in the inorganic, mental, spiritual and non-bacterial spheres the stuff is supreme."

A Homeopathic journal of the day outlined how to administer this new cure: "Take 0.5 cc of blood from the patient's vein into a sterile glass syringe containing 4.5 c.c. of freshly distilled cool water. Incubate for 24 hours at 37 degrees C. then take 0.5 cc of this incubated solution into another syringe and keep diluting it until you have a 1:1000 saturation. But to get the full formula just send Dr. Rogers $100 in cash."

On November 9, 1915, the *Chicago Herald* reported that a woman who was a plaintiff in a $20,000 suit against Rogers, based on charges of malpractice, "got service on Rogers by throwing a brick through the plate glass in his front door. The Deputy Sheriff of Cook County had apparently failed for four or five months to get service on Rogers."

Dr. Rogers was a very active practitioner who founded many quasi-medical organizations–organizations which he used to promote whatever projects and schemes he was engaged in at the time. He used testimonials extensively to proclaim the virtues of Auto-Hemic Therapy. Consider Case No. 7176 in the treatment of laziness. "A man, considered the laziest person in his community with a habit of drinking *30* whiskies a day, took the serum. He stopped drinking, shaved himself and changed from a bum into a sober, clean, wholesome, bright & honest workman."

Frigidity was cured in a young woman with a morbid dislike of her husband. Within a week of taking the serum she "became normal." At $100 per treatment, paid in advance without exception, this was an expensive therapy in 1920–especially as the patients seem on the whole to have been from the lower socio-economic classes. Their stories, were it not for the tragic element in the background, would be amusing. But they are tragic, as ultimately are the stories of so many desperate people who encountered quacks with their devices and hollow promises.

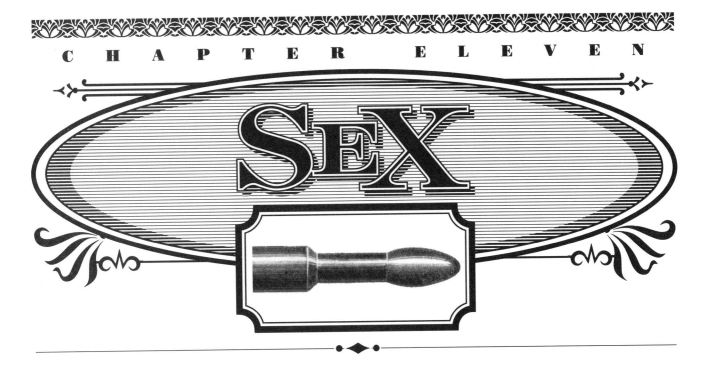

SEX EX MACHINA.

Until 1984, the literature about health fraud and quackery contained no reference to sex and sexuality other than to condemn the ever-present manhood cures and the few equivalent nostrums for women. The great quackbusters like Dr. Arthur Cramp and Dr. Morris Fishbein at the AMA Investigative Bureau never condemned a device solely as a sexual aid or sexual toy. Indeed, devices explicitly labeled as sexual aids would have been immediately banished from the marketplace as obscene! These devices had a better chance for survival by claiming to be cure-alls–no matter how preposterous the health claims may have been.

In 1986, Rachael Maines completed a research fellowship at the Bakken Library and Museum in Minneapolis, Minnesota, and in its 1986 newsletter published an article suggesting that in the early 1900s doctors had treated "hysteria" in women by bringing their patients to orgasm. Ms. Maines stated that the doctors were much relieved by the invention of the electric vibrator for the time it saved when dispensing the treatments.

Ms. Maines has expanded her thesis in her book, *The Technology of Orgasm.* She traces how, as houses became wired for electricity, the vibrator left the doctor's office and became a medical appliance for home use–heavily advertised in the back pages of women's magazines. Ms. Maines' is the

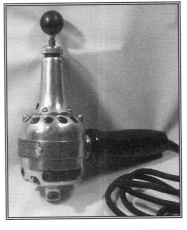

THE WHITE CROSS ELECTRIC VIBRATOR ALLEGEDLY IMPROVED CIRCULATION AND RELIEVED BOTH ACUTE AND CHRONIC AILMENTS THAT HAD THEIR ORIGIN IN "CONGESTION" OR "POOR CIRCULATION." EARLY 1900s.

first book written which explores the sexual use of a quack or fringe medical device.

Vibrators were not the only sexual toy in the history of quack medical devices. We have watched many of our visitors stroll through the Museum of Questionable Medical Devices and come across these risqué appliances or their pictures. Invariably, the museum visitors' eyes open a bit wider and in a moment, there is a smile or a chuckle or an outright guffaw as the sexual nature of the devices becomes readily apparent. Clearly, the purveyors of sexual gadgets in the late nineteenth and early twentieth centuries, censored by obscenity laws, tried to obscure the real purpose of their devices in the general confusion of the quack device market.

207

The following is from the jacket copy to *The Technology of Orgasm*:

From the time of Hippocrates until the 1920s, massaging "hysterical" female patients to orgasm was a staple of medical practice among Western physicians. Hysteria, an ailment considered common and chronic in women, was thought to be a consequence of sexual deprivation. Doctors performed the "routine chore" of relieving hysterical patients' symptoms with manual genital massage until the women reached orgasm, or as it was known under clinical conditions, the "hysterical paroxysm." The vibrator first emerged as an electromechanical medical instrument in direct response from physicians who, far from enjoying the implementation of pelvic massage, sought every opportunity to substitute the services of midwives and, later, the efficiency of mechanical devices.

In *The Technology of Orgasm*, Rachel Maines offers readers a candid, often wryly humorous account of why such treatments were socially and ethically permissible for doctors and why women were believed to require them. The author explores hysteria in Western medicine throughout the

---

HOW TO MAKE A VIBRATING CHAIR

Fasten attachment R in hole F of the Vibrator like an applicator.

Put the Vibrator in clamp No. 9 and fasten the clamp to the back, side, front or anywhere on the chair. (A rocking chair is best adapted.) Be sure it is very tight before turning on the current.

For general stimulation and that tired feeling occupy the chair from one to two minutes daily. Lean backwards as much as possible.

ATTACHMENT R

CLAMP NO. 9

How to convert a rocking chair into a vibrating chair using the White Cross Vibrator.

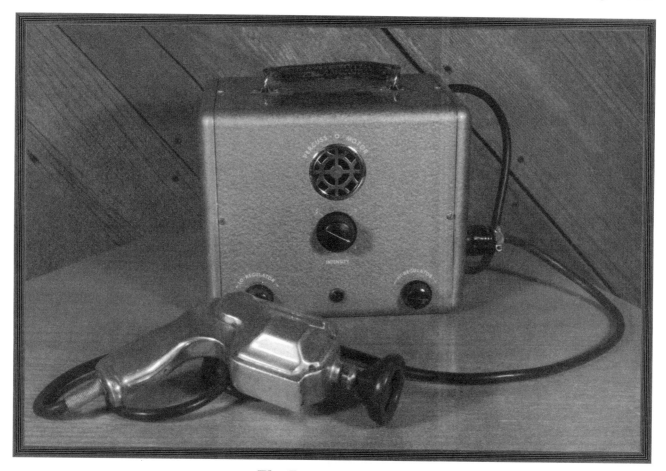

The Percusso Motor.
A very heavy duty vibrator used in Reflexology treatments.

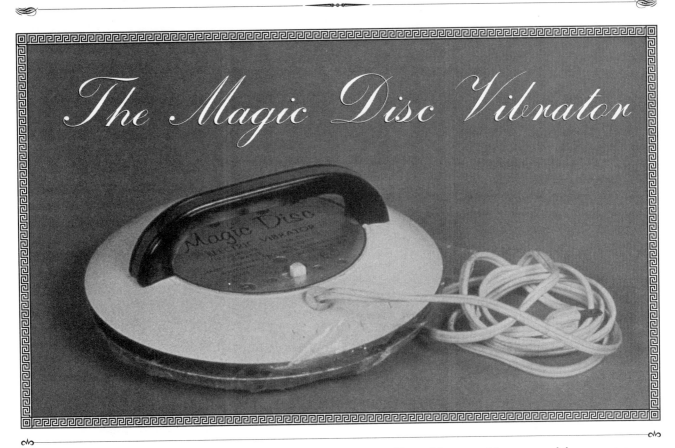

THE MAGIC DISC VIBRATOR, ALSO KNOWN AS THE HANDY HANNAH VIBRATOR, GIVES A GENTLE VIBRATION. LITTLE ELSE IS KNOWN ABOUT IT.

ages and examines the characterization of female sexuality as a disease requiring treatment. Medical authorities, she writes, were able to defend and justify the clinical production of orgasm in women as necessary to maintain the dominant view of sexuality, which defined sex as penetration to male orgasm—a practice that consistently fails to produce orgasm in a majority of the female population. This male-centered definition of satisfying and healthy coitus shaped not only the development of concepts of female sexual pathology but also instrumentation designed to cope with them.

Invented in the late 1880s by a British physician, the vibrator was popular with turn-of-the-century doctors as a quick, efficient cure for hysteria which neither fatigued the therapist nor demanded skills that were difficult to acquire. Some entrepreneurs even opened vibratory "operating theaters." Maines describes in detail the wide range of vibratory apparatus available to physicians by 1900, from low-priced foot-powered models to the Cadillac of vibrators, the Chattanooga, which in 1904 cost $200 plus freight.

Hysterical women presented a large and lucrative clientele for doctors, and vibrators reduced, from about one hour to ten minutes, the time required for a physician to produce results, significantly increasing the number of patients he could treat in the course of a single workday. These women were ideal patients in that they neither recovered nor died from their condition but continued

to require regular medical "treatment."

Maines traces the vibrator from its beginning as a sanctioned therapeutic instrument to its fall from respectability and disappearance from medical offices—after appearing in stag films in the 1920s—to its reemergence in the 1960s as a sex aid. In the preface, she entertains readers with her enlightening adventures in vibrator historiography.

The Lure of Sex Frauds

Nuxated iron, endorsed by Civil War generals (who lived to tell of their experience), was later advertised in the 1930s for "strength, energy, and power" with testimonials from heavyweight champion Jess Willard, who claimed his

The Vatican at Rome Recommends Nuxated Iron

If you lack BODILY or MENTAL VIGOR; If you are WEAK; NERVOUS or IRRITABLE, TRY NUXATED IRON TODAY.

Nuxated Iron CONTAINS ORGANIC IRON LIKE THE IRON IN YOUR BLOOD and LIKE THE IRON IN SPINACH, LENTILS AND APPLES.

NUXATED IRON also contains a remarkable product, brought to the attention of the French Academy of Medicine by the celebrated Dr. Robin, which represents the principal chemical constituent of active living nerve force FOR FEEDING THE NERVES, so that NUXATED IRON might be said to be both a BLOOD and a NERVE FOOD.

THERE ARE 30,000,000,000,000 RED BLOOD CORPUSCLES in your blood and each one must have iron.

Today about one person out of every three is said to suffer more or less from the great devitalizing weakness brought on by malnutrition or lack of sufficient nourishment; which is caused NOT BY LACK OF FOOD but often by LACK OF SUFFICIENT ORGANIC IRON in the blood to enable us to GET THE STRENGTH OUT of our food.

IRON IS THE MASTER PRINCIPLE OF THE BLOOD AND BLOOD IS LIFE. Our forefathers ate the husks of grains and the skins and peels of vegetables and fruits, rich in strength-giving organic iron, but modern methods of cookery throw all these things away — hence the alarming increase, in recent years, in Anaemia—iron starvation of the blood with all its attendant ills.

When, as a result of iron starvation, you get up feeling tired in the morning, when you find yourself nervous, irritable and easily upset; when you can no longer do your day's work without being all fagged out at night; when your digestion all goes wrong, or you have pains across the back, shortness of breath, heart palpitation or your face looks pale and drawn, do not wait until you go all to pieces and collapse in a state of nervous prostration, or until in your weakened condition you contract some serious disease, but consult your family physician and have him take a specimen of your blood and make a "bloodcount" of your red blood corpuscles or test the iron-power of your blood yourself by adding plenty of spinach, carrots, or other iron-containing fruits and vegetables to your daily food and take organic iron—Nuxated Iron—with them for a while and see how much your condition improves. Thousands of people have surprisingly increased their strength, energy and endurance in two weeks time by this simple experiment. But be sure the iron you take is organic Nuxated Iron and not metallic iron which people usually take and which is made merely by the action of strong acids on small pieces of iron --an entirely different iron from Nuxated Iron. The fact that you may have taken metallic iron without receiving any benefit does not prove that Nuxated Iron will not help you. Nuxated Iron represents organic iron in such a highly concentrated form that one dose is estimated to be approximately equivalent (in organic iron content) to eating

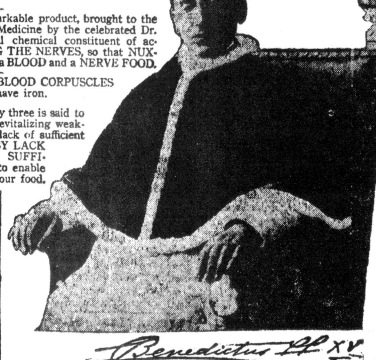

Benedictus PP XV

WHAT THE VATICAN SAYS ABOUT NUXATED IRON

"I am happy to inform you that your gift of Nuxated Iron has been accepted with particular gratitude by the Holy Father, who, persuaded by its beneficial effects, and AFTER HAVING IT SPECIALLY ANALYZED BY THE DIRECTOR OF THE PHARMACY OF THE VATICAN, formulates the most sincere wishes that your product may become famous and be as appreciated by the public AS ITS VALUE CERTAINLY MERITS."

(J. Tedeschini, Institute of the Secretary of State - Vatican)

"The composition of Nuxated Iron is such that the physiological and therapeutical effects cannot fail to be produced, as is usually the case in the prescription of pharmaceutical products of this kind,"

(F. Narciso Duribischeim, Director of the Pharmacy of the Vatican.)

half a quart of spinach or one quart of green vegetables. It is like taking extract of beef instead of eating pounds of meat. Nuxated Iron is used by over 4,000,000 people annually.

Beware of substitutes. Look for the letters N.I. on every tablet. Your money will be refunded by the manufacturers if you do not obtain perfectly satisfactory results. At all druggists.

"secret" was Nuxated Iron. When Jack Dempsey beat Willard, an equally big newspaper flyer claimed that Dempsey used Nuxated Iron. Some of the advertisements for the product touted its ability to improve a man's romantic energy. It is surprising then to discover that Pope Benedictine the 15th also endorsed Nuxated Iron! Our sample in the museum states that you should not take too much of it or you will have an unexpected event. It contains Nux vomica (strychnine).

At the turn of the century, there was a steady growth of sex aids, mostly for men, which were targeted to the widespread desire of the older male to achieve youthful sexual vigor. Of course, it can't be overlooked that the tremendous semi-legal sale of questionable products indicates

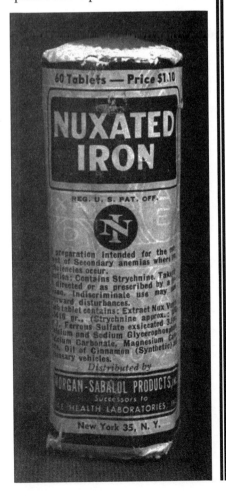

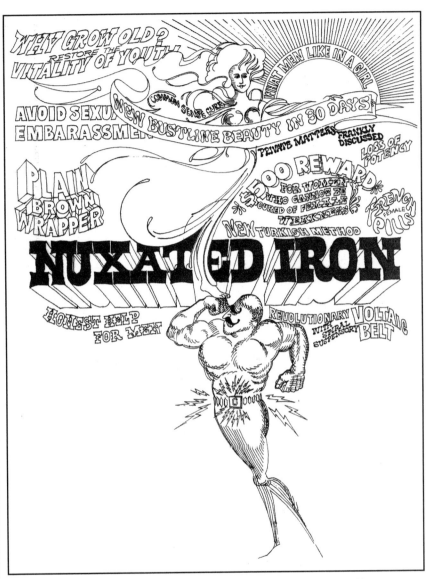

the real need, both social and individual, for more valid information and responsible attention to this area.

In a 1902 issue of *The American Journal of Clinical Medicine*, Dr. T. W. Williams writes, "Nothing affecting the life of man produces so much vice, degradation and secret misery as his sexual relations." However, he goes on to say, "Many houses can be brightened and inoculated with contagious joy by the rehabilitation of the sexual love of the head of the family."

To this end a number of mechanical devices were invented,

including a device by Dr. Williams called The Obturator. Dr. Williams was an early sex researcher, by no means a quack, who attempted to treat impotence using the scientific information of the time.

The Obturator was described as a valuable little surgical device made of soft rubber, the object being to close the return valve at the base of the penis that has allowed blood to return too fast (see attached sketch). A longer hose inflates the device, and the testicles slip between the ring to ensure a snug fit. Dr. Williams explained, "The instrument essentially facilitates the conditions for accomplishing coitus (impotence being for the one who suffers from it a physical and mental evil), its use rendering possible the accomplishment of a function natural and important for both body and mind and it can in general only operate favorably, unless one is misled by the artificial contrivance to excess in coitus, a circumstance, however, which should not be attributed to the instrument, but to the wearer!"

In 1920, W. T. Springer of Waterloo, Iowa, formed the Springer Treating Device Co. which made a device called Hyperaemia. He modestly claimed that

his invention was "The most wonderful discovery since the world began. From a state of gloom and doom to happiness and health." It was described as "four in one–Vacuum, Moist-Heat, Vibration and Electricity, all used in one application. This gives enforced circulation of blood to the parts in trouble, and the blood brought in this way to any weakened organ, causes the weakness to vanish and strength and vigor will follow."

The operation of the device was as follows: The hood-like appliance is filled with hot water and attached tightly to the patient. A wire from an induction coil

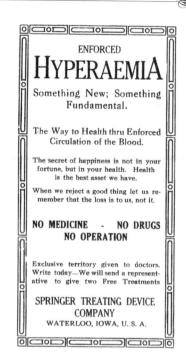
☞ Two Views ☜

of Dr. Williams' Obturator, which he described as a "valuable little surgical device."

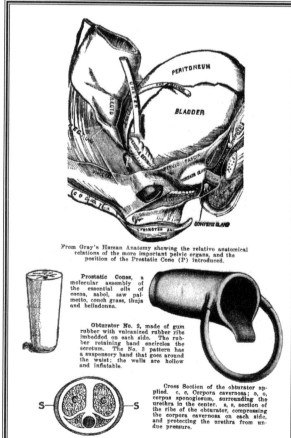

From Gray's Human Anatomy showing the relative anatomical relations of the more important pelvic organs, and the position of the Prostatic Cone (P) introduced.

Prostatic Cones, a molecular assembly of the essential oils of cocoa, sabol, saw palmetto, conch grass, thuja and belladonna.

Obturator No. 2, made of gum rubber with vulcanized rubber ribs imbedded on each side. The rubber retaining band encircles the scrotum. The No. 3 pattern has a suspensory band that goes around the waist; the walls are hollow and inflatable.

Cross Section of the obturator applied. c, c, Corpora cavernosa; o, o, corpus spongiosum, surrounding the urethra in the center. s, s, section of the ribs of the obturator, compressing the corpora cavernosa on each side, and protecting the urethra from undue pressure.

is misled by the artificial contrivance to excess in coitus, a circumstance, however, which should not be attributed to the instrument but to the wearer."

A-Body -double with air-space between.
C-Rubber Tube for inflating A. d e Valves.
B Rubber retaining band encircling scrotum

The Obturator No. 2

The obturator or penile Splint, made under my patent, is constructed in three different ~~sizes~~. The accompanying illustration shows one of the latest and more popular of these. ~~The No. 1 pattern is lighter and has no beak. The No. 3, or DeLuxe pattern, is constructed with extra elastic straps on each side and an elastic band which encircles the waist and buckles to the straps, preventing its coming off after the subsidence of erection, preferable, generally, for all night wear for this reason.~~

No. 1, 7½ inches long, No. 2, 3 inches. Either fits any sized organ.

with a battery is connected to the front of the metal hood and the olive tipped electrode coated with a little Vaseline and inserted in rectum 2 to 3 inches (for prostatic massage). The appliance is pressed to the body, completely covering the genital organs; so tightly that no air can pass between appliance and body. The end of the hose from the gauge is connected to the hole in the top of the appliance. Hot water is turned on or the hand pump is used to start the vacuum and then the electric current is turned on, starting at zero, and increasing to the level desired. The moisture within the metal hood enables the transmis-sion of an electric current which passes through the affected part.

Despite strenuous efforts, the author has been unable to locate any of these extraordinary and frightening devices.

Not surprisingly, the main promise of questionable devices for men—which come in infinite variety, evidently to match this quality in women—is for impressive sexual athleticism and, in the process, bolstering the sagging male ego.

Essentially, these work by extending, supporting, or strengthening the male organ. They take many forms, including splints,

continued on page 219

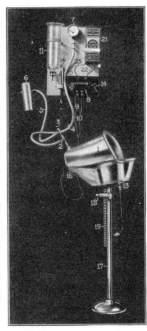

No. 1, The Appliance. No. 2, Connection for hose (No. 4) which connects with vacuum gauge No. 7. No. 3, Regulator Valve. No. 5, Hose from No. 3 to Pump No. 6. No. 8, Induction Coil. No. 9, Olive Electrode No. 15, used for prostatic gland. No. 17, Adjustment Screw on Induction Coil. No. 16, Cupping Glass. No. 12, Carrying Case. No. 14, Switch on Induction Coil. No. 18, Pedestal to hold Appliance. No. 11, No. 13, Stop to adjust Dark. No. 19, to any desired Pedestal. No. 20, Complete Sexual Treating Device with either Water or Hand Pump. Nos. 22 and 23, Connecting Wires from Dry Cell to Electric Coil. No. 21, Dry Cell.

THE STRINGER SELF TREATING DEVICE (BELOW) IS PROBABLY THE MOST BIZARRE SEXUAL AID EVER INVENTED. THE SMALLER PICTURE ABOVE IS THE OFFICE MODEL DESIGNED, INEXPLICABLY, FOR WOMEN!

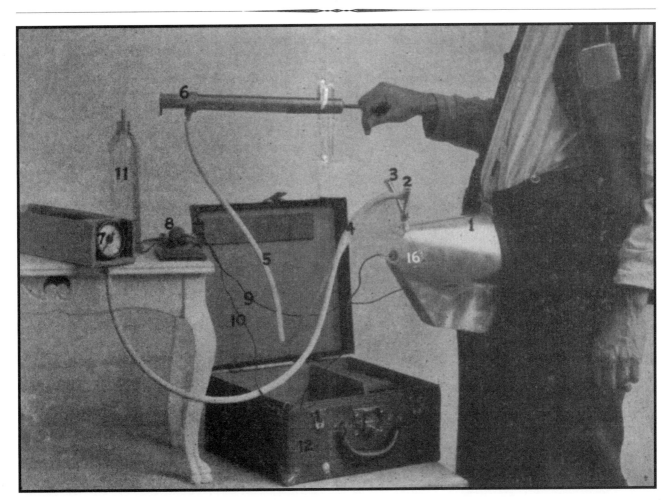

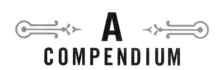

A
COMPENDIUM
OF ASSORTED
MALE
ORGAN
DEVICES

Presented for Your Entertainment

and Wonder!

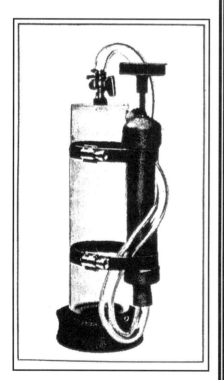

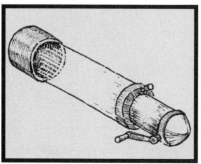

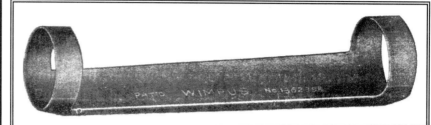

The "Wimpus"
An Aid to Impotents

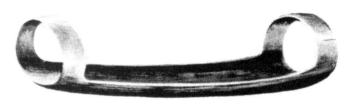

AN AID TO NATURE
The ERECTOR

Necessity is the mother of invention, and as an aid to nature we are offering for your serious consideration the facts about our surgical appliance that is sold under the registered trade name of "ERECTOR."

The Erector is not a "cure." Briefly, it is an ingenious appliance which when used, simply by virtue of its construction, supplies the necessary rigidity to make penetration. The fact that it has won great favor among men in all walks of life is sufficient evidence of its merits and efficacy.

Embarrassment, which is occasioned entirely by false modesty, is the only impediment to frank discussion and quick relief for most of these troubles. Mortification and despair are the penalty if you are not man enough to seek relief from your misfortunes.

When the natural organs, from general debility, excesses or other causes, become impaired, human ingenuity is compelled to devise some adjunct by the aid of which the organ can register something like its normal efficiency.

IMPORTANT

For men that would like to purchase this appliance for future use—the **ERECTOR** is hermetically sealed in plastic

A New Road to "Strongville"

If You Want to Get Back Your Pep, Vim, Vigor, and Vitality, the Greatest Boon in Life, Send for the Potentor.

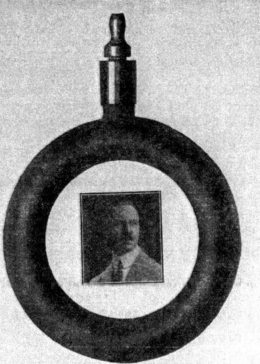

If you have tried the rest, now try the best. A new invention. Guaranteed efficient, warranted harmless.

Worn without the slightest discomfort like a suspensory. A boon to mankind. U. S. Patent applied for.

THE POTENTOR
Dr. Kratzenstein, the noted Nerve Specialist. Inventor.

THE POTENTOR

is designed to stimulate pep, vim, vigor and vitality, and corrects what has gone wrong. The systematic use of this mechano-therapeutic apparatus exercises its healing influence through elastic pressure on the spermadic cords, also through hyperemia on Dr. Bier's principle of congestion. In this way the testes receive an increased blood supply, get better nourishment, and are stimulated in a natural manner to produce a greater secretion of hormones. These hormones are eagerly absorbed by the blood, forming its most important nourishment when the blood gets these strong ingredients again, increased vigor, vitality and better nerve control are the results and all organs are benefited.

GREATER EASE OF ACTIVITY

Shortly after wearing the Potentor one should experience a feeling of well-being, GREATER EASE OF ACTIVITY, bouyance, cheerfulness, more joy and interest. Potency is stimulated, circulation, innervation and metabolism should be greatly improved.

TESTIMONIALS

I have received a great many testimonials unsolicited, similar to the one given below, but what is of vital interest to you is what will the POTENTOR do for you? A SIXTY-DAY TRIAL WILL CONVINCE YOU!

THE ROBUT-MAN

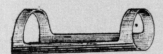

sizes 3½ to 6

This is a mechanical device for men which is used as an aid in performing the sexual act, where the erections are only partial.

If your glands are weak and you are unable to have marital relations use a ROBUT-MAN. It is made of a special hard rubber and can be obtained in the following sizes: 3½, 4, 4½ 5, 5½, 6. These prove marvelous, where a man fails to have firm erections and when bending occurs. This ROBUT-MAN prevents this and is worn as a splint on the organ. It is very easy to insert with this on, and is no inconvenience to the female either.

The ROBUT-MAN is cut out on the sides, held on the penis by several rings and serves as a splint by its rigidity on the bottom side. With the aid of this device, your organ can be inserted into the vagina, rigidly even though your organ is not completely erected. This device should be used for mild cases where there is but little erection.

You should use POWER PRESCRIPTION 7-11 or Formula 55 until your glands and erections become strong— as the above device is used naturally as a temporary aid in performing the act.

HOW TO FIND THE SIZE ROBUT-MAN YOU NEED

Hold the end of the organ (head) between your fingers. Pull the organ away from the body with a slight stretch. Now measure organ with a ruler from the back of the head of organ to the base. Be sure to measure the organ while not erected. It must be soft, and DO NOT include the head of the penis when measuring. The length in inches will be your size. For example, if your organ from back of head to base measures 5 inches, your size is 5. When ordering be sure to mention the size desired.

THE MONSTER AUTO-MAN

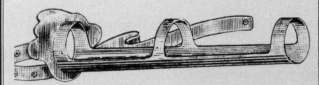

size 5½ inches long

Use An AUTO-MAN

This wonder device is used as an aid in performing the act, where there is NO ERECTION AT ALL.

This is a one-sided solid rubber device into which the male organ is placed into and held there by flexible rings and a rubber stretchable strap which is wound around the base of the penis. This device helps the male organ to become erected immediately and larger, by preventing the blood which is being pumped through the deep vessels from returning through the superficial blood vessels. This is accomplished by the winding around of the special strap at the base of the organ to the desired pressure. The tighter the strap is made, the stronger the erection. When nature fails entirely, use the WONDER MONSTER AUTO-MAN, the mechanical "penis".

This device may be worn without fear of injury whatsoever, It is perfectly harmless and may be worn with comfort and ease—it may be inserted into the female without any discomfort to her whatsoever. This device is of course intended for temporary erectional use, whereas the medicine POWER PRESCRIPTION 7-11 or Formula 55 is taken to build up the glands to permanency.

For immediate relations use the MONSTER AUTO-MAN, a great discovery, and should be kept on hand at all times, in case . . .

THE MECHANICAL PUMP DEVELOPERS

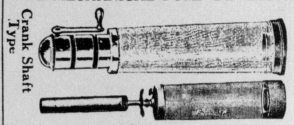

Crank Shaft Type

Piston Type

This developer is a vacuum pump instrument—it consists of a glass tube. Over one end is placed a rubber cap with a small opening into which the organ fits when placing same into glass tube vacuum. Over the other end of the tube is fitted a metal cap with a crank shaft or piston which by pumping creates a vacuum. When the male organ is placed into it, it draws more blood and keeps it in the organ thus causing an erection, By bringing more blood to the organ it improves the circulation, nourishes and massages it. The penis being made up of a network of spaces like a sponge is naturally apt to shrink when the circulation is poor. By pumping more blood into it, the size of the organ can be increased and better erections obtained.

Full directions accompany all our devices and instruments.

SPECIALISTS
APPROVE MECHANICAL DEVICES

For developing and maintaining erections.

States Dr. J. S. Wooten in the Texas Medical Journal:

"The mechanical devices for maintaining and developing erections function by compressing the veins and preventing their too rapid emptying, thus maintaining the penis in rigid state."

State Drs. J. Bray and O. Lowsley in a recent article in the Journal of the American Medical Association:

"It is advisable to employ mechanical contrivances for encouraging and maintaing erections, or splinting a soft penis so that intromission might be accomplished in the absence of erections."

State Drs. McDonald, Elder and E. G. Ballenger at a recent South Eastern Surgical Congress.

"For 15 years we have employed a vacuum pump in the treatment of the penis when subnormal in size—the patients with small organs usually showed improvement. Small penises soon become normal in size."

Space does not allow for many other quotations from Specialists.

Please do not write asking us our opinion about yourself as we maintain no correspondence department. Everything about our medicines and mechanical appliances is explained fully in our literature.

Yours for more pleasure and vigor,

PRESTO PRODUCTS

4328 N. KEDZIE AVE.   Chicago, Illinois.

USE THIS HANDY ORDER BLANK

TO: FRE-SAN PRODUCTS MFG. CO.
2903 MAYFIELD RD.
CLEVELAND, OHIO 44118

DATE: _____

PLEASE SHIP THE FOLLOWING:

QTY	SIZE	AMOUNT
	"C.T.D."- SMALL - 5" Long	
	"C.T.D."- SMALL - 6¼" Long	
	"C.T.D."- MEDIUM - 5" Long	
	"C.T.D."- MEDIUM - 6¼" Long	
	"C.T.D."- LARGE - 5" Long	
	"C.T.D."- LARGE - 6¼" Long	
	"C.T.D." LUBRICANT	
	TOTAL	

SHIP TO:

Name _____
Address _____
City & State _____
Enclosed: Zip Code _____
☐ Check   ☐ Money Order   ☐ Cash
REMARKS: _____

PLEASE CUT ON DOTTED LINE

DIRECTIONS FOR USING THE
"C.T.D." (Coitus Training Device)

1. Place BOTH elastic bands on the UNDER side of the "C.T.D." as shown in Fig. 1.

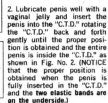

2. Lubricate penis well with a vaginal jelly and insert the penis into the "C.T.D." rotating the "C.T.D." back and forth gently until the proper position is obtained and the entire penis is inside the "C.T.D." as shown in Fig. No. 2. (NOTICE that the proper position is obtained when the penis is fully inserted in the "C.T.D." and the two elastic bands are on the underside.)

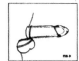

3. Take the two elastic bands as shown in Fig. 2 on the underside of the "C.T.D." between the fingers of both your hands and pull them back so that you can place the scrotum bag through BOTH elastic bands at one time. Pull BOTH the elastic bands up as far as you can behind your testicles as shown in Fig. No. 3.

We suggest that, if necessary, your wife also use the vaginal jelly or any other lubricant suggested by your doctor for additional lubrication to herself.

NOTE: Before using the "C.T.D." for the first time, cleanse thoroughly with soap and lukewarm water. When through using — repeat the same procedure and dry thoroughly.

CAUTION: FEDERAL LAW RESTRICTS THIS DEVICE TO SALE BY OR ON THE ORDER OF A PHYSICIAN.

Mfg. by
FRE-SAN PRODUCTS MFG. CO.
2903 MAYFIELD ROAD • CLEVELAND, OHIO 44118

Mfg. in U.S.A.   Patent Pending   Printed in U.S.A.

MALE IMPOTENCE
Can Now Be Alleviated
with the Use of Our
"C.T.D."
(COITUS TRAINING DEVICE)

Physicians have proven that in the majority of cases, if a male's confidence can be restored in reference to sexual relationship, then there is a better chance to help him with his impotency.

SINCE ITS INNOVATION THE "C.T.D." HAS PROVED BENEFICIAL TO THOUSANDS OF USERS AND HAS MET WITH WIDE APPROVAL BY MANY OF THE MEDICAL PROFESSION WHO HAVE PRESCRIBED OR DISPENSED IT.

Male impotency or the inability of the male to either initiate or satisfactorily terminate normal sexual intercourse is a frequent underlying cause of marital disharmony.

The current therapy of impotency, whether organic or psychosomatic in origin, has been sadly neglected and has proven to be in a great number of cases, ineffective, time-consuming and expensive. Now, however, all forms of impotency, whether due to premature ejaculation, premature senility, or simply impotency of psychological origin, are amenable to a new form of treatment, the "C.T.D." (Coitus Training Device).

The "C.T.D." offers for the first time a new, safe and dependable artificial device which can be effectively used in the above mentioned resistant or difficult to treat cases.

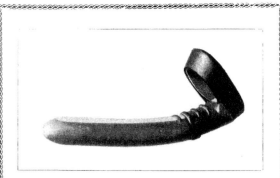

THE "A-VĀL"
PATENTED

DISTRIBUTORS
A-VĀL SPECIALTY CO.
NOT INC.
222 N. STATE STREET   CHICAGO, ILL.

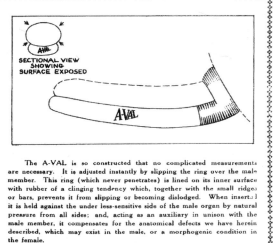

SECTIONAL VIEW SHOWING SURFACE EXPOSED

The A-VAL is so constructed that no complicated measurements are necessary. It is adjusted instantly by slipping the ring over the male member. This ring (which never penetrates) is lined on its inner surface with rubber of a clinging tendency which, together with the small ridges or bars, prevents it from slipping or becoming dislodged. When inserted it is held against the under less-sensitive side of the male organ by natural pressure from all sides; and, acting as an auxiliary in unison with the male member, it compensates for the anatomical defects we have herein described, which may exist in the male, or a morphogenic condition in the female.

The price is $15.00, prepaid, anywhere in the United States. Cash to accompany order.

DISTRIBUTORS
A-VĀL SPECIALTY CO.
NOT INC.
222 N. STATE STREET   CHICAGO, ILL.

VIEWS ON SEX HARMONY

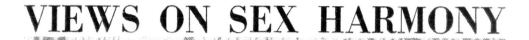

Sex is one of the most wonderful and beautiful things in the world and one must preserve it to maintain health and happiness in the home. The AID-MOR may help you do so.

The AID-MOR is not a gag or a joke. Its purpose is as old as time. It is made to aid married men in prolonging healthy marital relations and to help maintain the happiness of married couples. Medical journals have carried stories about articles of this nature before. The AID-MOR is primarily designed as an aid to the satisfaction of the female. It may be a big help to many elderly men and to many fat men for it will assist those unable to obtain suffcient erection for penetration.

There are periods that may occur in any marriage, where one partner's sex-desires lag behind the other's. Whether this happens from physical or psychological causes, the results are the same.

If the average wife is not being satisfied emotionally, she may be left in a nervous condition. This can be detrimental to her health and often becomes the cause of marital troubles. Many middle aged and elderly men often have intentions that are better than their techniques and congress frequently ends up with satisfaction only for the man. The AID-MOR will tend to alleviate this condition.

The AID-MOR is made from grease-resisting soft plastic, yet firm enough for its purpose. It is easy to keep in a sanitary condition, and can be used for years. THE AID-MOR IS NOT A CONTRACEPTIVE. It is solely intended as an aid to sex harmony in married life.

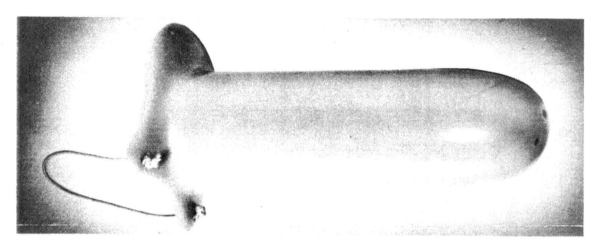

The AID-MOR is six inches long by one and one-half inches in diameter. This one size will answer for average married couples.

ABSOLUTE MONEY BACK GUARANTEE.

$10⁰⁰ EACH

Two for $16.00
Three for $21.00

To Order, use the coupon below, and the enclosed envelope. Make your check and money order payable to: MEDICAL SALES. Your AID-MOR will go out to you in a plain box on the day we receive your order. If, after using, you are not fully satisfied, return it for a full refund.

MEDICAL SALES CO., INC.
3220 Hudson Blvd., Jersey City 6, N. J.

Please send _____ AID-MOR(s). Enclosed is payment in full of $_____
(C.O.D.'s require a $3.00 deposit)

NAME_____
Please Print

ADDRESS_____

CITY_____ ZONE_____ STATE_____

NOTE: For fast air delivery add $1.00 extra per order.

suction devices, and even large plastic instruments which simulate the erect penis in every possible detail. Most are hard rubber or plastic, in simple or complex shape. They are fitted or strapped on; some use a pressure bulb. One, called a "hyperemator," was simply a small suction plunger that was more capable of harm than hardening.

The early mail order and diagnosis specials were replete with semi-plausible literature referring to physicians and sociologists with the old standby phrases like "The result of thirty years experience and research in a most vital area of human relationship is a line of personal products for men." One enterprising advertiser included a tape measure for men to check the results of the treatment.

Many of the devices were based on a way of interruption of blood flow to sustain erection when applied the base of the penis, similar in principle and results to using a rubber band or even downward pressure of the fingers. Some were based on the principle of exercise, as though the penis were a muscle.

Physicians were cautious about these devices since they tended to cause undue engorgement and soreness. It is also true that most of these devices were highly objectionable to women and thus interfered with the physical and emotional balance needed to achieve sexual response and mutual gratification.

Dr. Alfred Kinsey had good advice: ". . . good health, sufficient exercise, and plenty of sleep still remain the most effective of the aphrodisiacs."

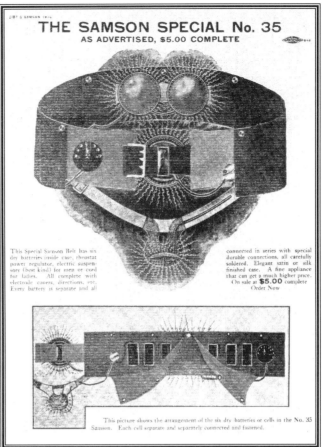

THE SAMSON SPECIAL No. 35
AS ADVERTISED, $5.00 COMPLETE

This Special Samson Belt has six dry batteries inside case, rheostat power regulator, electric suspensory (best kind) for men or cord for ladies. All complete with electrode covers, directions, etc. Every battery is separate and all connected in series with special durable connections, all carefully soldered. Elegant satin or silk finished case. A fine appliance that can get a much higher price. On sale at $5.00 complete Order Now

This picture shows the arrangement of the six dry batteries or cells in the No. 35 Samson. Each cell separate and separately connected and fastened.

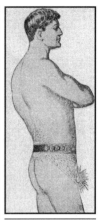

THIS PAGE: The Samson and Herculex electric belts sent current throughout the body to combat cases of sexual weakness, nervous debility, and prostate troubles. The current is passed into the sexual nerve center at the back—where it saturated the nerves leading to the sexual organs—and met the opposite pole in front, thus completing a circuit. This continuous flow to the sexual system occurred whenever the appliance was worn

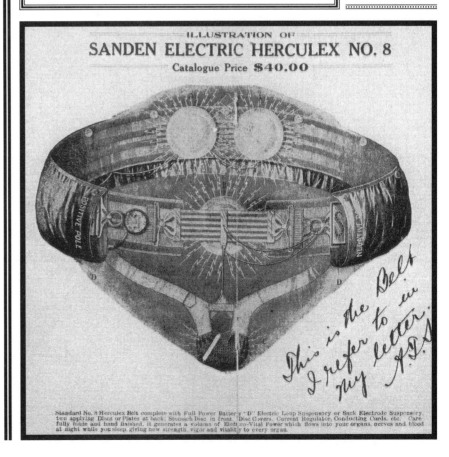

ILLUSTRATION OF
SANDEN ELECTRIC HERCULEX NO. 8
Catalogue Price $40.00

Standard No. 8 Herculex Belt complete with Full Power Battery "D" Electric Loop Suspensory or Sack Electrode Suspensory, two applying Discs or Plates at back, Stomach Disc in front, Disc Covers, Current Regulator, Conducting Cords, etc. Carefully made and hand finished. It generates a volume of Electro-Vital Power which flows into your organs, nerves and blood at night while you sleep, giving new strength, vigor and vitality to every organ.

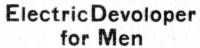
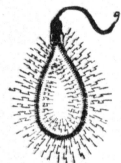
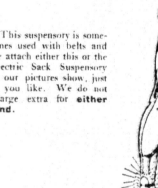
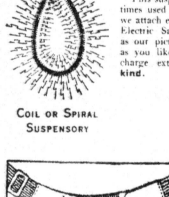
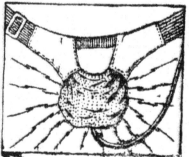
The Saddle

The Bono Drug Company, owned by Maurice Lundin, distributed three nostrums which the post office judged to be fraudulent and banned from the mails in 1929:

✳ French Pep Tablets, for internal consumption, were an impotence remedy which also claimed to cure an enlarged prostate, "kidney trouble," and "bladder trouble." The ingredients were extract of damiana, asafetida, bromides, aloin, and zinc phosphide.

✳ French Pomade, applied locally, was to be used in conjunction with the French Pep Tablets. This was a petroleum jelly salve laced with red pepper, menthol, and citronella.

✳ Bonol Balsam, a baldness cure applied to the genitals, contained petroleum jelly, salicylic acid, and sulfur.

Like many quacks, Mr. Lundin had a strong entrepreneurial bent and his activities were not solely limited to nostrums. He also operated The Saddle Company of Nashville, Tennessee, which produced a rubber device called The Saddle. The Saddle was an impotence device sold via mail order around 1930. It retailed for $10 (despite a price stamp of $19 on its jewelry box-like case), a price which included a "Tube of Ointment" valued at $1.

Advertising copy for The Saddle was fairly discreet:

Just as our eyesight becomes weakened, or our hearing is getting poor, so other parts of our

What Is

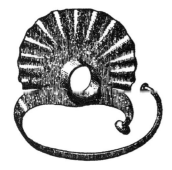

The Saddle?

"THE SADDLE"

is a surgical device, intended to assist men in protecting themselves from becoming "too old."

It is fully protected by patents issued by the U. S. Government and abroad.

Before giving any further description we would, however, like to say a few words as an introduction.

The subject matter at hand, although a very serious one, is rather delicate to handle, as we will meet on the one side prudery and on the other side licentiousness, both equally obstructive when any delicate subject is discussed, even in the most serious and scientific manner.

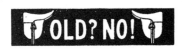

WHOLESALE AND RETAIL DISTRIBUTORS

THE SADDLE COMPANY

1703 EASTLAND AVE.
NASHVILLE, TENN.

bodily make-up cease to function the way nature has intended. Rheumatism may force one man to use a walking stick, and compel another to employ an ear phone. The Saddle should be looked upon in the same matter of fact way as we look upon a pair of eyeglasses or a set of false teeth—as an assistant to nature and conjugality. . .

The SADDLE conforms with the anatomical constructions of the body and assists where nature is weak. It makes it possible for an otherwise weak and incompetent organ to again comply with the demands of nature, provided there is any vitality left to build on. The SADDLE when used according to directions will, through its elastic pressure, give the whole organ an increased supply of blood, which will give better nourishment to the testes and other parts, thereby causing a greater secretion of hormones. This again will result in increased vigor and the strengthening of the whole organ.

But not discreet enough. The Saddle was judged obscene by the U.S. Postal Service and banned from the mails.

Be a Manly Man!

Here is the advertising copy for the Perfect Organ Developer:

It is impossible for a woman to love a man who is sexually weak. To enjoy life and be loved by women you must be a man. A man who is sexually weak is unfit to marry. Weak men hate themselves. Upon the strength of the sexual organ depends sexual strength, in both men and women, furnishing the ambition and energy for all the advancement in

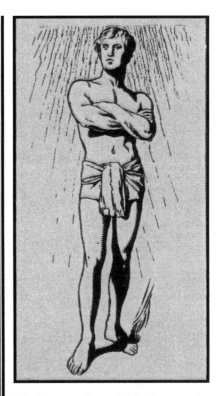

life. It is a well established scientific fact that the musicians, financiers and pugilists are men of exceptionally strong sexual power. Well developed sexual organs manifest themselves in the clear ringing voice, the glossy hair, the sparkling eye, the personal magnetism and force of character.

You know better than anyone can tell you whether you need this developer. You know whether you are at your best in mind and body, or if your sexual condition is perfect. That you may require the Perfect Organ Developer implies no guilt or sin. Men break down from overwork, care, worry, sickness and dozens of other causes. The sexual system is often the first to give away under strain owing to its intimate connection with the brain and nervous system. Men whose lives have been exceptionally pure may be found in this class of sufferers, but the necessity for proper treatment is just as great. To the man who is sexually defective this method of

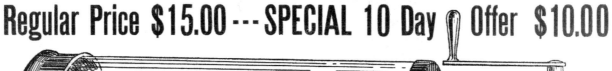
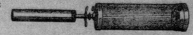
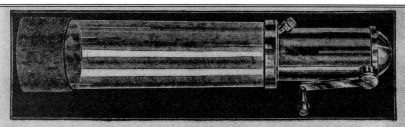
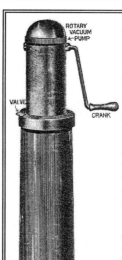

restoration is the very realization of the dream of philosophy and science.

Vital Power Vacuum Massager

"Organ developers" were the mechanical counterpart to the manhood nostrums which seemed to have their hey day during the 1920s. Few survived because the devices consisted of glass tubes connected to a power source.

The Vital Power Vacuum Massager contained a built-in hand crank. This device was produced by W. J. Lynch in Springfield, Illinois in 1921. The Perfection Developer, manufactured by Walter H. Hartman d.b.a. the Hart Company, was a glass cylinder attached to a pump. A bicycle pump was used by the Vital Gland Power Company for their device. This company used testimonials from men in their 80s to promote their product while their sales force was almost entirely young women. In 1923, the Vital Gland Power Company realized sales of $173,407. The devices were denounced by the AMA Investigative Bureau and these companies were barred from using the mails by the U. S. Postmaster General.

Doc Brinkley: Pumping Up the (Sexual) Flat Tire

Dr. John Romulus Brinkley would feel right at home in the age of Viagra and the World Wide Web. Doc Brinkley was the first to exploit mass media for a forthright public confrontation of impotence and to reach the impotence mass market. An experienced radio personality, he waged an astonishingly successful independent populist campaign for governor of Kansas, though

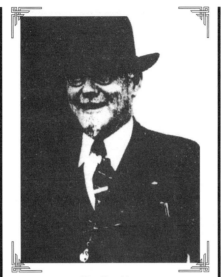

Doc Brinkley

Brinkley lost the election. While Dr. Brinkley lacked e-mail and a website, he was the unparalleled master of "interactive" radio for the 1920's health care consumer. Yet when he is remembered, it is generally with ill-will, for Doc Brinkley may have been the greatest quack of the twentieth century.

Brinkley, born to Appalachian poverty in 1885 and orphaned in early childhood, never finished

high school. Nonetheless, he obtained three medical degrees. Two were from bogus medical diploma mills, the Bennett Medical College of Chicago and Eclectic Medical University of Kansas City, and the third, from the University of Pavia, Italy, was annulled. Brinkley's loss of a temporary California medical license in 1922 culminated in the filing of criminal charges for alleged conspiracy to violate California medical laws. Brinkley was never tried on this charge for the governor of Kansas refused to extradite him. (Dr. Brinkley did have a criminal record for selling alcohol during Prohibition; he served no jail time.)

In 1930, the Kansas State Board of Medical Registration revoked Doc Brinkley's Kansas medical license. Dr. Brinkley refused to let his lack of education and licensing prevent him from practicing medicine; between 1930 and 1941, he operated clinics in Del Rio, Texas, and Little

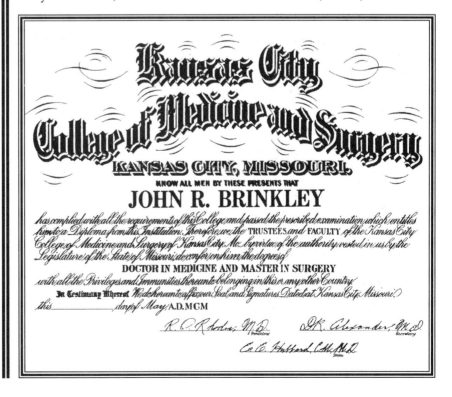

Rock, Arkansas. Indeed, his earnings during the Great Depression are estimated to have exceeded $12 million.

The fortune was born in Milford, Kansas where John Brinkley and his second wife, Minnie Jones, settled in 1917. The second Mrs. Brinkley was also an M.D. with a bogus medical diploma. In 1918, an elderly farmer sought help for impotence from Doc Brinkley. Brinkley's cure, described by Morris Fishbein of the AMA, was "the alleged sexual rejuvenation of the male by the (also alleged) implantation of goats' testicles into the human scrotum." The farmer was a satisfied patient: he reported complete recovery after two weeks and the birth of a son after a year! They called the baby boy "Billy."

Demand for the goat gland procedure was intense! Doc Brinkley's fame grew and in 1922, he performed the operation on Harry Chandler, publisher of the *Los Angeles Times.* Chandler's printed praise for the procedure was the cause of Dr. Brinkley's troubles with the California authorities. Back in Kansas, Doc Brinkley moved into a new field: radio. He founded KFKB (Kansas First Kansas Best), the first radio station in the state. Broadcasts from this 1,000 watt station carried to surrounding states: John Romulus Brinkley had found his advertising medium! Programming at the station was eclectic—country music, fundamentalist preachers, professors from a local college.... And three times a day, Doc Brinkley broadcast his own show, "The Medical Question Box."

Listeners mailed in health questions and Dr. Brinkley answered them on the air. The Doc soon branched out with a new

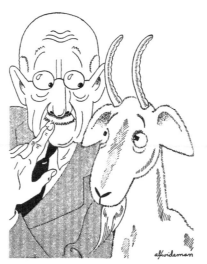

Neither goat glands nor any other glands will bring the Ponce de Leon fountain of youth to the senile.

venture, his own line of prescription medicines with no names, just numbers. Dr. Brinkley typically prescribed his own medicines on air as this excerpt from an April 1, 1930, broadcast exemplifies:

"Here's one from Tillie. She says she had an operation, had some trouble 10 years ago. I think the operation was unnecessary, and it isn't very good sense to have an ovary removed with the expectation of motherhood resulting therefrom. My advice to you is to use Women's Tonic No. 50, 67, and 61. This combination will do for you what you desire if any combination will, after three month's persistent use."

"The Medical Question Box" was an opportunity to push the "Goat Gland Cure," which Doc Brinkley did unreservedly. Late at night, he asked the men "Do you wish to continue as a sexual flat tire?" The number of goats used at the Brinkley Clinic climbed to 40 to 60 a week. The charge for each operation was $750 – paid in advance.

Initially, Brinkley filled his on-air prescriptions by mail order. He found this inefficient and so

organized the Brinkley Pharmaceutical Association—a network of druggists in several states who would fill prescriptions with Brinkley's formulas and pay Brinkley a commission. By 1930, the Brinkley Hospital was paying KFKB $2,000 to $5,000 a month for advertising. Commission fees from the pharmacists, another $9,000 a month, also went to KFKB. The Brinkleys owned only a third of KFKB stock, but their minority position would fail to shield the station's license.

Trouble began in 1928 when Dr. Morris Fishbein and *JAMA* exposed Dr. Brinkley for the questionable goat gland cure and for "blind prescribing." Though Fishbein was a ferocious anti-quackery advocate, he spent the next 13 years trying to quash Brinkley. Twice Brinkley sued Fishbein and *JAMA* for libel. Brinkley lost both times, but the cases and appeals lingered in the courts for years.

Dr. Brinkley tried to increase the power of KFKB to 5,000 watts and incurred another enemy: the *Kansas City Star* which owned a rival Kansas radio station. The *Star* investigated Dr. Brinkley, and in early 1930 ran an exposé calling Doc Brinkley "the master charlatan and lost manhood quack of Milford, Kansas." Dr. Fishbein again went on the attack with spring articles in *Hygeia* and *JAMA.* He also appeared that summer before the Kansas Medical Society, which petitioned successfully for the revocation of Brinkley's medical license.

Undaunted, Doc Brinkley used his radio station and his private plane to conduct a write-in campaign for himself as governor. He promised to return Kansas to the people—some suggest he wanted to appoint a new medical licensing board. In the midst of his election campaign, the Federal Radio Commission refused to renew the KFKB broadcast license on the grounds that "the operation of Station KFKB is conducted only in the personal interest of Dr. John R. Brinkley. While it is to be expected that a licensee of a radio broadcasting station will receive some remuneration for serving the public with radio programs, at the same time the interest of the listening public is paramount . . ." Dr. Brinkley lost

the election (and went on to lose again in 1932 and 1934).

Dr. Brinkley relocated to Del Rio, Texas, across the border from station XER in Villa Acuña, Mexico. He cut a deal with the Mexican government and was allowed to increase XER's power from 75,000 to 500,000 watts– making it the most powerful radio station in the world! Unfettered by U.S. regulation, Doc Brinkley's signal could be heard throughout the Mississippi River Valley and sometimes reached New York! Again, radio advertised Brinkley's

clinic, moved from Kansas to Del Rio in 1933, and Brinkley's newest prescription, "Formula No. 1020." In 1937, the AMA published a chemical analysis of the product: one part indigo to 100,000 parts water. Dr. Fishbein acridly wrote, "The kind of genius capable of taking a body of water like Lake Erie, coloring it with a dash of bluing and then selling the stuff at $100 for six ampules represents a type which all the world up to now has never been able to equal. John R. Brinkley is the absolute apotheosis in his

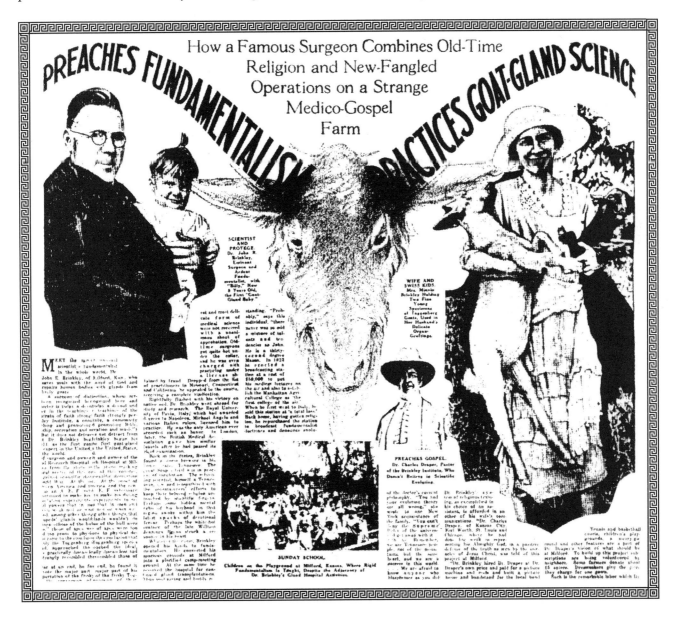

field. Centuries to come may never produce again such blatancy, such fertility of imagination, or such ego."

The tide again turned against Brinkley after 1937. Fishbein kept up the pressure in AMA publications. The U. S. government continued to try and persuade Mexico to shut down Brinkley's transmitter. Competition from other charlatans, especially native Texan James Middlebrook, hurt Brinkley financially. The Brinkley Clinic moved to Little Rock, Arkansas. The federal government charged Brinkley for $200,000 as Brinkley was making costly settlements in wrongful death suits.

In April 1941, the Mexican government shut down the Villa Acuña. Doc Brinkley had a massive heart attack followed by a leg amputation and two more heart attacks. The U.S. Postal Service charged Brinkley with mail fraud. He was never prosecuted. The June 13, 1942 *JAMA* reported "Dr. John R. Brinkley, 'goat gland' specialist, died May 26 at a hospital in San Antonio. Newspapers report that he had been under treatment for a heart ailment since the amputation of a leg in Kansas City, Missouri last winter. He was 56 years of age."

The diploma on page 223 was issued by the Kansas City College of Medicine and Surgery, which was in existence from the early 1900s until October 1923, when a *St. Louis Star* reporter wrote in a famous exposé that he had bought a license to practice medicine for $1,000.

The reporter, Harry Thompson, also received a bogus high school certificate issued by the Missouri examiner of schools, Professor W. P. Sachs, who made a full confession to the state prosecuting attorney: "My traffic in fraudulent educational credentials began about eleven years ago when a ring was organized. I sold approximately 3,000 of these certificates directly or indirectly to persons who could not have passed the examinations but later became doctors of medicine."

The ring leader of the diploma-mill operation, Dr. Adcox, paid $5 each for the certificates issued by Professor Sachs and then sold them for $200 apiece. Dr. Adcox and Dr. Alexander, the "Secretary" of the college, also provided the prospective "physicians" with a bogus medical school transcript and the answers to the licensing board's examinations in either Connecticut or Arkansas, which they had purchased for $1,000. One of their more famous students was none other than "Dr." John R. Brinkley.

Ralph Voight of Kansas City, one of the other ring leaders, reported that although he had accomplished the impossible on a number of occasions, by far the hardest job of his life was when he "took forty-two boobs to New Haven to get licenses for them. Assisted by a couple of other smart guys who knew their stuff, the three of us sat up all night in the Hotel Garde writing answers. It was a tough job, we prepared forty-two different sets of answers, one for each boob, and all they had to do was go into the examination room and copy the answers in their own handwriting. Only one failed to get his license—a dumb bird who could not copy his paper."

Following the *St. Louis Star* exposé, 167 physicians who had been certified by the Connecticut board lost their licenses, and the ring-leaders of the bogus Kansas City College of Medicine and Surgery went to prison.

The Prostate Gland Warmers

Probably nothing causes visitors to the Museum of Questionable

The temperature of the prostate gland warmer is regulated by the light bulb in its circuit. We use a 25 watt bulb for demonstration; a 100 watt bulb provides significant heat.

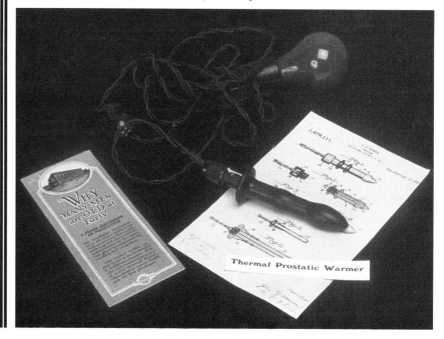

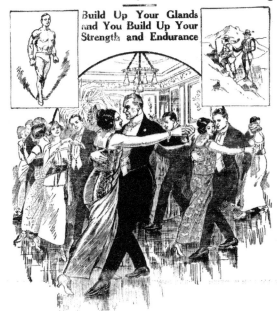

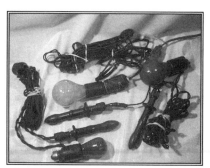

Three prostate gland warmers on exhibit in the museum.

Medical Devices to wince more than looking at the three Prostate Gland Warmers and the Recto-Rotor prostate poster (see end of chapter).

The devices were made by The Thermalaid Method Inc., successors to The Electro Thermal Co. of Stubenville, Ohio. The devices manufactured by this company are the only ones to be awarded a U.S. Patent, #1,279,111, assigned to John G. Homan. In the patent, Mr. Homan clams that "If a rectal dilator is used it will furnish a constant heat to the rectal anatomy, causing a gentle stimulation of the capillary blood vessels and the resultant improved local nerve condition. The reflex nerve action also has the effect of stimulating, through the abdominal brain, those centers which have the tendency to bring about normal healthy conditions, thus relieving an aggravating cause of several diseases . . . four watts is in nearly all cases sufficient to produce all the temperatures that can be borne!" The attached page from the patent shows five drawings of tips, none of which were used in the original patent.

The Thermalaid is essentially a rectal dilator consisting of a hard rubber unit to be inserted for the application of heat. The models in our display have a light bulb in circuit that regulates the wattage. Other models offered for sale used batteries rather than house electric current.

The Thermalaid and its cousins all were sold under the claim, either expressed or implied, that they would cure prostatic hypertrophy and diseases of the prostate. It was also recommend as a cure for constipation, hemorrhoids and, by implication, as a sexual stimulant. The Company also put out an "Electro-thermal Vitalizer," which was for the use of women and was to be inserted into the vagina.

Sales were made by the methods common to mail-order quacks, namely advertising in such newspapers and magazines as were willing to split the profits of quackery with the makers of these devices. Their advertisements also carried the usual number of testimonials. Dr. C. Herbert John of

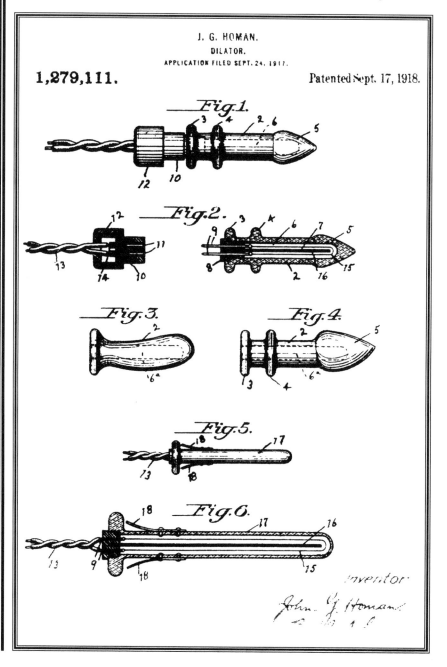

Order Blank on Reverse Side
MODELS

Model A THERMALAID is for use on electric light service only. A ten-foot cord with switch and suitable controlling apparatus is furnished.

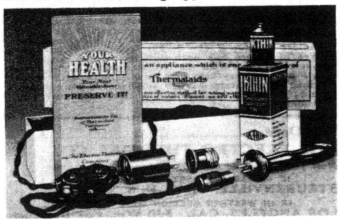

Model A

Our most popular and most widely used model because of its compactness and convenience. It may be used any time or place where electric light is available. Either 32, 110, or 220 volts can be used. Model A is neatly packed in a secure carton and enclosed in a second shipping box which has no advertising on it.
Carrying charges prepaid. INSURED. Price $20.00.

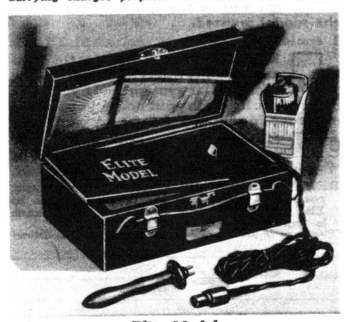

Elite Model

Elite Model THERMALAID operates from dry batteries and is for use where electric light current is not available. It is contained in a beautiful Keratol-covered carrying case with nickeled latch and leather handle. All models are equally efficacious, the selection being governed by whether or not electric current is available. This is a practical, durable, simple, economical outfit. Elite Model is securely packed with no advertising on the shipping carton.
Carrying charges prepaid. INSURED. Price $25.00.

LITHO IN U S.A.

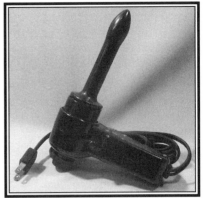

The Dial–A–Thon.

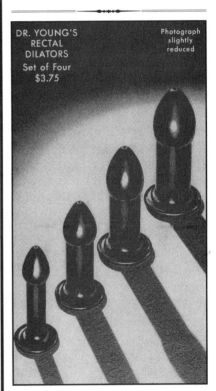

DR. YOUNG'S RECTAL DILATORS
Set of Four
$3.75

Photograph slightly reduced

Two Views of Dr. Young's Rectal Dilators.

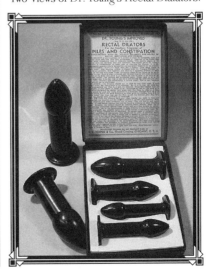

Chicago, follower of Albert Abrams, the King of American quackery, featured prominently in these testimonial ads. The Federal Trade Commission issued a cease and desist order in November of 1936.

The G-H-R Electric Equipment Company of Grand Rapids, Michigan also produced a popular device, The G-H-R Electric Thermitis Dilator. This company was particularly known for "scare ads."

The Lamothe Surgical Corporation produced the Recto-Rotor Lubricating Dilator, and claimed it would cure a man's lack of virility and give him high spirits and power. It allegedly prevented "incompleteness and prematureness of the climax in the procreative act. This directly affects the nervous system and upsets the whole procreative order, often preventing the individual from accomplishing the act at all." It was used with an ointment to produce all of the results promised. A physician, Dr. John F. G. Luepke, discovered that the company had wrongly listed him as endorsing the product. This so outraged him that he was able to

continued on page 233

The AMA campaigned to expose the fraudulent promises made by both the Thermalaid Co. and the G.H.R. Electric Dilator Co., sponsors of this advertisement. In 1941, the *AMA Journal* congratulated the Federal Trade Commission for issuing a cease and desist fraud order barring these advertisements.

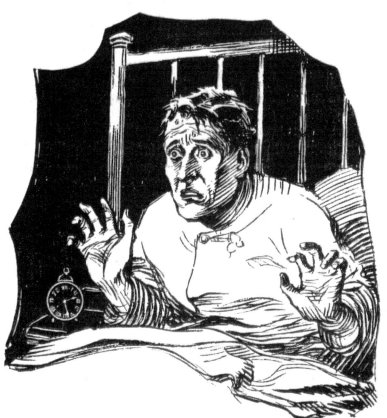

ARE YOUR NIGHTS LIKE THIS

Do You Know The Cause of Your Trouble?

NERVES Do Not Get A Chance To Rest When Your Sleep Is Broken

YOUR Opportunity Both Men and Women can Benefit By This Great Aid

WHY PERMIT YOURSELF TO GROW OLD

When Science has Discovered a Way Out

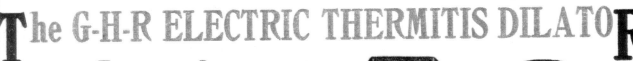
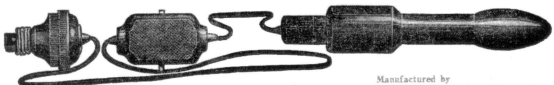

its healing, soothing and cooling Unguent exudes from the vent holes. By turning the knurled edge between the fingers a gentle massage is obtained, as well as the right exercise for the flabby muscles of the anus. Partly by this massage, and partly by the gentle cooling produced by the Unguent, an immediate reduction of the inflammation of the prostate and rectal canal is effected.

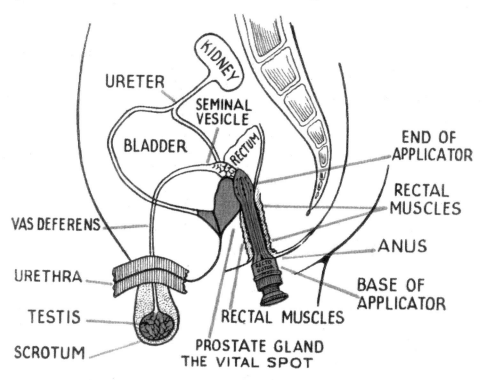

THE MALE PROGENITALS

Difference Between Efficient and Non-Efficient Dilators

The ordinary smooth dilator cannot break up the fecal matter in the rectum. It does not massage; it does not lubricate; and all the ointment comes off at the edge of the anus where it is not needed; whereas EZO UNGUENT oozes through the vent holes in the RECTO ROTOR and is applied directly to the tissues. The corrugation in our RECTO ROTOR gently lubricates, massages and dissolves the waste matter in the rectum, making it easy to expel and helps NATURE do her work.

A GRATEFUL RELIEF IS FELT INSTANTLY

Close examination of the original picture reveals that "Lamothe Surgical Corporation" is written in with white ink!

get the Post Office to shut the company down in 1932. Dr. Luepke acknowledged that the ointment had astringent and soothing properties, but in 1932, in an angry letter to the investigative unit of the AMA, he wrote "but that it would cure piles together with the friction movement of the applicator or reduce an enlarged prostate gland is a lie. The contrary is true! This friction is no massage—it is a harmful manipulation."

The accompanying photo shows the new company headquarters at 25 West Broadway, New York. It appears to be a five story building with the company name over the first floor. Closer examination of the picture, however, indicates that the name was drawn on the photograph—a common practice among quacks.

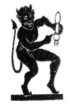

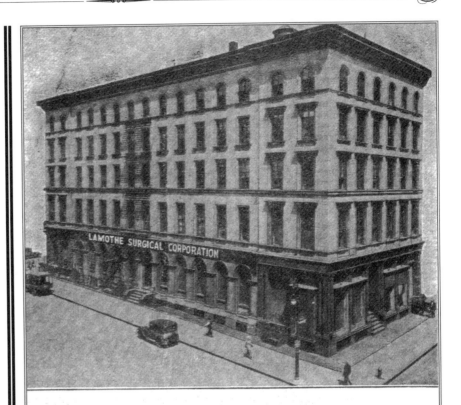

OUR NEW HEADQUARTERS
AT 25 WEST BROADWAY
NEW YORK CITY

Our out-of-town patrons are cordially invited to visit us when in New York and we will furnish a car for a visit to the many places of interest in New York and vicinity. If possible, advise us about a week in advance to enable us to make reservations for you.

P. H. LAMOTHE, President.
Lamothe Surgical Corporation.

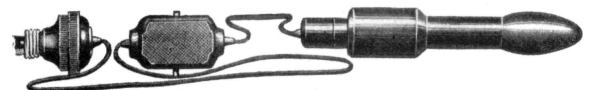

Be True to Yourself Always

The G-H-R Electric Thermitis Dilator

Is Used By Men and Women The Most Sensational Offer Is Herewith Explained

IN A CLASS BY ITSELF —
The RECTO ROTOR
THE LATEST AND MOST EFFICIENT INVENTION FOR THE QUICK RELIEF OF
PILES, CONSTIPATION AND PROSTATE TROUBLE

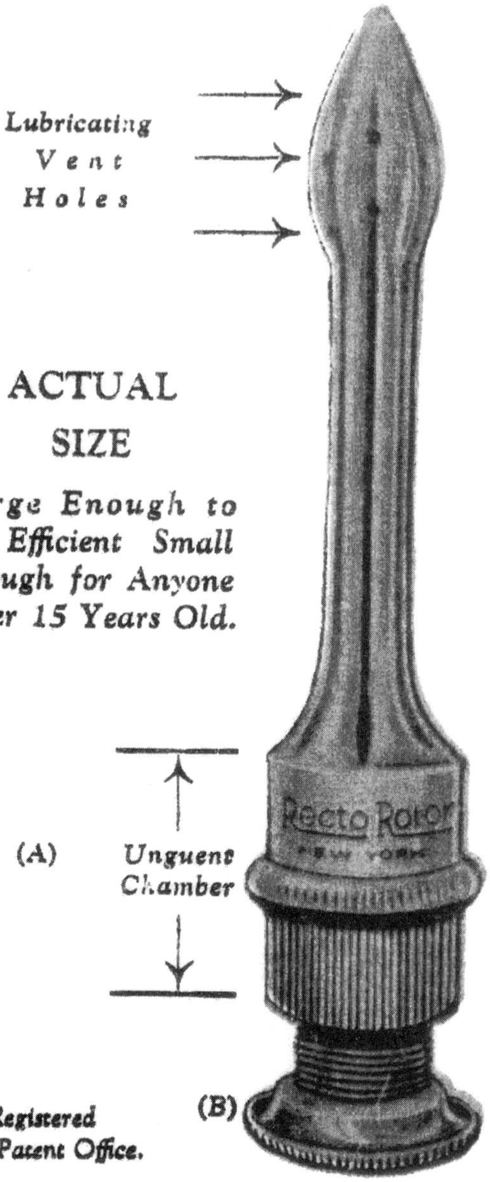

Lubricating Vent Holes

ACTUAL SIZE

Large Enough to be Efficient Small Enough for Anyone Over 15 Years Old.

(A) Unguent Chamber

(B)

Registered U.S. Patent Office.

The RECTO ROTOR is the only device that reaches the Vital Spot effectively. This picture tells its own story. Note especially those little vent holes in the nozzle through which the unguent inserted in the chamber below (a) may be forced out by turning the knurled cap (b). No other appliance in the world is so constructed: none other able to reach the Vital Spot to such good purpose.

The RECTO ROTOR obtains its amazingly quick results without the use of medicine, electricity, operations, or massage by an attendant. It gets results because of its scientific construction. It is made for the purpose of relieving congestion in the prostate gland, lubricating the colon and massaging the muscles of the rectal region. It is used by the patient himself in the privacy of his own home.

The RECTO ROTOR Lubricating Dilator is the only improvement ever made on the common "dilator" which hitherto was the most successful appliance for the relief of Piles and Constipation.

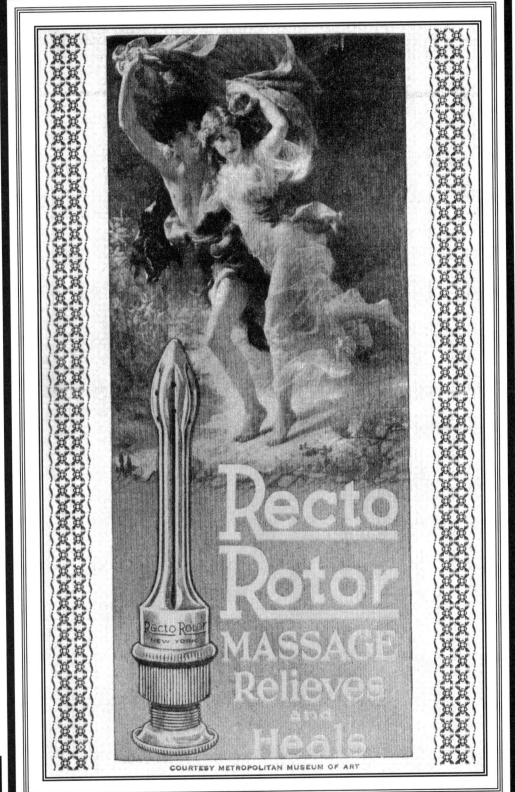

COURTESY METROPOLITAN MUSEUM OF ART

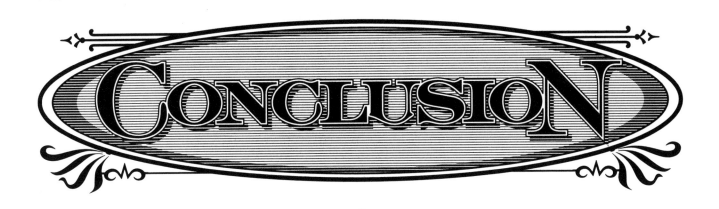

CONCLUSION

"In the foregoing pages, a number of the humbugs by which the public have been gulled have been separately examined, with the view of exposing in the sun-light of truth their heinous character and their mischievous tendency. And a feeble attempt has been made at remonstrance and expostulation with the infatuated dupes of these flagrant delusions. But there are a great variety of examples no less to be deprecated because of their intrinsic vileness, and most deplorable consequences, to which no allusion has been made, although the citizens are greedily bolting them down with equally marvellous gullibility. Nor is it possible to keep pace with the rapidity with which new and successful humbugs are introduced among us."

Humbugs of New York
David Meredith Reese, M.D.

1838

ABOUT THE AUTHOR

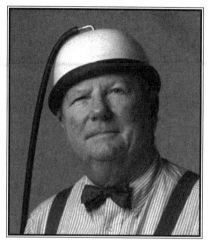

HUMBLE DEBUNKER OF MEDICAL QUACKERY.

Bob McCoy is the founder of the Museum of Questionable Medical Devices in St. Anthony Main in Minneapolis. This is the nation's largest public display of "quack" medical devices and was founded in 1987.

Mr. McCoy's past occupations include soap salesman, mill steel salesman (for 20 years), and family planning clinic administrator. He is a hobby printer, licensed humanist minister, and a member of the Committee for the Investigation of Claims of the Paranormal. It is as a skeptic that he has worked to expose health fraud, and the museum is an entertaining and informative means of doing just that.

He has demonstrated devices from the museum on many TV shows, such as David Letterman, Conan O'Brien, Good Morning America, and Today, as well as shows on the Discovery Channel, A&E, Travel Channel, and Minnesota Public Television. He has also participated in numerous radio talk shows, and been featured in dozens of national and international magazines and newspapers.

He is married with three grown children and five grandchildren.

Books Available From Santa Monica Press

The Book of Good Habits
   Simple and Creative Ways to Enrich Your Life
by Dirk Mathison
224 pages $9.95

Café Nation
   Coffee Folklore, Magick, and Divination
by Sandra Mizumoto Posey
224 pages $9.95

Collecting Sins
   A Novel
by Steven Sobel
288 pages $13

Health Care Handbook
   A Consumer's Guide to the American
   Health Care System
by Mark Cromer
256 pages $12.95

Helpful Household Hints
   The Ultimate Guide to Housekeeping
by June King
224 pages $12.95

**How To Find Your Family Roots and Write
Your Family History**
by William Latham and Cindy Higgins
288 pages $14.95

**How To Win Lotteries, Sweepstakes, and
Contests in the 21st Century**
by Steve "America's Sweepstakes King" Ledoux
224 pages $14.95

Letter Writing Made Easy!
   Featuring Sample Letters for Hundreds of
   Common Occasions
by Margaret McCarthy
224 pages $12.95

Letter Writing Made Easy! Volume 2
   Featuring More Sample Letters for Hundreds of
   Common Occasions
by Margaret McCarthy
224 pages $12.95

Nancy Shavick's Tarot Universe
by Nancy Shavick
336 pages $15.95

Offbeat Food
   Adventures in an Omnivorous World
by Alan Ridenour
240 pages $19.95

Offbeat Golf
   A Swingin' Guide To a Worldwide Obsession
by Bob Loeffelbein
240 pages $17.95

Offbeat Marijuana
   The Life and Times of the World's Grooviest Plant
by Saul Rubin
240 pages $19.95

Offbeat Museums
   The Collections and Curators of America's Most
   Unusual Museums
by Saul Rubin
240 pages $19.95

Past Imperfect
   How Tracing Your Family Medical History
   Can Save Your Life
by Carol Daus
240 pages $12.95

Quack!
   Tales of Medical Fraud from the Museum of
   Questionable Medical Devices
by Bob McCoy
240 pages $19.95

The Seven Sacred Rites of Menopause
   The Spiritual Journey to the Wise-Woman Years
by Kristi Meisenbach Boylan
144 pages $11.95

Silent Echoes
   Discovering Early Hollywood Through the Films of
   Buster Keaton
by John Bengtson
240 pages $24.95

What's Buggin' You?
   Michael Bohdan's Guide to Home Pest Control
by Michael Bohdan
256 pages $12.95

ORDER FORM
— 1-800-784-9553 —

	Amount
The Book of Good Habits ($9.95)	_____
Café Nation ($9.95)	_____
Collecting Sins ($13)	_____
Health Care Handbook ($12.95)	_____
Helpful Household Hints ($12.95)	_____
How to Find Your Family Roots and Write Your Family History ($14.95)	_____
How to Win Lotteries, Sweepstakes . . . ($14.95)	_____
Letter Writing Made Easy! ($12.95)	_____
Letter Writing Made Easy! Volume 2 ($12.95)	_____
Nancy Shavick's Tarot Universe ($15.95)	_____
Offbeat Food ($19.95)	_____
Offbeat Golf ($17.95)	_____
Offbeat Marijuana ($19.95)	_____
Offbeat Museums ($19.95)	_____
Past Imperfect ($12.95)	_____
Quack! ($19.95)	_____
The Seven Sacred Rites of Menopause ($11.95)	_____
Silent Echoes ($24.95)	_____
What's Buggin' You? ($12.95)	_____

Shipping & Handling:

1 book—$3.00

Each additional book is $ .50

Subtotal _____

CA residents add 8.25% sales tax _____

Shipping and Handling (see left) _____

TOTAL _____

Name_____

Address_____

City_____ State _____ Zip _____

❏ Visa ❏ MasterCard   Card Number_____

Exp. Date _____ Signature _____

❏ Enclosed is my check or money order payable to:

Santa Monica Press LLC
P.O. Box 1076
Santa Monica, CA 90406

www.santamonicapress.com

1-800-784-9553